AUTISM
CAUSES
UNVEILED

The Hidden Traumatic Brain Injury at Birth
Causing the Autism Epidemic.

By

DINESH DANNY

Printed in the United States of America

First Printing, 2025

ISBN - 978-1-7366047-1-7 (paperback) | 978-1-766047-2-4 (e-book)

More about autism and the author at -
www.dineshdanny.com, www.autismpi.org,
autismcausesunveiled.com, autismwhistleblower.com

ACKNOWLEDGMENTS

I would like to thank my wife and my two special needs boys for the time spent away from them while I wrote this book. They are the reason I wrote this book, but they also paid a hefty price in terms of my time and attention on them.

This book would not have been possible without the help of other impacted parents who gladly shared their stories with me, including answering some detailed questioning, helping to establish many of the paths to brain damage at birth and conclusions arrived at in this book. The parents who have undergone this journey before us have been our heroes and source of inspiration.

I would also like to thank the many wonderful nonprofits and websites out there for the plethora of good advice and knowledge they share, and in particular the many autism and mental health organizations for all the good work they have engaged in, trying to rid the world of autism.

PREFACE

As you might have guessed from the title, this book is a whistleblower to the true cause of the meteoric rise of the autism epidemic which is being kept under wraps by certain elements of society. This epidemic is a medical malaise that has been unleashed on populations mostly in the western world while catching up in the rest of the world where medical treatment gets modelled on western medical systems, medications, procedures and protocols. As a software engineer and parent with 2 boys on the autism spectrum, I am actually an outsider to the medical world, yet this is what allows me to tell you the story as it is, unfettered by the need to be bound by medical boards and professional interests. I am a whistleblower not because what I am revealing is not known, but because it is being kept under wraps by a media warfare being waged against impacted parents by the entities involved in the coverup.

It was a quirk of fate, an accident from over fifteen years ago, that profoundly changed our lives as new parents. It took us nearly a decade to fully understand its impact. My wife and I were blessed with two boys, born in 2007 and 2009. Our first son was hyperactive from his first steps. At three, we noticed his advanced reading skills contrasted with his limited speech, we later realized he was reading without comprehending; he struggled with responding to simple yes/no questions and remained hyperactive. I remember he had to be strapped down to that little chair even to get through testing. Evaluations confirmed our fears: autism. We hoped our second son would be spared, but at age three, he too was given the dreaded diagnosis.

Like numerous other parents whose children are diagnosed with autism, our lives were turned upside down. This was a complex problem made even more challenging with not just one but two boys on the autism spectrum. Over the past decade I left no stone unturned trying to find the cause of the problem so that we could pursue a solution. Doctors mostly pointed at genetic and environmental causes, which I believed for a while, but I was never totally convinced. It wasn't until a brain MRI scan of my second son gave me a light-bulb moment and I suddenly realized exactly what had happened. Piecing together events and incidents from the past, I was able to determine that the cause of their condition was the traumatic brain damage they had suffered at birth from Pitocin abuse in labor. Fingers have been pointed at Pitocin before, but here I was, staring at actual proof of the traumatic damage caused by the abuse of the drug and dealing with its consequences on a daily basis.

This book aims to clarify autism from an observant parent's perspective. I believe only parents, who have spent years observing their children from pregnancy through birth, diagnosis and beyond, are truly qualified to understand its causes in their child given all the possible causes. In keeping with the complex nature of autism, with multiple possible causes, I have endeavored to explore a wide range of topics that are, in my view, essential to understanding its origins. You will find detailed discussions of birth injury, labor drugs, the intricacies of brain science, the role of viral latencies, the brain immune deviation (ACAID phenomenon), the information revealed by MRI scans, the mechanics of contraction forces during labor, relevant anatomical details, the complexities of the legal battles surrounding this issue, and much more. It is my hope that by bringing these diverse areas of knowledge together in a single volume, I can provide a more holistic and helpful understanding of this devastating condition. Ultimately, understanding the cause of the autism epidemic requires nothing more than the convergence of known established facts presented in this book.

While the story of the birth of my two boys unfolded in the United States, it could have very well happened anywhere in the world. Everything in this book except the section on legal recourse applies to readers across the globe.

CONTENTS

INTRODUCTION

O ne of the most pernicious aspects of autism is that it doesn't just impact kids – the diagnosis strikes unsuspecting parents as well when they begin to notice their kids are not developing like all the other kids around. It knocks down the natural pride and joy parents have about their children and naturally raises the question of why autism struck their family. These kids look very normal in the early stages of development but then do not develop the increased focus with age and the language skills which are the highest order skills in human beings requiring maximum connectivity and coordination of multiple areas of the brain fails to develop properly. These kids mostly stay at the 3–6-year-old level of maturity for the rest of their lives, unable to live independent lives. While there are kids that make progress with early interventions, these are mostly kids with very mild affliction and even there the recovery is never fully complete. For the more severely impacted, parents often observe retrogression of skills; it seems to happen with nearly every viral encounter. Hard won skills slip away, a struggle that continues throughout their lives. This makes it impossible to outrun the grasp of autism with any intervention whatsoever in these cases. This is because the causes underlying the condition are complicated, with many factors at play. But that's exactly what we'll unravel, step by step, throughout our journey in this book.

Defining Autism

The first step to solving a problem is to accurately define the problem itself. Unfortunately, in the case of autism, this definition has been a challenge of epic proportions and a topic that has been constantly evolving.

The word autism is derived from the Greek word "autos," meaning "self" (like "automatic" means "by itself"). It was first used by Dr. Eugen Blueler in 1908 to describe the symptom of a schizophrenic patient that seemed drawn inward into himself and trapped in his own world.

The word has since been extended to childhood development symptoms where children refuse to interact and learn from the world around them, but instead get "drawn into" themselves. The International Classification of Disease (ICD) coding system developed by the World Health Organization classifies autism under the umbrella of Mental, Behavioral and Neurodevelopmental disorders. The Diagnostic and Statistical Manual of Mental Disorders (DSM) in the US defines autism as a "neurodevelopmental disorder that is characterized by impairments in communication and social interaction as well as patterns of restrictive, repetitive interests and behaviors during early childhood" (DSM-IV). The subsequent edition (the 2013 DSM-V) places more emphasis on the social communication and repetitive behavior aspects.

Yet the symptoms of autism are multiple and varied – in fact so many and so disparate the condition itself is called a spectrum disorder and is characterized by a set of nonspecific disorders in development. The most significant symptom is the lack of verbal development, which reduces the ability of the child to engage in social interaction. This results in them withdrawing into their own world and can lead to the development of obsessive and repetitive behaviors. Autism therefore correctly understood is a set of developmental disorders beginning in early childhood.

The fact that autism begins right from birth naturally skews the general perception of the causes of autism as genetic. Yet while there are some genetic causes that create the symptoms that fall under the vast umbrella of behaviors covered by the autism spectrum, they only constitute 10% or less of the total cases of "autism-like" symptoms out there. The other 90% of the cases are relegated to "unknown" causes that are currently under research – research designed to show that they are genetically caused as well.[1.1] Doctors seem to be trained to reinforce the claim that "nobody knows what causes autism" when what they really are saying is "nobody knows the genetic causes of autism.", because the birth injury causes are very well documented but not widely known.

Diseases, Disorders and Syndromes

Conventional science classifies medical conditions into categories based on our current understanding of the condition. Diseases by definition are conditions with a cause known to medicine i.e. the etiology of disease is fully understood. A disorder on the other hand is a condition with a standard set of symptoms where not every symptom occurs in every instance and very little is known about the causes. A disorder describes disruption of the normal or regular functions in the body or a part of the body. A syndrome is simply a set of symptoms which often occur together. By itself a syndrome cannot be classified as a disease or disorder. A syndrome could be caused by one or more diseases or disorders. For example, the Downs Syndrome is a well-known set of physical and mental conditions and is the result of a genetic disease caused by an extra chromosome in the 21st pair of chromosomes. Classification of diseases, disorders and syndromes in the world of psychiatry is even more controversial given that medical understanding of mental conditions is still rudimentary.

The Real Cause of Autism

Unfortunately, researchers looking into autism have knowingly or inadvertently created an elaborate web of diversions that obscure the truth regarding the causes of autism. There is a presumption that all autism has genetic roots. This results in the current research model focusing on identifying genes and pathways and mechanisms so complex that even the current scientific community struggles to comprehend them, let alone the average family impacted by autism's effects. While many genetic diseases create brain function deficits, the converse is not true. Most kids diagnosed with autism do not have any genetic disorders.

For a long time, the story of childhood autism in the western world has been a mystery mired in the complexity of brain development. Our understanding of autism is restricted by our limited knowledge of the intricacies of brain functioning and human intelligence. But as much as some people would like you to believe autism is some freak occurrence of nature, the cause of autism is in fact a story of deception, incompetence and moral turpitude of certain parties involved in perpetuating a lie that has managed to confuse the general population for decades. As I will elaborate on over the next few chapters, the overwhelming majority of cases of autism are the result of medical mistakes causing hypoxic or traumatic brain injury during birth.

A multitude of scientific studies and immense resources have been dedicated to research on this topic, but the truth is well known to certain groups. As I went about talking to other impacted parents and medical professionals trying to uncover evidence for my own situation, I found their experience corroborated my own findings. I also discovered that there is a surprising number of people even in the medical profession who know or have a hunch about the causes of autism but just don't say it loud enough – either because they are not impacted or because there is not enough evidence and it is against their professional pursuit to stand up and say the truth "as is" and incur the wrath of medical boards and other authorities. There is history of retribution on medical practitioners that don't toe the official line and that is not lost on current practitioners. This is why the truth has to emerge from an unlikely quarter, an engineer like me, with a background in research.

While the evidence of Pitocin and other labor drug abuse remains hidden in plain sight, there is a lot of misinformation that prevents the truth from emerging. In this book I explain why the diversions are misleading. I have outlined the effects vaccines have had and their role in compounding the autism epidemic brought on by pre-existing brain injury by way of a "vaccine double whammy" on the developing brain. I am not in favor of, or against vaccines as taking sides only results in inflaming an already charged debate. Instead, I have tried to explain the conditions under which vaccines might be considered risky and capable of stopping brain damage recovery permanently. These conditions are already outlined in every vaccine label, but parents don't get a chance to look into these and pediatricians are only told of the 'mild' side effects. It is something people on both sides of the vaccine argument need to look into.

I know there could to be naysayers wanting to attack this book on some irrelevant technicality. Most of these naysayers have conflicts of interest and reflexively defend their fellow practitioners. To them and to the reader I point out that all the material in this book is based on baseline facts established by the

Pitocin labelling and ACOG directives to Hospitals and Hospital protocols which existed until about 2018, in addition to facts gleaned from scientific papers or other publicly available material from sources like the US National Institute of Health. In some cases, I have offered plausible explanations for actual observed facts in the real world. I am not looking for academic confirmation of many of these points laid out in this book, since they are all established facts borne out by decades of experience. I have in some cases deliberately avoided getting bogged down by the complexity of the science involved. The actual answers are truly quite simple. These low-stakes science arguments almost always result in inaction and continuation of status quo. Our effort on the parent-side of the equation must be designed to establish and catalog causes of autism and establish legal evidence where necessary.

Proving the cause of autism in a US court has remained an elusive target for many parents, who know in their hearts and minds that birth injury caused their kids' condition but are unable to come up with the evidence to prove it. Legal recourse for parents and their children who were impacted by Pitocin abuse is both fair and necessary. Compensation for those lives impacted by malpractice is non-negotiable, but parents should know that the statute of limitations for proving cases of childhood autism in US federal courts is 18 years from birth. Most state laws are even more limiting in many cases. The need for individual cases vs mass torts and a legal catch-22 introduced in 2018 is preventing lawyers from taking up these cases and these have been major roadblocks for parents already dealing with a lot with their kids. The retrospective research and data collection efforts of autismpi.org outlined towards the end of this book could offer a way forward. and I urge parents to take a closer look at it and participate in this massive data collection effort.

PART I

Understanding the Brain

The brain is the command and control center for the whole body, making it the most complex and least understood of all organs. Our brains make us who we are: our memories, our unique capabilities, our personalities, our intelligence, our consciousness and a lot more. The processes that drive and control these aspects of brain functioning lie at the junction of many different branches of science, including biochemistry, biophysics, and molecular biology.

The most significant naturally occurring risk to brain health in a person's life is the birth process. It presents a dual possibility of brain damage from lack of oxygen and from traumatic injury occurring from being pushed out head first. While natural brain processes are only now being understood, the processes of damage and recovery are still under study. Autism is a brain development disorder and it is critical we start our journey to understand its causes with studying the brain.

CHAPTER 1

Brain Development

A utism is an affliction of the brain, so let's begin with a pseudo technical exposition on the human brain and the aspects important to brain functioning and development. If you are a parent of a kid with autism you are almost required to become an amateur brain researcher if you would like to understand what your child is going through. Unfortunately, a lot of impacted parents continue to remain unaware of the true reasons for their children's condition in the midst of all the misinformation and diversions out there. A good understanding of the human brain is essential for understanding the afflictions that can come about as a result of disturbance or damage to any of these very delicate and complex mechanisms.

Our knowledge of the human brain continues to improve with time and some of these facts continue to evolve. What's presented in the following chapters is mostly at the structural and functional levels. Even if you know quite a bit of detail about the brain, I hope there are some details here that may be new and help with an understanding of mental health problems and symptoms that have now become a growing concern in the US and other countries in the world. This basic knowledge is also critical to understanding the terminology used by doctors, medical reports and medications when trying to understand the diagnosis and treatment options in mental health challenges like autism.

Childhood Brain Development

Out of all the living creatures out there with well-distinguished brain structures, there exists one critical factor that separates human brains from all others. And that is the fact that the human brain is an unfinished organ at birth. A newborn calf or fawn can walk right within a few minutes of birth, while the human baby is completely dependent on its parents for years. In fact, 18 years of parental care for human beings is the longest in the animal kingdom. That time also correlates directly to the time it takes the human brain to reach full maturity.

The fact that the human brain is not at an advanced stage of development at birth should not be seen as a deficit. That fuzzy undeveloped brain in the early stages of human life is the reason that allows the human brain to learn a lot more from environmental inputs. This prolonged development time also affords humans the higher skills of language, art, higher cognition, memory, personality, and fine motor skills that are ultimately more advanced than the rest of the living beings on this planet. But the processes that lead to all these remarkable skills also makes the human brain the most complex system and the least understood organ in our body.

At the most basic level, while every organ is vital to the human body, the brain is simply the most critical organ. People die when the brain is dead. Being the command and control center, it powers our consciousness, every subconscious occurrence and every conscious movement or thought. This amazing feat is accomplished by about a 100 billion neurons in the brain, working together to make our conscious movements and actions as well as our subconscious and autonomous activities like breathing and digestion possible. Our knowledge of the brain in relation to those higher skills has been constantly evolving and is now vastly improved from where we were a few decades ago.

From the time of birth, the brain increases by about 4 times in volume until age 6. Even then it's only 90% complete, with full structural maturation occurring well past adolescence. In the early childhood stage, there is a high level of experience-based development of the brain. Audio visual coordination, attention span, motor development and fine motor coordination are all learned skills. The acquisition of these skills in turn helps develop the neural network of the brain further, strengthening certain connections while eliminating others. All this growth over a prolonged period of time results in the development of what is arguably the most complex biological unit known to nature.

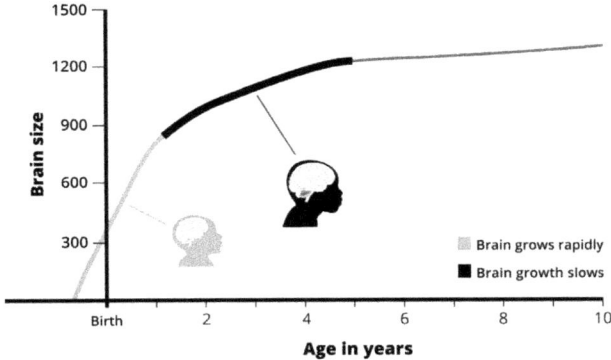

Fig. 1.1: Brain Growth with Age

Stages of Brain Development

Brain development happens in stages, with later stages building on the foundation built in the previous stages. In the first stages the sensory pathways of vision and hearing are established, followed by language and then higher-order cognitive skills such as critical thinking and reasoning. Strong foundations in the early stages makes for better higher-order skills later. The illustrated chart in Fig. 2.2 from the Harvard University Center on the Developing Child details the various stages of brain functional development as a function of the rate of neuronal connections formed with time.

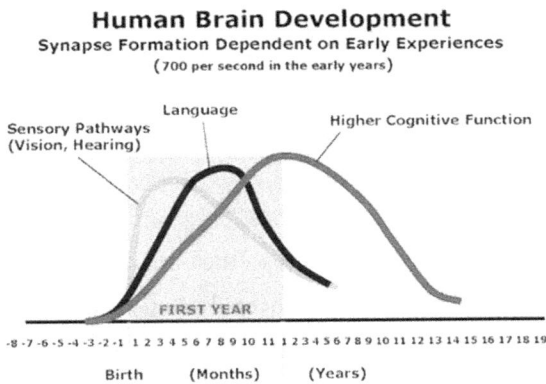

Fig. 1.2: Brain functional Development with time showing neural connections for different brain functions develop sequentially.

Notice how neural connection development really takes off at birth and the maximum rate of development is achieved in the first year of life in a specific order. Experiential learning after birth increases exponentially reaching a rate of about 700 synaptic connections established per second. Neuronal connections relating to the sensory pathways of hearing and vision are the first ones to be established. Language skills are built on top of the sensory pathways of hearing and vision and higher cognitive skills like focus and problem-solving follow language learning. A disruption in the initial development of sensory pathways interferes with the subsequent development of all other skills including language and problem-solving.

Brain Functional Areas

The brain has three main parts: the cerebrum, cerebellum and brainstem. The cerebrum and the cerebellum are divided into 2 lobes each and they are all attached at the brain stem.

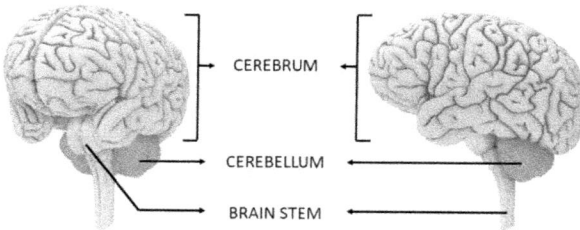

Fig. 1.3: Three main structural parts of the human brain.

The brain stem is the relay center for the Cerebellum and cerebrum taking their messages to the rest of the body through the spinal cord. Additionally, the brain stem is responsible for controlling the autonomous functions of the body including breathing, heart rate, digestion, sleep and wake cycles and many other functions key to the basic functioning of the human body.

The lobes of the Cerebellum are located on the rear side of the head, tucked just under the cerebral lobes. The main known function of the cerebellum is the coordination of various muscle groups to help maintain posture and balance. Shifts in balance are detected and coordinated by the cerebellum to ensure smooth movements. The cerebellum also coordinates eye movements and is involved in motor learning like in learning to ride a bicycle or playing an instrument. Recent research has also suggested a cerebellar role in thinking and mood, although this functionality hasn't been fully explored by scientists.

The cerebrum is the largest part of the brain and is composed of right and left lobes called hemispheres. It performs higher functions like interpreting touch, vision and hearing, as well as speech, reasoning, emotions, learning, and fine control of movement. These are also the functions that are impacted in autism. The following picture gives a good idea of the various areas of the cerebrum and the functionalities they control.

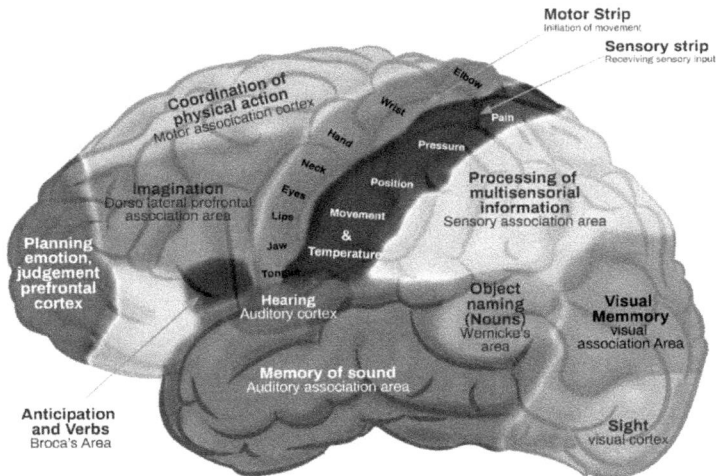

Fig. 1.4: Cerebral functional areas

Notable special areas and features of the brain and their functions are shown in Fig. 1.4. Notice how the following main functional areas are surrounded by other areas that support the association and coordination of these senses:

Main Function Area	Surrounding Support Area / Memory
Sensory strip	- Sensory association area
Motor strip	- Motor association coordination area
Hearing	- Auditory association area
Sight	- Visual memory and association area
Planning/ Emotion	- Imagination, prefrontal association

As we will discuss in upcoming chapters, the cerebrum, being the largest, outermost region of the brain, makes it the most susceptible to traumatic damage particularly during birth, when a baby makes its way out of the mother head first. The higher-order functions controlled by the cerebrum are also the same found deficient in kids impacted by the autism spectrum disorder. Deficiencies in auditory and visual processing, lack of fine motor skills and slow processing speeds, are all telltale signs of damage to the cerebrum.

Key Take Away: The human brain is the most complex and least understood of human organs. Brain development occurs in stages, with every stage of development being the foundation of the next stage. The first two years of life represent the period of maximum brain development, and 90% of the brain is developed by age 6. Damage to the main underlying networks of the brain is largely irreparable. Any damage to the brain at birth means subsequent development is significantly hindered.

CHAPTER 2

Brain Functioning

B rain substructures like neurons, grey and white matter, the myelin sheath, and neurotransmitters play an important role in understanding neurodevelopmental disorders. Let's look at these in a little more detail.

Neurons

The neurons that make up the brain are of various shapes, sizes and types that serve varying functions in the brain. Outside of the central nervous system, neurons are found all over the body in the peripheral nervous system, the enteric nervous system and every other part of the body that the brain controls either autonomously or voluntarily. In the brain, neurons work together forming neural networks that are responsible for all the higher-order functions that the human brain is exclusively capable of like speech, learning, thinking and imagination.

Neurons are specialized cells with very distinct shapes that are designed for the creation of networks to pass chemical and electrical signals. The diversity in the structure of neurons is so large these cell types are still being discovered. Unlike other cells, neurons never divide, and neither do they die off to be replaced by new ones. They usually cannot be replaced after being lost, although there are a few exceptions. There are also neuron support cells, called the neuroglia or glial cells, that help regulate the chemical environment of the brain. The main signaling neurons are thought to be of the most common multipolar neuron structural type, with a branched cell body and a single elongated cable-like structure called an axon, which also has a branched end to it. The human brain is estimated to have about 100 billion neurons and as many as 20 to 50 times more glial cells supporting the functions of these neurons.

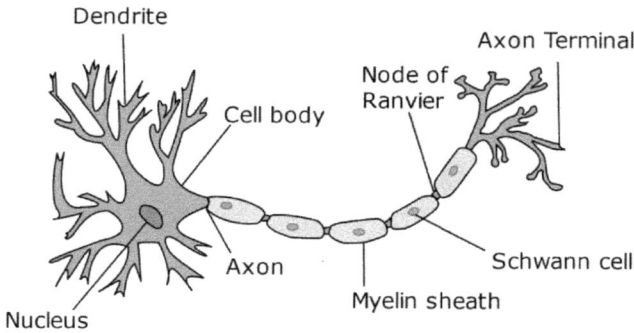

Fig. 2.1: Diagram of a Typical Neuron

Dendrites are an arbor of receptacles around the cell body of a neuron that help receive information from other neurons. Each neuron has a single long fiber called an axon. At the tip of the axon is a growth cone that serves to guide the axon to targeted brain regions. Once the axon reaches the target site, synapses, or points of connection, form between the axon and the target.

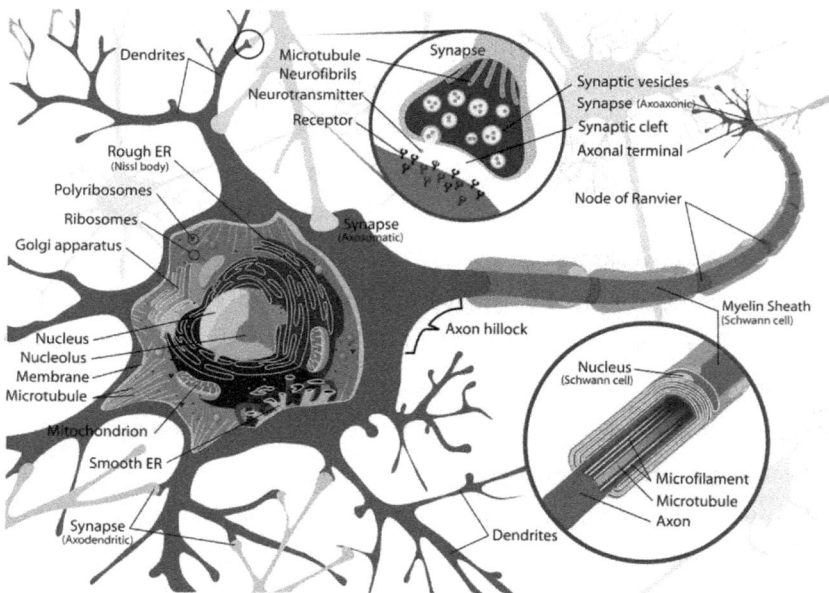

Fig. 2.2: Diagram showing a 3d cut section of a neuron cell with synaptic connections to other neurons and myelin sheath highlighted.

Bunches of neurons together form the nervous system. Neuronal axons can range in length from less than a millimeter to a meter or more. The longest axons run down from the brain into the spinal cord and beyond.

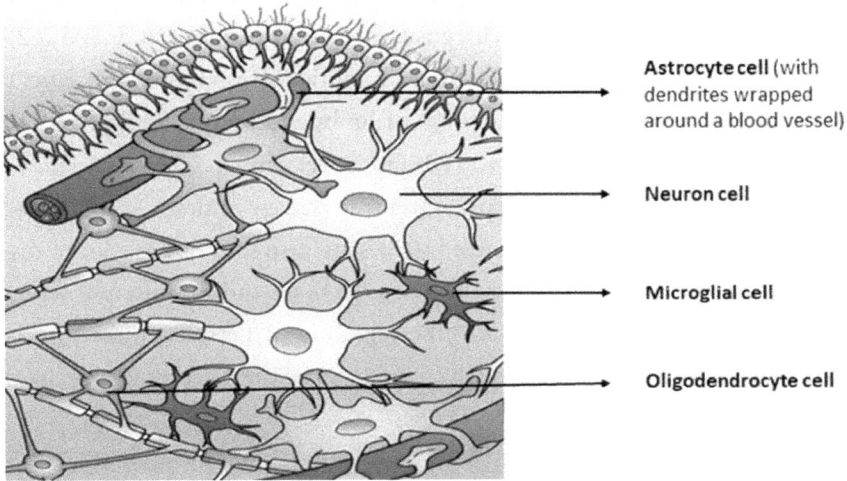

Astrocyte cell (with dendrites wrapped around a blood vessel)

Neuron cell

Microglial cell

Oligodendrocyte cell

Fig. 2.3: Illustration of the three different types of glial cells found in the central nervous system.

In the brain, neurons with long axons are encased in a fatty substance called myelin, which is what makes the brain's white matter white. Myelin acts as insulation for axons, helping signals transmit over longer distances. For this reason, myelin is mostly found in neurons that connect different brain regions, rather than in the neurons whose axons remain in a local region. An axon typically develops side branches called axon collaterals, so that one neuron can send information to several others. These collaterals, just like the roots of a tree, split into smaller extensions called terminal branches. Each of these has a synaptic terminal on the tip. Groups of axons are organized into tracts by glial cells which help connect areas of the grey matter to other areas, whose coordination is necessary to carry out brain functionality. Every aspect of this intricate web of neurons and supporting cells helps conduct important brain functionality. Damage to any of these fine structures can result in loss of connectivity between areas and impact one or more aspects of brain functionality depending on the area of damage.

Different parts of the brain that serve different functions use this network of connections to communicate with other functional parts of the brain. Working together these neuron networks coordinate between our various senses and regulate our responses to sensory inputs that include visual recognition, imagination, auditory senses, olfactory (smell), gustatory (taste) and the rest of about 20 senses known to modern science including equilibrioception (sense of balance), proprioception (awareness of the position of limbs and body), vestibular sense (ability to feel velocity), thermoception (ability to feel temperature), kinaesthesia (sense of movement), and chronoception (sensing passage of time). It is believed some ancient civilizations were aware of 300+ senses, so science has a lot to discover yet about the working of the neurons in the brain and the different senses they support and coordinate. Clearly the relationship between these mostly unknown senses and the neurons involved ought to be pretty complex and hard to decipher.

Grey versus White Matter

The cerebral cortex, the outer folded body of the brain, shows two distinct areas of coloration when sectioned out: the grey matter and the white matter. While grey matter is more pinkish-white in reality, grey is the name that has stuck. The difference in coloration is due to the difference in composition of the two areas. The grey matter is mostly composed of the body of the neurons, the dendrites, synapses and axon terminals, while the white matter is composed of the myelin-coated axon parts of the neurons.

Grey matter can be structurally further differentiated into multiple layers based on the type of neuron types that predominate in that layer. The grey matter is richly supplied with blood vessels due to the enormous needs for oxygen and energy to carry out the brain's mental processes. This makes the grey matter more susceptible to hypoxic damage under conditions of oxygen deprivation, an event we discuss in chapter 5. Grey matter in the various folded areas of the brain is connected to grey matter in other areas of the brain through the axons of the neurons in them. These distinct connected grey matter areas work together in groups with every group enabling a certain higher-order function. This coordination of the various grey matter areas is important to higher-order functions of the brain such as memory, language, imagination, critical thinking, etc., and damage to this area has corresponding impacts on these cognitive capabilities.

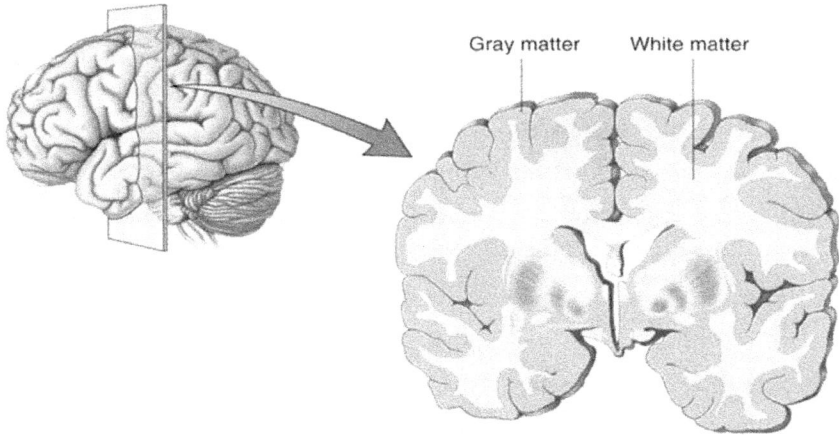

Gray matter   White matter

Fig. 2.4: Grey vs White matter.

White matter is made of the long axon fibers of the neurons in the grey matter. The white matter takes up three fourths of the volume of the cerebrum, which highlights the importance and sheer complexity of wiring in the brain that they represent. These axons are coated with myelin, a mixture of proteins and fatty lipids, that helps conduct nerve signals and protect the axons. This fatty myelin is also the reason for the whiter coloration of the white matter. Nerve signals travel between different parts of the grey matter and up and down the spinal cord through groups of axons called tracts that connect them. Damage to the white matter in the brain can result in severing of these connections and leads to loss of coordination between grey matter areas that is crucial to a lot of higher-order functioning. In case of white matter damage, the resulting inability for various areas of grey matter to coordinate might explain why individuals on the autism spectrum lack broad interests and tend to favor narrow areas of interest. The lack of conversational skills in autism might also be a result of this, since conversation involves interpreting language, understanding verbal and nonverbal cues, memory recall and correlation, which requires using different parts of the brain all at once in real-time.

Myelination

Most of the development in the early stages of childhood brain development involves the creation of pathways between the various functional areas of the brain and the myelination of the neurons connecting these pathways. Structural maturing of individual brain regions and their connecting pathways is required for the successful development of cognitive, motor, and sensory functions. Such growth is eventually responsible for a smooth flow of neural impulses throughout the brain, which allows for information to be integrated across the many spatially segregated brain regions involved in these functions. The speed of neural transmission is an important factor, and this depends not only on the junctions between nerve cells called synapses but also on the structural properties of the connecting axon fibers. Critical axon structural properties include their diameters and the thickness of the special myelin insulation around many fibers. Large groups of myelinated axons, which connect various regions in the brain, appear visibly as "white matter." Axon tracts of the major pathways carrying impulses in the human brain continue to develop throughout childhood and adolescence.

The nerve impulse is a rapid propagating wave, approximately 1 millisecond in duration, of chemical depolarization followed by repolarization. While it is really a transmission of a chemical impulse or action potential, the neuron axon can be thought of as behaving as an electrical transmission line whose cross-sectional diameter is an important determinant of impulse propagation velocity. The larger the diameter, the greater the velocity of propagation. Correspondingly, the myelin sheath that surrounds certain types of axons is a periodically interrupted type of electrical insulation, and its presence represents a substantial increase in pulse propagation velocity over that of a bare axon of the same diameter. The breaks in the myelin insulation, called the "Nodes of Ranvier," represent ion rich areas that help bolster the speed and strength of the nerve impulse.

Myelination is thus a major aspect of the workings of neural circuits. Any disturbance in the myelination process due to certain genetic conditions is known to lead to neurological disorders grouped under the heading of leukodystrophy. Such disorders are rare but have a genetic etiology. Unlike autism, which is a childhood developmental disorder, leukodystrophy conditions can be triggered even at later ages and is identifiable in an MRI scan. As rare as they are, at least 23 different known subdivisions of leukodystrophy are known to exist. Multiple Sclerosis (MS) is another disease that results from de-myelination of nerve cells. MS is caused by the body's immune system attacking the myelin sheath, causing damage to the brain and the rest of the nervous system. All this goes to prove the importance of myelination in the functioning of the brain and central nervous system – and how damage to these areas could have significant neurological impacts.

Neuron Fiber Lengths

Neurons make up most of the cerebellum (lower lobes at the rear of the head close to the neck) and cerebrum (2 upper lobes) of the brain. They are of different types and varying lengths and are often a source of confusion when trying to understand brain morphology and functioning. Not all neurons in the brain have the typical structure of a cell body with a very elongated axon attached. About 80 percent of brain neurons have very short axons, almost not distinguishable from the dendrites. The rest of the 20 percent have longer axons of varying lengths and traverse across the brain connecting its many regions. These longer axon neurons are also the ones whose axons are protected by the myelin sheath so they can transmit the action potentials across without loss.

Longer neurons are of particular interest due to the possibility of damage and a lesser possibility for recovery from damage. It is common knowledge that damage to the neurons of the spinal cord is the cause for paralysis in case of injury below the point of damage and such damage is mostly irrecoverable. The longest neurons in the body are those that run from the base of the spinal cord to the toes and are about one meter long. Those that run from the brain into the spinal column are also known to be very long. How long are the longest neurons in the brain? The answer depends on the location and function of the neuron within the brain, with lengths reaching the entire width of the two lobes of the cerebrum connecting areas in the left lobe of the cerebrum to areas in the right lobe for example. Neurons that project from the brain down into the spinal column are also very long.

Analysis of data from the neuromorpho.org database compared to the results of other scientists has allowed researchers from aiimpacts.org to arrive at the following conclusions for various neuron lengths in the cerebral and cerebellar brain areas:

Table 2.1 – Neuron lengths by location and type

Connection type	Average length per neuron (mm)	Contributing neuron types	Sources of evidence
Cerebellar, short-range	5.7 - 6.1	Granule (~70%), stellate, basket, Purkinje, Golgi	Morphometry
Cerebral, short-range	14 - 20	Pyramidal (2/3rds to 85%), stellate	Fiber density in rats, morphometry
Cerebral, long-range	100	Pyramidal	Width of corpus callosum, relationship between brain volume and global connection length

Source: aiimpacts.org

As seen in Fig. 2.5, the corpus callosum and anterior commissure are the neuron fiber bridges that connect the two hemispheres of the cerebrum. The projection fibers that constitute the internal capsule are neuron axon connections that connect the outer cerebral areas to the basal ganglia. The basal ganglia are the motor control centers which help decide between the various responses to the sensory inputs received.

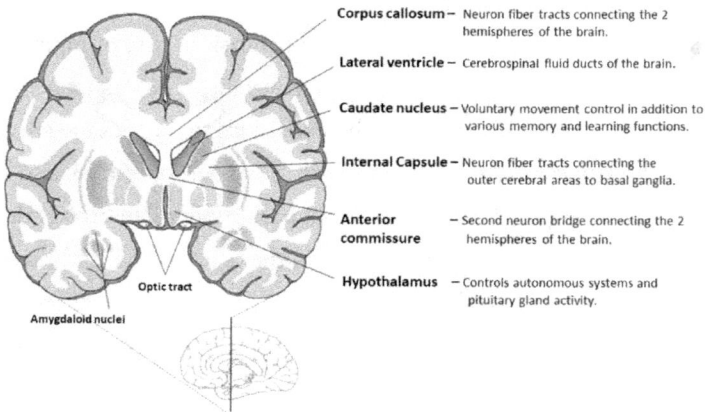

Corpus callosum – Neuron fiber tracts connecting the 2 hemispheres of the brain.

Lateral ventricle – Cerebrospinal fluid ducts of the brain.

Caudate nucleus – Voluntary movement control in addition to various memory and learning functions.

Internal Capsule – Neuron fiber tracts connecting the outer cerebral areas to basal ganglia.

Anterior commissure – Second neuron bridge connecting the 2 hemispheres of the brain.

Hypothalamus – Controls autonomous systems and pituitary gland activity.

Optic tract

Amygdaloid nuclei

Fig. 2.5: Coronal or frontal cross-section of the brain, showing important neuron fiber connections of the brain and white matter functional control areas.

Traumatic damage to some of these longer length fibers in the deep brain areas can happen during birth as a baby's head makes its way out of its mother. For example, damage to the caudate nucleus is reported to result in loss of motivation, obsessive-compulsive disorder and hyperactivity. Even the smallest of scars in the brain can lead to negative outcomes for those babies impacted by trauma. Sometimes the damage is so small that it not visible in MRI images, due to the limitation of about one millimeter resolution of MRI, but the adverse effect on development is very real. This rarity of MRI visible scarring has also been one reason the traumatic brain injury at birth has remained hidden in most instances of autism.

Neurotransmitters

Neurons are connected to each other by special junctions called synapses. The synaptic junction allows action potentials to be transmitted to the target neuron using chemical molecules called neurotransmitters. The key concept to the synapse is that the neurons don't touch each other but have a very small gap between them called the synaptic cleft. Communication across this synaptic cleft is controlled by these neurotransmitters. Every neuron is connected to about 1000 other neurons. So, for the 100 billion neurons in the brain, there are about 100 trillion synaptic junctions.

Recall that proteins are made up of long chains of basic building blocks called amino acids. Neuro transmitters are singular amino acids or amino acid like compounds which convert the action potentials at the synaptic junctions between neurons into chemical messages triggering specific actions in the next connected neurons. The influence of the neurotransmitter on the next neuron or muscle could be excitation, inhibition or moderation.

Neurotransmitters are synthesized by the neurons at the axon terminals and stored in synaptic vesicles at these synaptic junctions. They are released into the synaptic cleft when an action potential is received from the axon and work to excite, inhibit or modulate receptors on the muscle or neuron they are connected to. They often trigger a response in the post synaptic cell. The synapses and neurotransmitters ensure that signals travel in only one direction. They also allow for signals to be amplified or moderated, and working with other neurons they this can result in amplification or reduction of impulses. Overall, this can allow for complex signaling and a wide array of behaviors to emerge.

While there are hundreds of neurotransmitters in the brain, there exist 6 major neurotransmitters. The table below shows main neurotransmitters their functions and the results of their deficiency or excess.

Table 2.2: The Main Neurotransmitters

Neuro-transmitter & Effect	Function	Deficiency	Excess
Glutamate (Excitatory)	Primary excitatory neurotransmitter of the nervous system, controls all behaviors, learning, memory	Insomnia, concentration problems, mental exhaustion, low energy	Hyperactivity, anxiety, pain amplification, Neuron damage
Dopamine (Excitatory or Inhibitory)	Neuromodulator involved in voluntary movement, pleasure, motivation, learning	Parkinson's Disease (initiating movement), depression	Schizophrenia
GABA (Inhibitory)	Major inhibitory neurotransmitter, controls all behaviors including anxiety, motor control	Huntington's Disease (destruction of GABA neurons), loss of motor control	Inhibits brain function
Serotonin (Inhibitory)	sleep, memory, mood, pleasure	Depression	Prozac works by blocking re-uptake of serotonin
Endorphins (Inhibitory)	Inhibiting pain	Hyper-sensitivity to pain	Insensitivity to pain
Acetyl - Choline (Excitatory)	Muscular movement, memory, cognitive function	Alzheimer's Disease, paralysis (botulism)	Convulsions

As you can see these neurotransmitters can have opposite effects of excitation and inhibition. Some of the commonly paired neurotransmitters include Serotonin and Melatonin, Dopamine and Norepinephrine, and GABA and Glutamate. Additionally, neurons allow for co-transmission of more than one neurotransmitter from a single neuron. This makes it possible for even more complex behaviors to emerge.

Once the neurotransmitter has acted on the receptacles of the subsequent cell, it needs to be quickly eliminated so the next cycle of excitation or inhibition can begin. The brain has very efficient methods to perform this elimination including diffusion out of the synaptic cleft followed by absorption by glial cells, enzymatic breakdown by astrocytes, and re-uptake or re-absorption of the neuro transmitter back into the pre-synaptic neuron. Thus, the complex biochemistry of these small amino acid molecules called neurotransmitters plays a very critical role in the functioning of the brain.

A significant portion of medications for autism and psychiatric disorders involve medication that tries to address supposed deficiency or excess of neurotransmitters. They are sometimes useful but outcomes very unpredictable due to the complex nature of neurotransmitter interactions. Psychiatric medication to this day is mostly trial and error. Individual reactions to specific medication need to be very carefully monitored if such a medical path is pursued.

Key Take Away: We have looked into the functioning of neurons, their physical structures, chemical and electro chemical signaling, using neurotransmitters. We considered the different excitatory and inhibitory effects of neurotransmitters. Other components of the brain physical structure like grey and white matter, myelin, all play very critical roles in the proper functioning of the brain.

CHAPTER 3

The Protected Brain

T his chapter examines common protective bodily functions which tend to be performed slightly differently in the brain, compared to how they are performed in the rest of the body. This is due to the special status of the brain as the most important organ of the body. Just like understanding the development of the human brain is essential for understanding the afflictions that can come about as a result of disturbance or damage to any of these very delicate and complex mechanisms, it's important for parents of children on the spectrum to grasp how damage to brain function can impact their child – and why the brain by design is unlikely to repair itself as fast as (or as much as) other parts of the human body.

The Blood Brain Barrier

The blood brain barrier is a specialized protection mechanism around the blood vessels supplying the brain that regulates the flow of nutrients to and from the brain. This affords the brain an additional layer of protection from an infectious disease or other metabolic toxins. Inflammation in the tight cranial space can lead to neuron damage, and so this mechanism limits brain inflammation by limiting both disease vectors and immune cells from entering brain tissue. Additionally, being a very active environment, the brain needs a lot of efficient, active transport of nutrients (including removal of waste products). The blood brain barrier is designed to do just that with specialized layers of endothelial cells, astrocytes (support neurons) and pericytes (substrate cells).

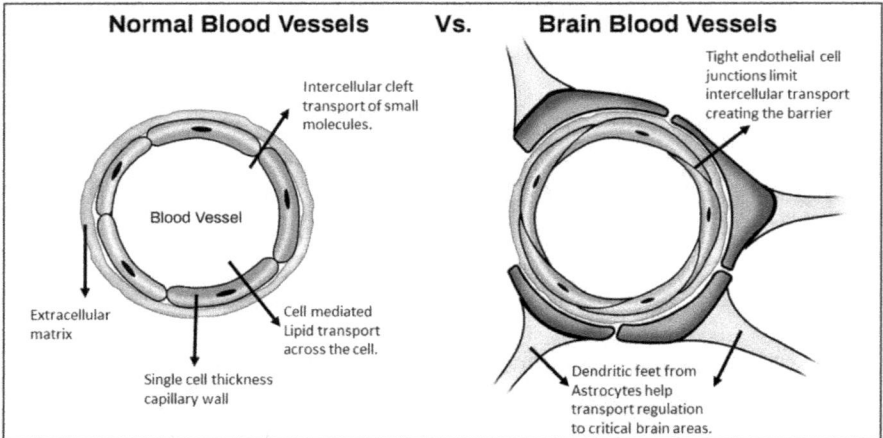

Fig. 3.1: Blood Brain barrier. Notice the tight overlap of the endothelial cells in the brain blood vessel (right) creating the barrier. The astrocyte feet also modulate the uptake of molecules into the brain across the barrier.

Endothelial cells make up the walls of all blood vessels in the body. However, the endothelial cells in the blood vessels of the brain are special as they are bound together with tightly overlapping cell walls called "tight junctions." These tight junctions only allow for very selective transport of molecules between the cell walls of adjacent cells. The endothelial cells are wrapped by a layer of cells called pericytes that typically bind them to the surrounding tissue. However, inside the brain these are bound to specialized astrocyte neurons that excel at controlling the transport of nutrients into and out of the brain tissue which is made up of glial cells and other types of neurons.

As I discuss in detail in later chapters, the blood brain barrier is a very important and distinguishing feature of the brain because while it is mainly beneficial due to the protection it provides from external threats, it also presents a challenge when treating brain conditions. Medicines meant to treat the brain may not make it past the blood brain barrier. Alzheimer's is suspected to be caused by plaque buildup in the brain from the inability to drain certain substances out across the blood brain barrier. Brain injury can compromise this barrier and this limits the ability of the central nervous system to heal itself. This is one of the reasons brain damage is actually permanent in many cases.

Brain Immune Privilege

Certain organs in the human body seem to have evolved such that they are able to tolerate the presence of foreign substances (antigens) inside of them. The presence of antigens inside of these organs doesn't evoke the typical immune response that happens everywhere else in the body. This includes the eyes, testicles, placenta and fetus and the central nervous system (CNS). These organs are said to have immune privilege, as typical immune responses in these areas could be more damaging than useful; hence evolution seems to have taken a path to allow these organs to stay outside the bounds of the immune system.

Originally the entire brain was thought to be immune privileged by virtue of the blood brain barrier. It's now been proven that the brain immune privilege is limited to certain parts of the central nervous system. The brain has a different type of immune response from the typical peripheral immune system response. While immune cells are typically not allowed past the blood brain barrier, at times of need, there is complex signaling that allows certain special immune cells across the perineal, endothelial and astrocyte layers and enter the brain vascular regions.

The exact working of the immune system is not fully understood and still a subject of intense research. There is an enormous amount of complex physiology involved in the inner working of the immune system in higher-order vertebrates. The major organs involved in immunity include adenoids, bone marrow, lymphatic system, spleen, thymus and tonsils. In very simplified terms, there are 2 layers of immunity. The innate immune system consists of the skin, stomach acid, enzymes found in tears and skin oils, mucus and the cough reflex and is the first line of defense. Innate immunity also includes cell mediated defenses like regular white blood cells that engulf and digest invading pathogens and the lymphatic system that creates and maintains these white blood cells. The key distinguishing feature of innate immunity is the fact that this defense is not against specific pathogens, but directed toward a broad range of common antigen (foreign body) characteristics learned over the course of evolution. The innate system also has ways of triggering the adaptive immune system when unable to take care of the situation by itself.

Active immunity is the second line of defense against the pathogens of the outside world. The active part of innate immunity involves two kinds of immune patrol cells, macrophages and dendrites found at the tissue level. Macrophages are cells that engulf and digest identified pathogens and dendritic cells are cells that attach to the pathogen and inactivate them or return to the lymphatic system with a template of how the foreign body can be attached to. When innate immunity fails to stop invading microbes, the adaptive immune system is called into action by dendrites returning with templates for attacking the foreign body or pathogen (antigen). The adaptive immune system is a more directed response to the specific antigen consisting of white blood cells created in the lymphatic system. At this point the body tissue level response turns into a blood cell, whole body response. The white blood cells of the adaptive immune system are of 2 types the B-cells (plasma cells) and the T-cells. The B-cells have a large number of receptors that bind to specific antigens. Once bound the B-cells return to the lymphatic system to create more copies of themselves. These then go out to bind more antigens and present them to T-cells for further action. They do this presentation by introducing binding proteins called antibodies into the bloodstream so more antigens can be identified and removed. The subtype of T-cells called the killer T-cells are responsible for removing the antigen cells from the system using an antibody dependent digestion mechanism. They are generated in the lymphatic system in response to the antigens bound by the B-cells. This dual response with directed antigen response, from the lymphatic system is the signature response of the adaptive immune system.

This very simplified version of the entire immune response system is captured in fig 3.2:

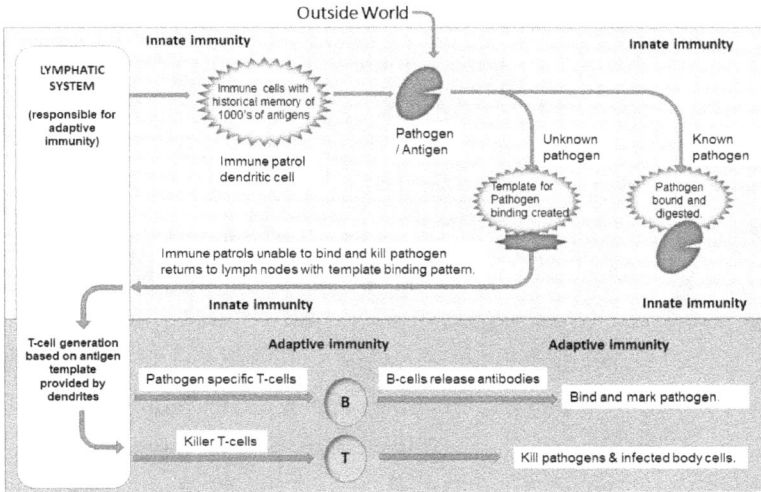

Fig. 3.2: A simplified view of the immune system showing innate immunity, adaptive immunity and their relationship to the lymphatic system.

The immune system is very complex including certain other proteins like cytokines, interferons that I have not discussed here for the sake of simplicity. The actual roles of certain organs, cell types and proteins in the immune system are still being discovered and identified.

The ACAID Phenomenon

The blood brain barrier seems to offer a separation of the brain immunity from the rest of the immune system. But recent discoveries suggest there is still interaction of the brain with the B-cells of the immune system. The brain lacks a lymphatic system, but there is evidence of the brain tissue draining antigens into the cervical lymphatic nodes found in the neck. The immune system response to antigens coming from the brain is heavily skewed toward the B-cell response. This avoidance of the T-cell response in the brain is what makes the brain immune response different from elsewhere in the body. In fact, re-introduction of the same antigen in other parts of the body after a previous encounter in the brain also leads to the lack of a T-cell immune response. Originally observed in the anterior chambers of the eyes, this phenomenon is called ACAID (Anterior Chamber-Associated Immune Deviation).

ACAID is a phenomenon of immune suppression that is known to exist in many mammals (starting with mice all the way to higher primates). It was first noticed when corneal transplants were observed to be the least rejected transplant by the immune system. The eyes are an immune privileged organ protected from the immune system by the blood-retinal barrier. This is because evolution has over long periods identified that a typical immune response in some areas of the body is actually more detrimental than useful. It is observed that introducing an antigen (foreign particle) directly into the anterior chamber of the eye results in immune suppression for that antigen in the rest of the body. Research is underway to look into ways of taking advantage of this phenomenon to treat autoimmune diseases, organ system transplant rejects, etc. These are the positive aspects of the ACAID phenomenon. However, if foreign organisms directly invade these immune privileged organs (perhaps via damaged areas in the barriers that typically protect them), then they might end up obtaining immune suppression in the rest of the body, leading to chronic illnesses that are hard to treat.

The white matter of the brain is one area where the blood brain barrier creates a different immune environment. Not much is known about ACAID immune suppression in the case of white matter, as human testing for something like this is not possible. Nevertheless, this phenomenon of ACAID combined with a compromised blood brain barrier in subjects with brain damage might actually play a role in why viruses might survive in some other parts of the nervous system and continue a chronic, low grade, long term adverse impact on the affected individual. In the rest of the brain tissue, glial cells form part of the regular response in addition to the innate immunity afforded by the blood brain barrier, and there is interaction between the neuronal and immune systems (particularly at the cellular level where the glial cells aid in the removal of antigens, astrocytes aid in the transport of antibodies and B-cells across the blood brain barrier). There is also evidence of B-cell response, but the inflammatory T-cell response has not been found in the brain. But the white matter of the brain is the only area that is totally immune privileged – and therefore cordoned off from easily repairing itself – or ridding itself of viruses as well.

Neuroplasticity

Neuroplasticity is a word coined in recent times to describe how the brain and its connections are constantly changing as a result of external stimulus and environmental input. Practicing certain activities is known to reinforce the corresponding areas of the brain where the functionality resides. We all recognize the saying "practice makes a man perfect." Apparently, the reasoning behind it is neuroplasticity – the rewiring of your brain to do that task perfectly. The proportion of grey matter and synapses in the various areas of the brain may also change over time corresponding to the activities the individual predominantly engages in.

Another area where neuroplasticity helps is the possibility of recovery from injury. Studies on monkeys and mice have demonstrated the ability of their brains to recover from injury over long periods of time. It's been demonstrated they develop the same functionality of the damaged area of the brain in areas adjoining the damage with adequate external stimulation. This ability of healthy individuals to recover from damage seems to occur at all ages except in individuals past the age of 70 or so, where genetic damage becomes more significant and reduces the chances of neuroplastic recovery.

However, the ability of the brain to heal itself due to neuroplasticity is also misunderstood. It is far from the truth that the brain can heal itself. The extent of damage and location of the damage plays an important role in any possibility of recovery from injury. Scar tissue occurring from damage is known to inhibit regrowth of neurons in the scar and surrounding areas. It represents a major challenge to recovery. In cases of significant scarring damage to the brain or other parts of the CNS, the damage is usually permanent given our current knowledge of brain healing and treatment options. Also, if the ability to recognize and respond to external stimuli is lost as a result of damage, the ability to recover is lost as well.

Traumatic Brain Injury (TBI)

The brain is the most fragile of all living tissue, with a very fine and intricate neuron structure in the white matter. It is also the most sensitive to changes in oxygen levels and oxygen supply. The brain requires about 15% of cardiovascular output in adults – a number known to be even higher in children. The system is so critical that the 2 main arteries supplying the anterior brain and the posterior brain and brain stem back each other up, through the bilateral communicating posterior arteries.

Hypoxic brain injury happens when there is an insufficient supply of oxygen reaching the brain tissue. This results in neurons dying out from lack of oxygen causing permanent brain damage. It is called cerebral hypoxia or cerebral anoxia. Hypoxia can happen to a fetus at or near birth due to many causes, but it is mostly related to the constriction of blood supply to the fetal brain. Any constriction of blood supply to any part of the body is called ischemia. So, it is not surprising that brain injury at birth is referred to as hypoxic-ischemic injury. It can be caused by any one of many causes that can reduce blood flow to the fetal brain.

Many natural pregnancy complications related to birth cause hypoxic brain damage, resulting in neurodevelopmental disorders ranging from cerebral palsy to high functioning autism. Hypoxia or loss of oxygen to the fetal brain can be due to low maternal blood pressure, placental detachment, inflammatory disease in maternal pelvis constricting blood flow to placenta, and blood clotting complications. Other birth complications like placenta placement, cord compression, nuchal cord and other less common malformations of blood vessels can lead to hypoxia as well. And it is also the case that extensive and prolonged contractions – particularly when artificially induced at a high frequency– can create pressures that choke off blood supply to the fine capillaries of the brain.

Extensive damage to brain tissue can also occur as a result of the pressure on the brain violent contractions can cause:

- ▸ Pressure can cause physical trauma to the long axons of the neurons in the white matter, which are only a few nanometers thick and fragile enough to break.
- ▸ Excess pulsating pressure at the same points for a long time can also cause the cell bodies of the neurons and glial cells to get damaged from the physical trauma.

When the brain is injured due to external trauma to a point where its functioning is adversely impacted, it is said to have sustained a TBI.

Of particular interest in the case of autism is the possibility of traumatic brain injury at birth. There are three causes of TBI at birth:

▸ Large head of the baby or small maternal hip (cephalopelvic disproportion);
▸ Rupture of prematurely fused skull plates (craniosynostosis) driving fragments into the brain during birth;
▸ Force of contractions hammering the fetal head against a non-effacing, non-compliant cervix.

The damage from TBI can be to the grey matter, the white matter or both. As neuron bodies in the grey matter have their axons projecting into the white matter and damage to any part of the neuron results in that neuron dying out, the damage permeates the entire brain regardless of where the damage originates.

At this point it should be clear that despite neuroplasticity, damage to the brain could be particularly debilitating due to the body's inability (by design) to repair those regions. The most serious problem with brain trauma at birth is that it can be distributed over large areas of the brain. Such brain injury results in neurodevelopmental delays and disorders that I will argue later are often classified as autism. Additionally, scar tissue is associated with seizures and complications with motor control while preventing the regrowth of neurons making such damage permanent.

Gut Brain Axis - The Second Brain

The human gut has up to 200 million neurons which form an important part of the digestive system. This is so important that it is considered its own separate part of the nervous system called the 'enteric nervous system'. The guts form the basis of the fight vs flight response, so the neurons of the guts might actually be involved in the 'gut instincts' that people frequently talk about!

The gut–brain axis is the biochemical signaling that takes place between the gastrointestinal tract and the central nervous system. Key to this signaling is the chemicals created by the microbes of the gut. Hence the term has now been expanded to be called the microbiome gut-brain axis. Research interest was sparked by a 2004 paper from Kyushu university Japan showed mice with a sterile gut environment were more prone to higher stress responses.[3.2] Subsequent microbiome research, mostly done in mice has shown the importance of the gut biome in the normal functioning of the brain.

Exciting new relationships about the gut flora or microbiome and a person's mental and physical health are being discovered fairly frequently these days. This is leading to more acceptance and common use of probiotics and pre-biotics as health supplements in our times. The consumption of foods for their probiotic value like yoghurts and fermented foods are known in many cultures around the world.

Gut dysbiosis is a common symptom in many individuals suffering from autism. Numerous autism treatments also focus on alleviating the gut-dysbiosis in autism as a pathway to helping alleviate autism symptoms. There is also evidence that victims of traumatic brain injury invariably end up with gut problems and there are reasons for why this is the case. I will reveal the reasons and true causes for these relationships in the upcoming chapters.

Key Take Away: The immune process works differently in the brain than elsewhere in the body due to the low tolerance for swelling and also due to the protection of the blood brain barrier. This brain immune privilege, combined with the ACAID phenomenon, might actually be detrimental if invading antigens gain entry into the brain through compromised blood brain barrier areas as in instances of traumatic brain injury. And traumatic brain injury can be brought about by the force of contractions hammering the brain against a non-compliant cervix.

PART II

Autism and TBI at Birth

Traumatic Brain Injury is always a possibility during childbirth although the reasons for its occurrence has evolved alongside the evolution of birth aid techniques. It has historically been the major cause of mental retardation throughout history. A baby making its way out of the mother head first has always been a brain damage risk. The natural birth process has developed so as to minimize this risk. When this natural process is interfered with, it is sometimes a recipe for disaster. In short, your brain health and intelligence are in large part determined by how you were born – literally.

CHAPTER 4

The Perils of Childbirth

I am a parent of two boys on the autism spectrum and have been in the unique position that only autism parents find themselves in: of having front row seats to the events that unfolded in the lives of their kids, right from pregnancy and birth to their diagnosis and treatments. To explain why the causes of autism are not primarily genetic but instead are the result of birth complications, which result in birth injury often from medical interventions and drug injury at birth, I want to share with you some of the basics I needed to learn in order to look past the deceptions we have been fed. It takes a certain level of understanding of the many factors that impact autism to see the real reasons behind it, and the first and foremost of those is understanding the perils of childbirth.

Childbirth Then and Now

Throughout time, the birth of a child is a happy occasion for the entire family and a cause for celebration in all traditions of the world. The arrival of that bundle of joy changes the lives of a couple forever, propelling them forward to a new stage of life as parents – a stage which has the potential to fill the new parents' lives with joy and laughter and brings a certain meaning and purpose to life.

However, historically things have never been this simple. There were times not so long ago when women did not go to the hospital to have a baby. Childbirth was fraught with danger to the lives of both the mother and the child. A woman who survived her first pregnancy was thought to have been reborn. In peaceful societies of ancient times, where men were not dying in wars and conflicts, the male-female ratio was tilted heavily toward men simply due to the fact that a significant population of women died due to complications of childbirth. Even until a century ago, pregnancy was so much of a risk that entire traditions and customs about what happens if a mother dies in pregnancy were observed. One remarkable success of modern medicine has been the ability to reduce the risk of childbirth, to a point where pregnancy is considered a mostly secure and safe process, with very little or no risk to life at any point. A lot of this success can be attributed to the mastering of safe C-sections.

The C-section is one of the first surgeries of modern times. Originally, C-sections were a last-ditch effort to save the baby while the mother was left to die. With the arrival of modern medicine came the option of anesthesia and surgery where the mother was sewn back up and lived. In the last 50 years, the whole birth process has become much less of a risk after the development of the standard C-section delivery using modern surgical techniques.

All this begs the simple question: do animals die during pregnancy and birth? The answer is yes. The birth process can be a challenge for first-time mothers everywhere in the mammalian kingdom, although it depends a great deal on the size of the newborn relative to the mother and the length of the labor. Animals are known to go through pain during labor, although labor in animals is much shorter than in human beings. Certain species are known to lose 15-20% of first-time mothers to delivery-related deaths—a number similar for humans until the advent of modern times and advances in C-section delivery.

The Birth Process

Like the rest of the newborns in the mammalian world, human babies are born coming out of the birth canal head-first (the exceptions to this are the water-dwelling mammals like dolphins and whales whose calves come out tail first, which helps prevent the possibility of drowning/suffocating as they get pushed out slowly). Nature and evolution have taken care to ensure that delivery does not hurt the baby in any way. The child is kept protected inside the amniotic sac surrounded by amniotic fluid inside of the mother's uterus to ensure its safety (think airbags protecting passengers in an automotive crash). Such is the level of protection provided to the baby by the natural design. Nature has perfected this process over hundreds of thousands of years making sure it is almost flawless. That is not to say breech births – where the baby comes out legs first – do not happen on some rare occasions both in human beings and in the animal world. But even in such cases techniques have been developed by traditional midwives to ensure the safe delivery of the baby.

The birth process is by itself a miracle of nature. But the safe protection of the baby also means the child has to break or pass through several barriers head first to arrive into this world. These barriers are:

▶ Amniotic sac and fluid-filled amnion;
▶ Cervix uterus wall; and
▶ Pelvic bones.

The schematic diagram below shows the "head-on" task for the baby to be born

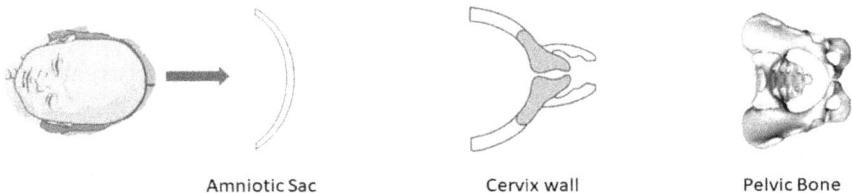

| Amniotic Sac | Cervix wall | Pelvic Bone |

Fig. 4.1: The Three Barriers to Birth

Overcoming each of these barriers is challenging. The pressures the head is subjected to during the birth process can lead to brain injury depending on the size of the baby's head and the pliability of the cervix wall. It should be noted that the birth process has historically been the leading cause of brain damage and mental retardation in infants and in extreme cases can even result in the death of a baby. Loss of oxygen to the brain from reduced blood flows during contractions is another danger that has to be navigated in a successful birth.

While fraught with dangers, the labor process itself (as shown in Fig. 1.2) occurs naturally in what is under normal circumstances a positive feedback loop:

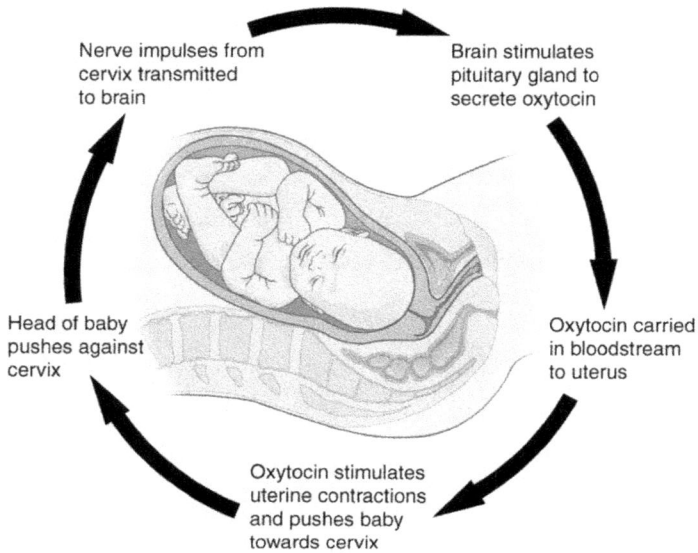

Nerve impulses from cervix transmitted to brain

Brain stimulates pituitary gland to secrete oxytocin

Head of baby pushes against cervix

Oxytocin carried in bloodstream to uterus

Oxytocin stimulates uterine contractions and pushes baby towards cervix

Fig. 4.2: The positive feedback loop in birth.

The first contractions of labor squeeze the upper end of the uterus called the fundus, pushing the baby toward the cervix at the lower end of the uterus. The cervix contains sensitive nerve cells that monitor the degree of stretching. These nerve cells send messages to the brain, which in turn causes the pituitary gland at the base of the brain to release the hormone oxytocin into the bloodstream. Oxytocin causes stronger contractions of the smooth muscles in the uterus, pushing the baby further down the birth canal. This causes even greater stretching of the cervix. The cycle of stretching, oxytocin release, and increasingly more forceful contractions leads to the effacement of the cervix and the baby is released into the birth canal, ready to be pushed out.

However, this positive feedback process doesn't happen as smoothly as this description might make it seem. Enormous changes in the mother's body are required to expel the baby at the end of pregnancy. And the events of childbirth, once begun, must progress rapidly to a conclusion or the life of the mother and the baby are at risk. Unfortunately, most of the literature out there does not elaborate on these risks and the potential for lifelong consequences (particularly for the baby) when this rapid progress requirement is not observed religiously.

The Three Stages of Labor

The process of labor is divided into three stages in the medical literature.

First stage: This is the longest-lasting and arguably most significant stage of labor. It lasts from the time of onset until the cervix is completely dilated to 10cm. Medical science divides the significant activities that happen during this stage into 3 phases.

▸ **Phase 1** (Early Labor):
Onset of labor contractions until the cervix is dilated to 3 cm.

▸ **Phase 2** (Active Labor):
From 3 cm dilation until the cervix is dilated to 7 cm.

▸ **Phase 3** (Transition):
From 7 cm dilation until the cervix is fully dilated to 10 cm.

This stage also includes the rupture of the amniotic sac in the initial stages of labor and the baby making its way past the first 2 barriers that keep it safe inside the mother during pregnancy.

Second stage: The period after the cervix is dilated to 10 cm until the baby is delivered. This is the pushing stage where the baby needs to be pushed out through the birth canal past the pelvic bone structure. This can result in the "crowning" of the head where the disjointed bones of the baby's skull deform to take a conical shape allowing easier passage through the birth canal.

Third stage: Delivery of the placenta, which includes the whole placenta organ along with the umbilical cord and the amniotic sac.

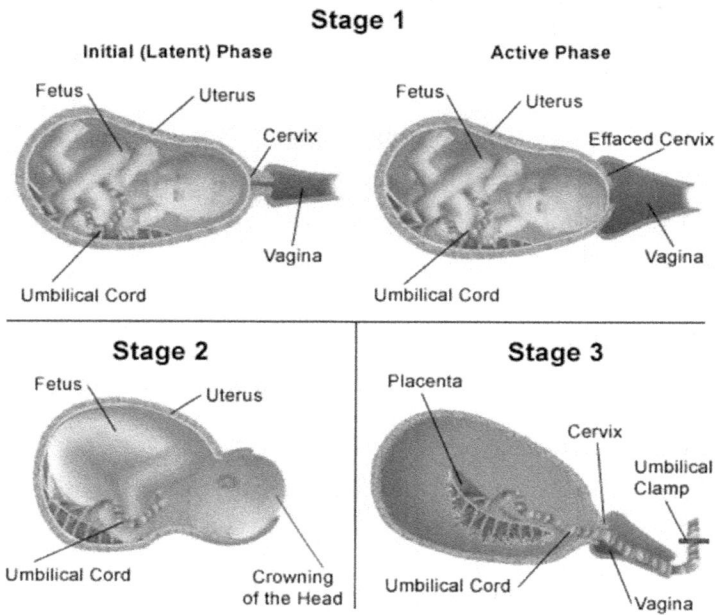

Fig. 4.3: Diagrammatic description of the 3 stages of labor.

While these stages are a generalization, every birth story is unique and no two deliveries go exactly the same. But in the vast majority of cases this seemingly enormous task of breaking and passing through these three barriers head first happens without a glitch. The water breaks, causing the uterine contractions to go faster, which in turn causes the thinning out and disappearance of the cervix wall. The baby can then be pushed out by the mother through the pelvic bone structure to be born into this world.

But this process has always been fraught with danger and has historically been the biggest source of maternal and fetal deaths. The amniotic sac is a tough membrane that typically remains intact until the end of the pregnancy, but there is the danger that it could break prematurely. Once the amniotic sac is broken it's advisable to deliver the baby sooner than later. The uterus cervix wall may also refuse to dilate and efface. This is where induced labor comes into the picture. A third complication can arise involving the bones of the mother's pelvis (including the pubic bone), which are designed to give to allow a baby to pass through. But sometimes the baby can remain stuck in the tight opening of the birth canal, necessitating a C-section. Finally, the baby's head is capable of deforming to take on a conical shape as it makes its way through the birth canal. This is due to flexible skull bones and disjointed skull plates, both of which can be damaged in delivery. In short, despite all these bodily adaptations in both the mother and the baby, birth remains a very challenging endeavor. The fact that most pregnancies go off without a hitch due to modern science means that these challenges are not given their due importance – obstacles that when not surmounted result in life-changing consequences for some newborns and their families.

Challenges for Mothers During Birth

Some of the major challenges for mothers include long labor times, large infant heads, and narrow maternal hips. Then there are these other rare complications that can happen where the mother's life can be in serious danger. Although considered rare, the occurrence of some of these complications has been on the rise. Typical complications have been overcome by modern medications and diagnosis methods, but some un-anticipated issues like blood clotting and amniotic fluid embolism that are very hard to detect continue to pose a risk. Table 1.1 outlines some of these major risks.

Table 4.1: Risks to the mother during pregnancy

High Blood pressure	Pre-eclampsia is a pregnancy complication characterized by high blood pressure and signs of damage to other organ systems like the liver and kidneys. It's essentially a sign of the mother's organs working harder to keep the fetus supplied with blood and nutrients compensating for a weaker attachment of the placenta to the mother's uterus.
Placenta issues	Abnormal placement or growth of the placenta in the womb can pose a serious risk to the mother and baby at delivery. For example, placenta praevia is a condition where the placenta attaches on the lower end of the uterus where it can interfere with or even block the cervix preventing vaginal delivery. Other placental complications can occur when the placenta attaches itself at the site of a uterine scar from a previous C-section or fibroid removal. Such an attachment can be deeper than typical complicating birth and postnatal recovery.

Hemorrhage	Excessive blood loss during and after childbirth, where the site of placental attachment to the uterus leaves a gaping wound that requires quick closure. Uncontrolled blood loss might require the removal of the uterus (hysterectomy) to save the mother's life.
Blood Clots	Blood clots in the legs or lungs (also known as thromboembolic conditions) are a leading cause of illness associated with pregnancy and birth and can be life-threatening.
Sepsis	Sepsis is an infection of the blood that can develop before or after the baby has been delivered. Infections can be more severe in pregnancy, when women may be at particular risk of infection of the womb or birth canal and after delivery, with the site of placental attachment at particular risk for infection. This was a leading cause of maternal deaths before the advent of antibiotics.
Amniotic Fluid Embolism	A very rare complication of pregnancy in which amniotic fluid, fetal skin or other cells enter the woman's bloodstream and trigger an allergic reaction. Women with this condition may collapse suddenly during the birth of their baby and it often results in the death of the mother.

Challenges for the Baby During Birth

The list of things that can go wrong for a baby are actually longer and more common, and includes every risk to the mother (since the baby is completely dependent on its mother). Caregivers and doctors typically do not discuss many of these to newly expecting couples so as not to induce a lot of fear and anxiety during a time when they should be happy and excited. While arguably wise, doing so does not diminish any of these serious risks that are part of any pregnancy:

- Premature rupture of the amniotic sac;
- Premature placenta abruption (detachment from the uterus);
- Fetal Acidosis from placenta complications at birth;
- Premature contractions and birth;
- High blood pressure in mother;
- Uncontrolled gestational diabetes in mother;
- Umbilical cord around the neck;
- Kinked umbilical cord with fetal distress;
- Umbilical cord prolapse (cord stuck ahead of head during birth);
- Breech (baby does not turn to be head down);
- No labor past 40 weeks (leading to cord ripening and detachment, meconium poisoning).

Every one of these conditions can result in life-threatening circumstances for the baby. Even with modern medical interventions babies are still lost to these complications, with the risk of death is still much higher to a baby than the mother. There are consequences of permanent brain damage to a baby from each of these risks, which can cause lifelong disabilities. As I will argue, the milder effects will end up being called Autism, ADD, ADHD and so on, though the link between the two has been de-emphasized.

It obviously takes exceptional skill and judgment on the part of an obstetrician to navigate through these enormous complexities. The US is credited with having the most advanced health care system in the world. For the birth process, this means a wider array of drugs, a wider array of interventions, and consequently a greater possibility of drug side effects and medical errors. The US also has among the highest incidence of autism in the world. The correlation is no accident. Autism is considered a disease of the advanced western countries – the price of technological advancement, as the pundits like to put it. Contrast that with the lower or non-existent autism rates in countries where the only birth intervention outside of natural remedies is the C-section. The logical conclusion is that there's a correlation between birth practices and these autism statistics. Perhaps in many cases allowing the natural processes to take their course as in other countries is better than advanced interventions. There are also arguments made that countries with advanced medical facilities tend to save children that would have otherwise died during birth in countries with lesser facilities. But based on experience, many interventions in advanced countries are actually directed at low-risk pregnancies and so this advancement argument may not be valid. We will unravel the reasons behind these statistics in the US and other advanced countries, and explore solutions in the upcoming chapters of this book. A nice map of the autism rates in various countries of the world is available from a popular demographics site called worldpopulationreview https://worldpopulationreview.com/country-rankings/autism-rates-by-country#top-10-countries-with-the-lowest-autism-rates

Standard of Hospital Delivery Care

Perhaps these findings about birth practices don't appear as shocking when you consider the fact that the standard of hospital delivery care in the US is among the lowest in the industrialized world. The US has a very technologically advanced but inconsistent medical system. For every expert physician there is another medical professional whose bungling of care, outright disdain for the patient and sheer incompetence – combined with bureaucracy and the practice of defensive medicine – has led to a system that's expensive and ineffective. Medical malpractice is known to be the third highest cause of death in the US. That is in spite of heavy-handed tort reforms in the last couple of decades having significantly eroded patient rights resulting in a lot of malpractice remaining hidden.

Some of the failures in the US can be attributed to factory-style hospitals trying to optimize their patient care and the doctor interaction times, medical insurance controlling care, doctors practicing defensive medicine instead of learning the art of diagnosis by interviewing their patients. This results in doctors missing out on patients not falling into their standardized template of care. When care in the obstetrics front suffers, it points to systemic issues, particularly in the competence and training of OB/GYNs. Recent research shows that only about 2.3% of doctors are responsible for 38.9% of all medical malpractice claims and 94% of doctors had no claim against them[4.1]. We could expect these kinds of distributions might happen with OB/GYNs as well.

Key Take Away: Historically, brain damage at birth has been the single largest cause of mental retardation and lower brain functionality and IQ. Since a baby has to make its way out of the mother - head first, physical brain damage at this stage is a very real possibility, and birth injury is the primary cause for a whole host of mental disabilities in children. But modern medical advice has sought to downplay the brain damage risk to a baby during birth as a consequence of past experience with birth injury litigations, resulting in focusing autism research onto genetic and other non-controversial areas.

CHAPTER 5

Controlling the Uterus – Birth of Modern Obstetrics

In 1980 synthetic forms of the hormone Oxytocin by names Pitocin and Syntocinon were approved by the FDA for elective induction of labor. It marked the beginning of the modern era of obstetrics. An era where childbirth went from being the natural event that it was throughout human history to a medical event in the United States and most of the western world. The trend has since caught on in most countries around the world. As a result, natural, home-based births have become a thing of the past, largely due to the risk child birth poses to the life of the mother and the child. The ability to induce labor represented a significant advancement in the field, allowing for better management of labor and improving outcomes for both mothers and babies.

But, have outcomes really improved since the introduction of modern control of the uterus? That's a question we will look into during the course of this book. This great deviation from the natural process comes with its own risks. When these risks are not fully understood by individual obstetricians they could make serious mistakes that can result in negative outcomes of brain damage to the baby or even death to the baby, the mother or both.

This modern labor management technique allows full obstetric control of the contractions of the mother's uterus, thereby deciding when and how a baby is delivered. To understand labor, it is necessary to have some intermediate knowledge of the uterus, pregnancy and the natural labor process.

The Uterus

The uterus is an exclusively female organ found in all mammals and a feature that distinguishes mammals from other classes in the animal world. It is a hollow muscular organ located in the female pelvis between the bladder and rectum.

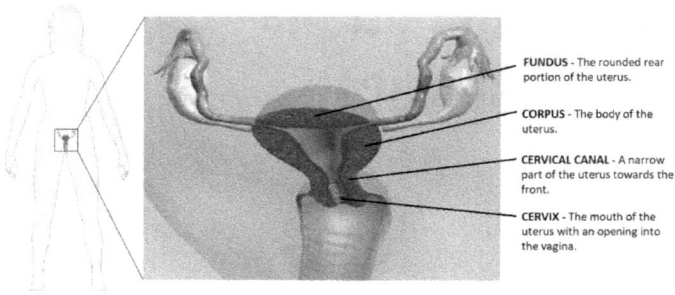

FUNDUS - The rounded rear portion of the uterus.

CORPUS - The body of the uterus.

CERVICAL CANAL - A narrow part of the uterus towards the front.

CERVIX - The mouth of the uterus with an opening into the vagina.

Fig. 5.1: Front cut cross-section view of the uterus

Functions of the uterus include nurturing the fertilized ovum that develops into the fetus and holding it till the baby is mature enough for birth. The human uterus is pear-shaped, about 3 inches long, 1.8 inches wide and 1.2 inches thick.

A typical adult uterus weighs about 60 grams. It increases in size and weight while stretching and growing to hold the baby during pregnancy. Just prior to birth, the mother's uterus typically weighs about 1.1 kg, or approximately 18 times the pre-pregnancy weight as it grows to support a baby averaging 3.5kg at birth.

Structurally the human uterus is divided into 4 distinct areas: the fundus, the corpus, the cervical canal and cervix as seen in figure 5.1.

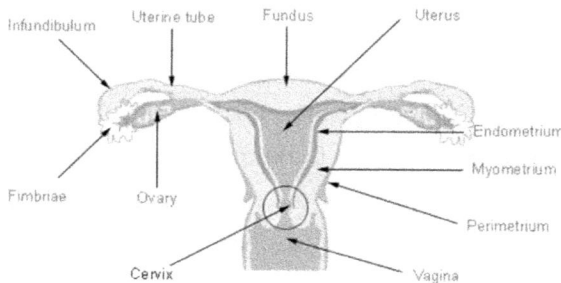

Fig 5.2: Cross-sectional diagram of the uterus, showing the three layers, endometrium, myometrium, perimetrium.

As seen in fig. 5.2 the uterine wall is made up of 3 distinct layers, with the innermost layer (composed of an epithelial and mucosal layer) called the endometrium. The inner endometrium is the functional layer of the uterus where the mucosal part of it gets sloughed off during the menstrual cycle. During pregnancy the endometrium, under the influence of the progesterone hormone, also creates the placenta and umbilical cord. The outer layer is called the perimetrium which is the lubricating layer around the uterus to reduce friction during movement.

The middle layer is the muscular layer called the myometrium. The myometrium is the smooth muscle layer of the uterus. It is the strongest muscle in the female human body by weight capacity and the force generated per cross-sectional unit area. It can stretch and contract with considerable force during childbirth. During childbirth, the uterus is capable of generating between 25 to 100 lbs (100 to 400N (Newtons)) of force with each contraction. The lower end of 25lbs is with induced contractions, while the higher end of 100lbs is expected with contractions combined with maternal pushing. Natural contractions are known to generate even less force than induced contraction. This is an enormous force acting on the baby although all this force is not transmitted onto the baby's head. Pressure transducers placed between the head and cervix tend to register a much lesser pressure compared to the force of contraction generated by the uterus. The reason being the force is spent in compressing the baby and placenta before being transmitted to the head. The cervix wall can also flex, so while force is still significant, babies can take quite a few of them without much damage. This is better explained with an example. Imagine trying to play a game of pool or billiards with tennis balls. Compared to the rigid billiards or pool balls, which are made of phenolic resin, the tennis ball can flex some. The result is, the tennis ball doesn't transmit all the force applied on it onto the next ball it strikes as it spends some of that force in flexing. The softer the ball, the less the force that gets transmitted across it. But the hard resin balls transmit almost the entire force and momentum onto the next ball they strike. So, modelling these forces in a birth situation has been a challenge that has still not been overcome. Contractions tend to spend some of that force squeezing the blood out of the placenta and compressing the body of the baby. But this is still a significant amount of force. To put this force in perspective, it is 3 to 12 times the weight of an 8-pound baby acting on the baby with a significant amount of it reaching the head. The birth process is hence at the intersection of the physics of the forces acting to push the baby through the cervical wall together with biochemistry of efface-ment (or dissolution) of the cervix itself during birth. The large range of this force also means the uterus under unfavorable conditions can deliver a crushing blow to a baby's head. Variables like the size and weight of the baby, the size of the head, etc., also play a role in how this force acts on a baby's head. A few hyper-tonic contractions on the high end of the range against a rigid non-effacing cervix can deliver a devastating blow, resulting in the death of the baby or causing sig-nificant brain damage.

The uterus is built strong and muscular exclusively for the birth process, but its strength can be a boon or a bane in the birth process and its characteristics vary widely in the population. The natural contraction response of the uterine myometrial layer is seldom dangerous to the baby, but artificial stimulation can cause an unpredictable contraction response, and is proven to be dangerous to the baby in many circumstances.

The Placenta

The placenta is a special temporary organ that develops during pregnancy inside of the uterus connecting the umbilical cord of the baby to the mother. The function of the placenta is to allow nutrient uptake, thermo-regulation, waste elimination, and gas exchange from the fetus using the mother's blood supply. It also responsible for the production of pregnancy related hormones and provides protection from infection for the fetus.

As seen in figure 5.3, the placenta accomplishes its functions by maximizing the area in contact with the maternal uterus and its rich blood supply using small finger like projections called the chorionic villi. These villi themselves have further substructures called microvilli which help increase the surface area in contact even more. Although they do not come in direct contact, through these structures in the placenta the maternal and fetal circulations meet to exchange gases and nutrients. The placenta also metabolizes a number of substances and can release metabolic products into maternal or fetal circulations. The placenta is also said to play a role in gene expression during pregnancy.

PLACENTA IMPLANTED ON UTERUS WALL

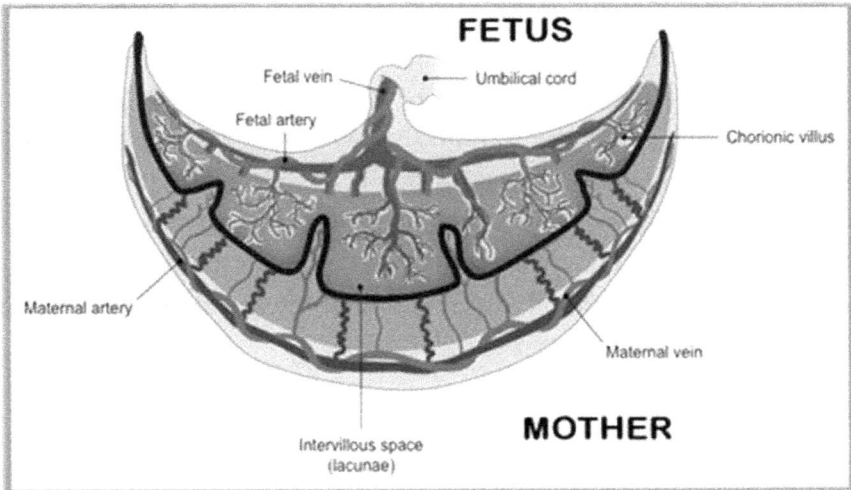

Fig. 5.3: Cross-section of the placenta and uterus wall at the site of implantation, showing the fine capillaries involved in the gas exchange between mother and fetus.

Given all this functionality, the placenta is potentially the most important organ of pregnancy, yet its typically not given due consideration unless there's a problem. Its position and strength of attachment to the uterus., play a significant role in many pregnancy complications. The placenta is designed to work between the systolic and diastolic pressure of the maternal blood to provide its nutrient and gas exchange functionality. This equilibrium is potentially disturbed when labor contractions begin.

When the delicate membranes of the placenta get squeezed by these forces meant to expel the baby from the womb, blood could get squeezed out of it, impacting the gas exchange and the amount of blood reaching the fetus. That's the reason there can't be more than a certain number (2-3) of contractions per 10 minutes. The issue is even more complex after the cushion of amniotic fluid is lost during labor.

The forces acting on the placenta during a contraction in the absence of amniotic fluid are a function of the force of the uterine contractions, the position of the placenta and the position of the baby and the umbilical cord. All these variables impact blood flow and oxygen supply to the baby. While it's typically not a problem with natural contractions, induced contractions (being much stronger) can result in loss of effectiveness of the placenta in keeping the baby adequately supplied. Hence for best outcomes it becomes paramount that once the amniotic fluid is lost, the baby is delivered in a very short amount of time. Because it depends on a slew of variables that can be different in every individual case, medical professionals disagree on exactly how long the fetus can survive without suffering brain damage. They typically point to the possibility of infection as the reason one can't wait for too long, but the reality of the situation is this disruption of blood and oxygen to the baby from the placenta that's the bigger cause for concern.

A Brief History of Labor Induction and Oxytocin

Different societies have evolved their own techniques to get the woman to deliver when a woman crossed 40-42 weeks of gestation with no indication of labor. Techniques varied from herbs and traditional medicines and gentle massaging to the beating of drums and firing of guns (remember the humorous phrase 'son of a gun'?). Certain ancient religions even have their own gods and deities that are dedicated to the pursuit of good birth whose blessings were believed to lead to a positive birth outcome for a pregnant woman.

Crossing this 42-week time limit is believed to be a risk to the lives of both the pregnant woman and the baby by modern obstetrics and its one size fits all approach. Historically, healthy women have stayed pregnant for 46 weeks or more while still delivering healthy babies, with the longest on record lasting over 53 weeks in 1945 (Beulah hunter – Los Angeles CA). But that said, pregnancy and childbirth were one of the primary causes of death for women in olden times. Then came the C-section, originally used as a last-ditch effort to cut open the mother to save the baby, and which over time was perfected to be safe for both the mother and child, becoming a life saver for women having difficulty delivering a baby.

In 1906 oxytocin and its uterine contraction property was discovered by British pharmacologist Henry Dale. It is named after the Greek word 'oxytocic' which means 'quick birth'. Oxytocin is a naturally occurring hormone produced by the hypothalamus area of the brain and secreted by the pituitary gland in mammals. It became the first polypeptide hormone to be sequenced and artificially synthesized by Vincent Du Vigneaud who was awarded the Nobel Prize in 1955 for his work.

The modern birth technique of induced labor became possible during the 1980s. The discovery of oxytocin at the dawn of the 20th century combined with advancement in electronics, sensors and techniques to monitor a woman's contractions during labor, fetal heart rate, etc., have given medical sciences the capability to safely deliver a baby without resorting to a C-section when labor doesn't occur naturally. Since the 1980's induced labor has become the de-facto method of managing labor in maternity wards across the US and has been gaining traction in the rest of the world as well.

Interestingly, oxytocin is a molecule that acts both as a neuro transmitter in the brain and as a hormone in other parts of the body. It does not cross the blood brain barrier making this dual functionality possible. The oxytocin from the pituitary gland is the hormone part of it, released into the bloodstream and circulated throughout the body. Inside the brain on the other side of the blood brain barrier, it seems to be produced in oxytocin-projecting neurons separate from the pituitary gland. While it is most commonly described for its hormonal effect of uterine activity stimulation in women, it is common to both genders for its neurotransmitter role inside the brain. Various scientific studies have concluded that oxytocin is involved in human emotions. It is thought to be released during touching, hugging and orgasm. It also seems to play an important role in social recognition and bonding and is thought to be involved in the formation of trust between people, kindness and general emotional stability. Research has further expanded the involvement of oxytocin to a wide variety of physiological and pathological functions such as sexual activity, penile erection, ejaculation, pregnancy, uterine contraction, milk ejection, maternal behavior, social bonding, stress and many more.

Suddenly oxytocin is becoming this touted cure-all love hormone, and even a cure for some symptoms of autism and schizophrenia due to enabling social bonding. But as any sensible physician would tell you, nobody should meddle with hormones due to enormous consequences they have on the body. The long-term effects of artificially meddling with hormones in the human body remains riddled with unknown dangers.

A Brief History of Pitocin

Synthetically produced oxytocin is marketed under the name 'Pitocin' in the US and under various other brand names in other countries. A simple trademark search reveals the Pitocin name itself was registered by Parke Davis & Co, in 1928 long before synthetic oxytocin was produced. Originally, Pitocin was the name given to naturally sourced oxytocin from pituitary glands of cattle gathered from cattle slaughterhouses. The new name was a move to get away from the negative attitudes that had developed toward its predecessor (named 'Pituitrin') which had quickly become the norm to help with labor after 1909 – within 3 short years of oxytocin's discovery in 1906. However, Pituitrin was impure, often contaminated and resulted in adverse outcomes for mothers and babies. Back then women were given one injection of it, and up to 50% of pregnancies where it was administered the result was massive unregulated contractions, uterine rupture and even the death of the child, mother or both. The newly named Pitocin was a more purified form of the same naturally sourced version that tried to address the contamination issues. Yet the mode of administration remained in the form of injections. As there were no good means to measure contractions in those early days, it was not known how long the hormone lasted in the bloodstream after injection and how long it brought on sustained contractions.

With the ability to synthesize Pitocin in a lab beginning in the mid to late 1950s, it was possible to obtain a pure form of the oxytocin hormone. However, its use in inducing labor remained dangerous and its record very spotty at best. While it was possible to induce contractions with it there was not a good way to control and monitor contractions. Due to the dangers involved, for a couple of decades Pitocin was only used as a drug of last resort when all else failed, with C-sections and forceps remaining the birth options of choice depending on where in the natural birth process progression was halted.

The 1960s and '70s marked an era of enormous progress in modern medicine when many new electronic sensors and other instrumentation came into being. The cardiotocograph or the fetal heart rate monitor was invented by Dr. Orvan Hess in the 1950's and refined further throughout the 60's and beyond. But the birth process was still more centered on "intervention when needed" rather than the managed birth process that it has since evolved into.

Things changed in 1980 when synthetic oxytocin drugs Syntocinon (now discontinued) and Pitocin were approved for induction of labor. Pitocin was approved by the FDA for "Initiation or improvement of uterine contractions, and control of post-partum hemorrhage." It was the harbinger of the managed birth process and the philosophy of "active management of labor" in delivery rooms across the US and the developed world (and catching on very quickly everywhere else). The Pitocin trademark as of 2025 is owned by PAR pharmaceuticals, but having become a generic drug, it is produced by many companies around the world.

Pitocin is considered a miracle drug for its use in stopping post-partum bleeding. The delivery of the baby and the placenta leaves a gaping wound in the uterus at the site of attachment of the placenta to the uterus. All that essential blood supply to the baby developed over the months of pregnancy needs to be quickly reversed, the bleeding stopped and the uterus returned to its pre-pregnancy size and state. Pitocin is capable of doing just that in its post-partum use. It is credited with saving millions of women from bleeding to death after childbirth in delivery rooms across the world, and is listed on the World Health Organization's (WHO) essential medicines list (EML) for this purpose.

But the effect of the synthetic version of the hormone on the mother's body before delivery and its effect on the baby, is a subject of controversy in medical and academic circles. Numerous doctors and nurses have suggested the uterine contractions brought on by the synthetic hormone are much more forceful than natural contractions; so much so that the label on the drug warns against such a possibility in certain individuals. But that has not impacted the popularity and widespread use of this drug, causing unfavorable birth outcomes that remain hidden to this day.

The Induced Labor Process

Synthetic oxytocin or Pitocin is the main anchor of the induced labor process. This refers to the intervention that is done when the natural labor process is stuck or when a pregnant woman is postdated beyond the delivery date without indication of labor. In delivery rooms across the world Pitocin is used for its uterine contraction property in an attempt by modern medicine to replicate the events that happen naturally in cases where birth doesn't seem to be progressing naturally. It is therefore important to look at some of the steps involved in labor in more detail.

Cervix ripening: The cervix plays the very critical role of holding the baby inside the mother as it grows and develops in her uterus. A strong cervix wall at the mouth of the uterus ensures the baby stays in for the full term of the pregnancy and avoids the end result of a premature delivery. As the end of the gestational period arrives, the cervix begins to ripen and dilate to make way for the baby to come out. This dilation process goes hand in hand with the beginning of uterine contractions and labor. The exact mechanism of how this happens naturally is not fully understood. One aspect of natural contractions is that they do not come on when the cervix is not ready, and this is again a natural protection mechanism for the baby inside. A cervix that is soft and pliable is considered ripe for delivery versus when it is hard and rigid, where it is considered non-compliant and unready for labor and delivery.

A rigid cervix is responsible for increased intrauterine pressure during contractions which is associated with reduced uteroplacental blood flow. When inducing labor contractions externally with Pitocin, if the cervix doesn't dilate at the appropriate time in spite of the onset of strong contractions it can result in crushing blows to the baby's head and reduced uteroplacental blood flow with every contraction, resulting in brain injury which later results in developmental disorders or even the death of the baby.

Given such importance of cervical ripening and cervix dilation and a history of neonatal deaths and other adverse outcomes (brain damage) due to lack of cervix ripening, modern medicine offers multiple techniques for achieving cervix ripening. As far back as 1964 Edward bishop set forth a pelvic scoring system to assess the readiness of the cervix for labor.[7.4] This is explained further in chapter 7. It takes into consideration cervical dilation, position, effacement, consistency of the cervix, and fetal station. The score ranges between 0 and 13: a score of 8 or better is favorable for induction, while a score of 6 or less indicates a need for preparation of cervix using the following techniques.

▶ *Stripping the membrane:* Effective only in a very small percentage of women, this technique involves running an exam finger between the lower edge of the amniotic sac and the internal cervix wall gently separating the two, which might stimulate labor and cervix ripening.

▶ *Cervical ripening balloon:* This is a more mechanical, non-chemical way of ripening the cervix, where a double-balloon is inflated from both the internal and external sides of the cervix wall. The resulting additional pressure specifically directed on the cervix wall causes the tissue to soften and ripen over time causing the thinning and effacement of the cervix. The balloon is kept inside for up to 12 hours or until it falls out by itself.

▶ *Ripening agents:* Certain chemical medications are available that can cause cervical dilation in a significant number of women. This includes Cytotec (misoprostol) and Cervidil (dinoprostone or prostaglandin E2) which can be administered in the hospital or outpatient settings. They come in tablet form that can be inserted into the vagina, taken orally or administered in liquid form alongside Pitocin during induction. When done ahead of induction which is the more appropriate way to do it, in postdated women, often, multiple doses over many hours are required to get the cervix ready for labor. Depending on the method used the baby might need monitoring in the hours following the administration of ripening agents.

Amniotomy: This refers to the act of artificially breaking the water or the amniotic sac in a pregnant woman mainly as a way to help labor along. The amniotic sac is composed of 2 layers. The external layer, which is attached to the uterus at the site of placental attachment, is the chorion, and the internal layer in contact with the amniotic fluid is the amnion. The amniotic fluid is comprised of a serous fluid initially, and later added onto through fetal urine as the pregnancy progresses.

Water break tends to happen naturally preceding natural onset of labor or water could break during labor. Amniotomy is known to have been practiced by obstetricians historically for a few hundred years for speeding up labor. In modern times, the use of fetal monitoring equipment requires an amniotomy. The fetal scalp electrode (for accurate fetal heart rate monitoring) and the intrauterine pressure catheter (to measure the strength of contractions used to monitor the baby in a cardiotocograph) do not work without the access provided by amniotomy.

Once amniotomy is complete it is important to deliver the baby within a set time (preferably 8 hours or less). The risk of cord compression, infection, etc., start climbing once the protection of the amniotic fluid is lost. Hence it is a natural bodily response to speed up contractions upon loss of amniotic fluid even without augmentation of labor. The speeding up is due to the positive feedback loop described in Figure 1.2 in chapter 1 due to the direct action of pressure transferred from the baby's head to the cervix rather than the even distribution of pressure that might exist in the presence of amniotic fluid.

Doctors don't seem to agree on a fixed time frame or an exact deadline from the time of water breakage/amniotomy to the time of delivery vaginally or through C-section for best outcomes. Estimates of this time vary widely among the medical community, between 8 and 72 hours. I believe this safe time limit is closer to 8 hours based on the experience of some parents I have talked to. Failure to deliver in that time could result in negative outcomes due to one or more of the following reasons:

▸ Uneven pressure on the placenta from contractions in the absence of amniotic fluid might result in unpredictable effects on the gas exchange of oxygen supply and carbon dioxide elimination from the baby;

▸ Uneven and unpredictable pressures acting on the umbilical cord could result in cord kinking and compression which will again interfere with the gas exchange between mother and baby.

▸ The direct pressure acting through the head of the baby against the cervix wall during contractions will result in irreversible traumatic brain damage if excessive contractions beyond labelled contraindication limits are allowed.

The above effects are unpredictable and easily constitute major risks as the time between loss of amniotic fluid and birth increases. There are cases where babies have been induced with Pitocin that had positive outcomes even though it took long hours, but upon closer scrutiny these are usually instances where the induction was done with the amniotic sac still intact. The entire dynamic changes once the amniotic fluid is lost for the reasons stated above.

Contractions: Uterine contractions are the main mechanism by which the baby is delivered at the end of pregnancy. While these may start spontaneously at or around 40 weeks in most women, both premature contractions resulting in premature birth of the baby and postdating of pregnancy where no contractions arrive even after 40 weeks of pregnancy are fairly common.

Contractions work when the endometrial muscles of the rear fundus side of the uterus contract, thereby propelling the baby headfirst through the cervical canal. Too little contraction force and there is no progress in labor, but too forceful a contraction and there could be head trauma to the baby, uterine rupture, reduced uteroplacental blood flow and even death. The force of the contraction is also a function of how soft (compliant) or rigid (non-compliant) the cervix is. A compliant cervix results in the generation of lesser contraction force, but there is still progress in labor.

The frequency of contractions is a factor that is controlled carefully while inducing labor. A maximum of 5 contractions per 10 minutes is medically allowed (normally 2-3 every 10 minutes). Anything higher and there is overstimulation called tachysystole contractions of the uterus. Another variable is the duration of a single contraction. When a contraction lasts longer than 2 minutes the condition is called

Uterine Hypertonus. When tachysystole or hypertonus conditions of the uterus exist (called hyperstimulation) there is not enough time for the placenta to recharge with fresh blood supply for the baby between contractions, resulting in low oxygen outcomes like hypoxia and fetal acidosis. These conditions typically lead to a non-reassuring pattern on the cardiotocograph, which needs to be quickly interpreted and the baby C-sectioned out.

Thus, any excursions in any of these controlled conditions in induced labor can result in brain damage to the child. So, it is important to monitor these parameters very closely when undertaking medically induced labor. Such monitoring is made possible in current times using a machine called the cardiotocograph, more commonly known as an electronic fetal monitor (EFM). It monitors both the fetal heart rate and the occurrence of uterine contractions in the mother.

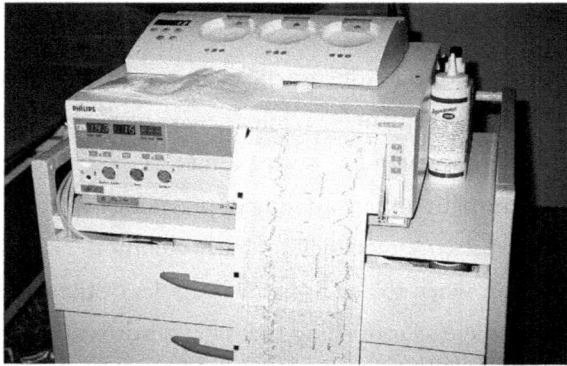

Fig 5.4: Typical cardiotocograph seen in delivery wards across the world.

Cardiotocograph (CTG) is the central monitoring device that records and displays information about the fetal heart rate and uterine contractions. It can receive information from various measurement sources, including:

1. Fetal Scalp Electrode (FSE): Provides a direct and accurate reading of the fetal heart rate.
2. Tocodynamometer (TOCO): An external sensor placed on the mother's abdomen that measures uterine contractions.
3. Intrauterine Pressure Catheter (IUPC): Provides a direct and accurate measurement of intrauterine pressure and contraction strength.

The availability of electronic fetal monitoring is the main reason induced labor is even possible. While this is a valuable tool in the hands of the OB/GYNs and maternity ward nurses, its interpretation is a subject of controversy as well. Court cases have been won and lost over their outputs and their correlation with outcomes for babies.

Electronic fetal monitoring: Electronic fetal monitoring is based on the principle that the fetal heart rate goes down during a contraction and recovers quickly after the contraction abates. If there is lack of swift fetal heart rate recovery after every contraction then the fetus is said to be in distress and doctors might force a C-section if the readings from the fetal heart rate (FHR) monitor show signs of fetal distress. However, the actual interpretation is a subject of controversy because of the possibility of errors in the instrumentation placement, positioning, quality of the signal, fetal position and so on. Initial monitoring before any cervical dilation is done with an abdominal monitor, and when the cervical dilation reaches 2cm or more then the head of the fetus is reachable and a fetal scalp electrode is placed on the scalp. Yet while the accuracy of readings is improved, the interpretation of what they mean and what really constitutes fetal distress is a totally different ball game.

Interpretation of monitor readings is a complex undertaking, and scientific papers continue to be published trying to bring clarity and accuracy to the process. The key to successful monitoring is to establish a baseline fetal heart rate, which is easy to do when contractions are few and far apart. The normal fetal heart rate is between 110–140 beats per minute. An abnormal condition is said to exist when the baseline heart rate is not within this range. Bradycardia is when the baseline heart rate is less than 110 bpm, and tachycardia occurs when the baseline heart rate is greater than 140 bpm. Each of these states is indicative of certain conditions like fetal heart issues, fetal malposition, maternal fever, fetal hypoxia, fetal anemia, amnionitis and many others which are cause for concern.

Doctors have created a three-tiered fetal heart rate interpretation system. Categories I and II are considered safe while category III represents fetal distress. The latter is mostly characterized by decelerations in heart rate from baseline between contractions. Understanding FHR flows may be beyond the understanding of typical parents, but delivery room doctors and nurses are trained for years to pay close attention and interpret those readings with their training and experience. They are expected to accurately identify fetal distress and other conditions, which they mostly do. But in instances where they don't act appropriately at the right time can end up causing irreparable brain damage, which can range from mild ADD issues all the way to quadriplegic cerebral palsy and even fetal death. Time is of the essence in some of these issues. Imagine what would happen to a person that suffocates for 10 minutes unable to breathe. They go into a coma from brain damage or die. That is exactly what could happen to a fetus in distress.

There are significant flaws in the current state of induced labor monitoring. Internal fetal heart rate monitoring is typically used during the inducing of labor. Fetal heart rate monitoring tends to give attending OB/GYNs the confidence that everything is going well during induction of labor even if that might not be the case. The basis of fetal monitoring is the belief that hypoxia or ischemia will cause fatal heart arrhythmias that can be detected and acted upon. When the brain is not receiving sufficient oxygen in its autonomous control regions of the brain stem the initial response is that it sends signals to the heart to beat faster to increase blood flow. But when the lack of oxygen persists it impacts the brain's ability to send out those signals and the heart rate might fall from baseline. At that point a lot of damage might have already occurred, particularly to neurons in the lobes of the cerebrum. A vast majority of babies C-sectioned out as a result of fetal distress are known to suffer from neurodevelopmental disorders, all of which fall under the umbrella of autism spectrum disorders.

The other issue is the traumatic injury that can be inflicted by Pitocin induced contractions. The brain doesn't sense pain upon damage to itself, unlike the way it can sense damage to other parts of the body. Electronic fetal monitoring has absolutely no way of monitoring traumatic injury outside of measuring the pressure of contractions. Fetal head compression and intracranial pressure are impossible to accurately measure. Upon loss of amniotic fluid this pressure is all directed at the fetal head trying to make its way past the cervix in the second stage of labor. The head-on contractions during this stage of labor end up pounding the brain in place as the brain has nowhere to go, nowhere to expand into unlike the pushing stage where the skull can change shape and elongate. So abusing labor drugs by use of excessive contractions to achieve cervical dilation can cause traumatic brain injury by shearing the fine axonal fibers of the neurons. The Pitocin drug label actually carries a warning against this kind of brain damage. Unfortunately, traumatic brain damage is not a parameter electronic fetal monitoring can actually warn against. Obstetricians that ignore this time and contraction limit aspect can end up causing brain damage in babies unlucky enough to come under their care. Unfortunately, there are no signs of fetal distress and so the fetal monitor in these cases actually provides a false notion of safety.

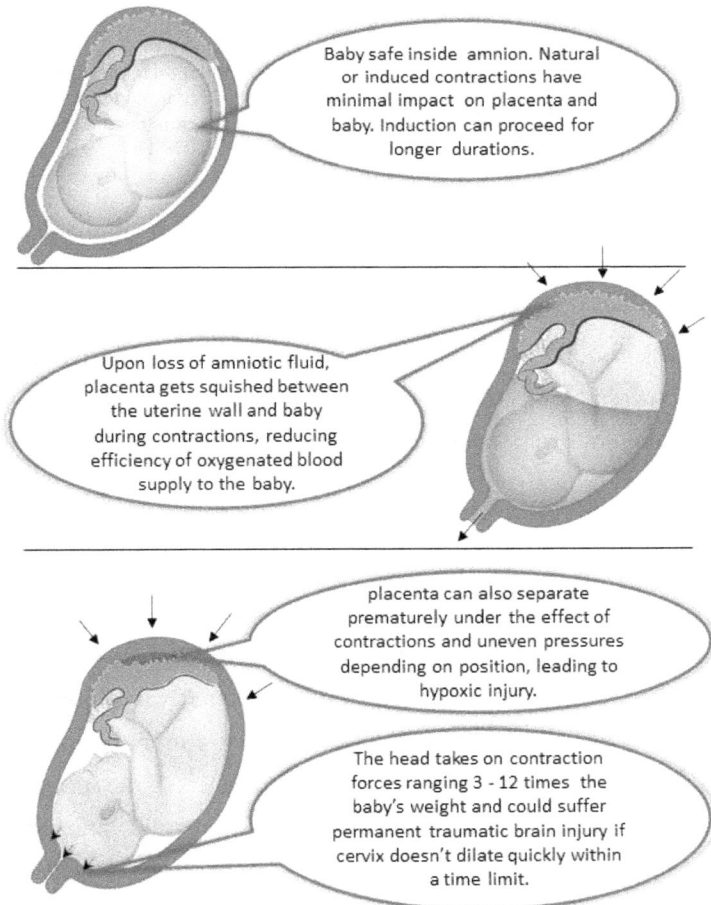

Baby safe inside amnion. Natural or induced contractions have minimal impact on placenta and baby. Induction can proceed for longer durations.

Upon loss of amniotic fluid, placenta gets squished between the uterine wall and baby during contractions, reducing efficiency of oxygenated blood supply to the baby.

placenta can also separate prematurely under the effect of contractions and uneven pressures depending on position, leading to hypoxic injury.

The head takes on contraction forces ranging 3 - 12 times the baby's weight and could suffer permanent traumatic brain injury if cervix doesn't dilate quickly within a time limit.

Fig 5.5: Amniotic Fluid and Induction

Table 5.1 Contrasting two kinds of induction.

Two Types of Pitocin Induction	
With Amniotic sac intact	**Post Amnion rupture**
Uniform distribution of pressure inside the amniotic sac.	Lack of fluid medium means pressure is non-uniform across various parts of baby and placenta.
Pressure from contractions transmitted to cervix through the amniotic fluid.	Pressure from contractions transmitted to the cervix through the head of the baby.
Pressure on the umbilical cord and placenta is fairly uniform and there is little risk of hypoxia or other damage.	Risk of hypoxia and ischemia from uneven placenta compression and cord compression is heightened.
When people say I was induced for 30 hours and still have a fine baby, this is the type of induction they are referring to.	This sort of induction for more than 4-6 hours (depending on contraction frequency and other variables) causes sure shot traumatic brain injury.

Pitocin administration: Pitocin is the drug of choice for inducing and controlling contractions. When a pregnant woman is postdated for delivery or when natural labor is stuck, delivery rooms default to using Pitocin for active intervention and management of labor. Most hospitals and obstetricians develop and follow their own methods of how induction is done. In a postdated woman the most commonly followed sequence of interventions would be as follows:

1. Cervix ripening
2. Pitocin administered
3. Amniotomy (if needed)

However, depending on the individual practitioner, the choices of cervix ripening time and technique, amniotomy timing, etc., may vary. In spite of all the monitoring and available techniques, obstetrics is still more of an art than science, and the experience, expertise, judgment and beliefs of the specific obstetrician determine the techniques followed and the outcomes achieved. As they always say, no two deliveries are exactly same.

Pitocin only lasts in the blood stream for three to six minutes, so when used for labor induction it is administered as an intravenous (IV) fluid. Nurses typically adjust the dosage within a set range to try and achieve the desired rate of contractions. Once the desired rate of contractions is achieved, they continue to monitor progress of cervical dilation with time. Induction works best when the cervix is ripe or already dilated some when induction is started. The fetal heart rate and any signs of fetal distress is then carefully monitored and any signs of fetal distress are addressed immediately with an emergency C-section. If progress of cervical dilation is not rapid enough after the start of Pitocin induction, induction needs to be stopped and a C-section needs to be performed.

Failure to perform a C-section at this juncture is unfortunately the biggest cause of obstetric malpractice in the US and the cause of autism in many children (including my own). This is also the Pitocin contra-indication described in the FDA approved Pitocin labelling comes in: "Where adequate uterine activity fails to achieve satisfactory progress." Numerous obstetricians who believe blindly in the virtues of Pitocin and have not taken the time to study the warning labels and tend to increase the Pitocin dosage rather than stop induction upon such contra-indication. In cases of low-risk healthy mothers and babies, there is typically no fetal distress, which is the only other reason for them to stop induction. OB/GYNs typically tend to proceed all the way in their zeal to avoid the C-section, causing irreversible brain damage as indicated in the Pitocin labelling.

Is Pitocin the only game in town to induce labor? Apparently not. There are other natural ways of inducing labor as described by the Global Library of Women's Medicine (GLOWM), the educational arm of the International Federation of Obstetrics and Gynecology (FIGO). On their site they describe the following non-medical means of inducing labor and cervix dilation:

- ▶ Sexual intercourse
- ▶ Breast stimulation
- ▶ Herbal preparations
- ▶ Homeopathic solutions
- ▶ Purgatives
- ▶ Enemas
- ▶ Acupuncture
- ▶ Stripping of the membranes

Expert OB/GYN's typically use some of these techniques like enema and striping of the membranes the night before the date they attempt induction, so as to make the cervix compliant, and it makes a world of difference to the final outcome for the baby.

Key Take Away:

▶ Modern childbirth has largely shifted from a natural process to a highly medicalized event, driven by the trend towards active labor management in hospitals.

▶ Concerns have arisen regarding the safety of these medicalized labor processes, leading to the establishment of guidelines for drug use.

▶ A critical flaw exists in current electronic fetal monitoring during induced labor: these monitors primarily detect hypoxic (oxygen deprivation) injury, but **fail to detect traumatic brain injury** that can occur when induction proceeds against a non-compliant cervix.

▶ The continued use of Pitocin beyond its indicated contraindications, particularly when the cervix is not progressing, has led to traumatic brain damage in babies, often subsequently diagnosed as autism.

▶ Brain damage from induction exceeding contraindications is especially severe when performed after an amniotomy (breaking the water), as the loss of amniotic fluid removes the natural cushioning protection, leading to uneven pressure dissipation.

▶ Chapter 7 and 8 will detail the specific point of Pitocin contraindication beyond which traumatic brain injury becomes irreversible

CHAPTER 6

Our Story - Memories Rekindled by an MRI Scan

L ooking back, I often ponder the events around the birth of my boys, wishing certain paths had unfolded differently. Life has since been thrown into such a chaos, that these days, all I yearn for is a quiet, uneventful existence. Yet, I realize that my extraordinary journey, with all its ups and downs, is the reason for my writing this book. Perhaps every experience, even the challenging ones, serves a purpose. Revisiting the old memories and experiences that forever changed my life and my wife's is never easy, especially those surrounding the birth of our children, which remain deeply painful. However, I feel compelled to share our story so that the unfortunate events leading to our family's current circumstances can reveal a truth that may help thousands of other children and their families avoid falling prey to obstetric malpractice during their birth causing brain damage that is later diagnosed as autism.

Delivery #1

In many ways, my wife and I were just like any other couple in America—a classic tale of young couple chasing the American dream while raising a family. We were both young, educated, and thriving in our careers as software engineers. Two years after we tied the knot, we decided it was time to start a family. However, pregnancy didn't come right away; in fact, it took quite some time. Finally, after two long years of waiting, my wife became pregnant, and we were ecstatic. The joy we felt was even greater, coming after such a long wait. We were on the verge of becoming the happiest parents imaginable—or so we thought. Life had a series of unexpected challenges in store for us. But at that moment, you would never have guessed what the future held. We were simply happy, eager parents preparing to welcome our little bundle of joy into the world. Nothing was more thrilling, and we spared no expense getting ready: we got a new crib, adorable décor, a car seat, stroller, everything 'baby', imaginable. As the due date approached, we even upgraded one of our cars to a spacious new minivan to bring our baby home.

We had a wonderful primary care doctor and my wife had picked a gynecologist – we'll call her Dr. S. – that our primary care practice recommended. She was a well-spoken pleasant doctor who did give us a lot of good advice on our pregnancy. She was obviously trying to do a good job in her profession. We had no reason to believe there was any incompetence on her part. But, years later, we recognize our pick of Dr. S. was a fateful decision that turned our lives upside down and something we'll regret for the rest of our lives.

The pregnancy itself was picture perfect. My wife had no morning sickness, no complications whatsoever, no diabetes, no blood pressure, no sickness or medication of any type. Dr. S. kept reiterating about how she would have to stay as active as possible and how staying active was very important to avoid the worst possible outcome in pregnancy: a C-section. My wife continued to religiously take her prenatal vitamins, we ate fresh healthy homemade food, went out on walks and did everything the doctor asked us to do. As the due date approached, the doctor checked her out and said the baby was head down, ready to come. At week 39 of the pregnancy there was still no cervical dilation and no sign of labor pains. Dr. S. at the point told us about the risks of going past the delivery date, including cord ripening and meconium being a risk. She also told us about how the baby might get bigger if we waited and then we'd be forced to have that dreaded C-section. She went on to introduce us to the concept of induced labor. She mentioned how it was a "safe and natural" method. She even explained how the pelvic bones are designed to expand to make way for the baby and how the baby's head could change shape to come out and how the brain was neuroplastic and recover from the changes. Dr. S. went ahead to schedule us for induction right on the due date, which we now know is something against the norm for a first pregnancy, where it is typical to wait 42 weeks in a healthy first pregnancy rather than induce right on the projected 40th week due date.

We showed up at the hospital at 8:00 am on the morning of the appointed due date. She was checked for a bit and induction was started. It went on for about 6 hours but nothing seemed to be happening – she simply wasn't dilating. Around midafternoon the nurse came by to say we were not ready to have the baby yet and that we should go home now and schedule again in a week or so if nothing changes in the interim. At this point my wife's water hadn't been broken and nothing had changed. We didn't quite understand what was going on but decided to follow the medical advice and packed up and left the hospital. I believe the nurses had intervened at this point to educate the doctor about the 2-week waiting period in case of first pregnancy and the Pitocin contra-indication after 6 hours of induction. I wish the nurses had explained better about the 2-week grace time over the 40 weeks in case of the first pregnancy, so it might have raised the alarm bells in our minds about the doctor. But they were not legally allowed to give medical advice in those times prior to the Affordable Care Act rule changes.

We were asked to pick a second appointment, which we chose that same weekend about 5 days later. Nothing had changed in those 5 days; she was still not dilated. This time, however, they used a speculum to open the cervix and forcibly broke the placenta water (amniotomy) early on to try to get the dilation going. Induction went on and on for a total of 12 hours until our boy was born. Finally, we held that bundle of joy in our hands and were ecstatic.

As first-time immigrants used to a totally different tradition, we couldn't quite buy into the concept of starting out kids in day care at 6 weeks. We wanted to make sure our precious newborn had more time at home, so we requested that our parents who were visiting from overseas to see their new grandchild to extend their stay by a few months. We did everything imaginable to give him a healthy start – we even stayed away from processed foods. All signs were good: our baby was growing very rapidly and at the 100th percentile on some measures in those initial months.

Trouble Begins

But as he started to grow up, we noticed our boy was hyperactive and hard to keep up with. As a baby he was always restless and wriggling, and from the time he learned to walk he would run everywhere instead. Unlike other kids, his first words at 5 months old were not 'ma' or any of its variants; instead, his first word was 'car,' and his fascination with mechanical objects (over people) persisted as he grew up. We did not know what to make of these differences, but since he was hitting or exceeding all his milestones of growth, we didn't think much of it, assuming instead that we had a precocious genius who was hard to keep up with. One other thing we noticed was his vision was a little poorer than it could be. He would look at things by putting them very close to his eyes. But they said he had to be four until he could be properly tested out and he would improve if we took him out to parks and tried to make him see longer distances, which we religiously did whenever we had a chance.

It wasn't until our older boy was age 3 when we finally reported back to the pediatrician that something was wrong. He was not talking like the other kids and wouldn't even answer simple yes-no questions (although he had quite a few words and was otherwise very active). He did fall sick occasionally, but he wasn't any worse than other kids and never needed medical intervention beyond simply taking some children's Tylenol. He had been in daycare since he was 9 months old, where they were engaging him in early learning. He should have picked up speaking but that wasn't quite happening. He could read from when he was two and a half and we thought he was just too playful and impatient to slow down and learn how to talk.

Around this time my wife quit her job to stay home and help the kids full time. It was tough to teach a kid that wouldn't sit or stand in one place. Finally, when he was 5, he was formally diagnosed by a special needs pre-school psychologist as falling on the autism spectrum.

In the meantime, his younger brother was also starting to show signs of not developing language. He was not speaking full sentences and at 3 years old he was also identified as having speech development delays and admitted to special learning school. Life suddenly became very busy with 2 kids on the Autism spectrum. We were running between various doctor offices, specialists, speech therapists, ABA therapists, and trying out various classes including swimming, karate, piano, and gymnastics. They simply did not fit into any group classes due to focus issues and their inability to listen and follow instructions. We left no stone unturned trying to help these kids, but were clueless as to what had happened to these otherwise very cute toddlers. Doctors were quick to say that autism was not very well understood and could happen due to hundreds of reasons. I was adamant about solving the autism puzzle for my kids but it was almost like we were hitting a wall and nothing positive was happening.

Finally, a diagnosis breakthrough came when a neurologist we had consulted ordered an MRI scan for our second little boy. The results were a total revelation, causing me to remember long-forgotten incidents that happened at the delivery room years earlier that led to the current situation. For the first time in years, I had conclusive evidence from the MRI of exactly what had gone wrong: our boys had suffered traumatic brain injury at birth.

What was it about the MRI report of my younger son that triggered my recollection? See for yourself:

Children's Medical Center Dallas
1935 Medical District Drive, Dallas, TX 75235 (214) 456-2814

Radiology Report

Name: DOB: MRN: :

Ordering MD: Location: Magnetic Resonance Imaging,

Exam Date/Time   Order Number   Accession Number
07/19/2016

Procedure: MR BRAIN W/O CONTRAST

Reason for Exam: EXT-Delayed developmental milestones

Current Symptoms:

Report:

EXAM: MR BRAIN W/O CONTRAST

HISTORY: 7 years -old Male with EXT-Delayed developmental milestones Delayed milestone in childhood

TECHNIQUE: Sagittal T1 weighted images, axial FLAIR images, axial DWIs, coronal T2 weighted images were obtained.

Additional sequences: None

Field strength: 1.5T

COMPARISON: None

FINDINGS:

The corpus callosum is normally formed and of normal thickness , the 4th ventricle is normal in position, and there is no tonsillar herniation. There is a normal T1 hyperintense neurohypophysis within the sella turcica. The optic chiasm, tracts, and nerves are normal. There are no congenital midline anomalies.

The axial images show normal ventricular size and configuration. No pathologic extra cerebral fluid collections are present. There is a normal volume of white matter which is appropriately myelinated for age. There are scattered small areas of abnormal T2 prolongation within the peripheral frontal and parietal white matter, with a slightly larger focus measuring on the order of 1 cm in the left parietal white matter. These likely relate to multiple foci of white matter gliosis from remote insult. There is no evidence of cortical dysplasia, mesial temporal sclerosis, mass lesion, or hemorrhage. The posterior fossa is normal.

1 of 2

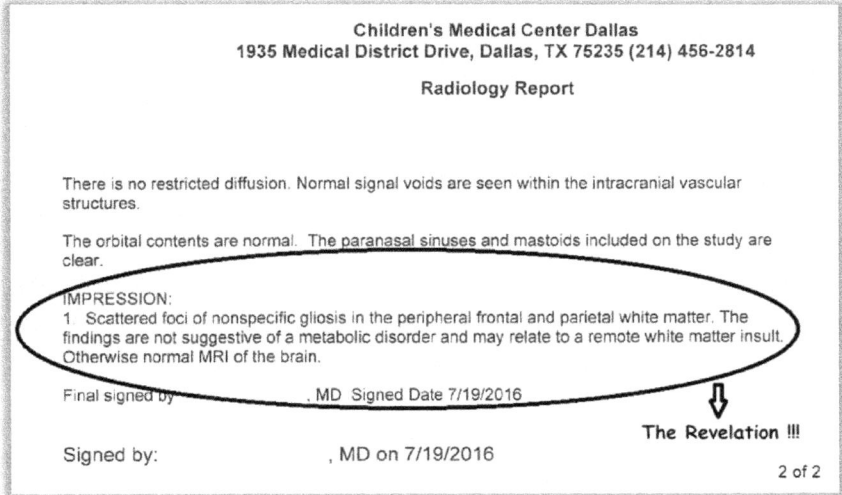

Children's Medical Center Dallas
1935 Medical District Drive, Dallas, TX 75235 (214) 456-2814

Radiology Report

There is no restricted diffusion. Normal signal voids are seen within the intracranial vascular structures.

The orbital contents are normal. The paranasal sinuses and mastoids included on the study are clear.

IMPRESSION:
1   Scattered foci of nonspecific gliosis in the peripheral frontal and parietal white matter. The findings are not suggestive of a metabolic disorder and may relate to a remote white matter insult. Otherwise normal MRI of the brain.

Final signed by   . MD Signed Date 7/19/2016

The Revelation !!!

Signed by: , MD on 7/19/2016

2 of 2

Fig. 6.1: MRI report of my second son at age 7

As you can plainly read, this report states there were impacts to the brain of my second boy due to white matter damage leading to a phenomenon known as gliosis. Gliosis is the general term for "nonspecific reactive change" of glial cells in response to damage to the brain. Gliosis involves the proliferation of several different types of glial cells, at the site of damage, including astrocytes, microglia, and oligodendrocytes. In its most extreme form, the proliferation associated with gliosis leads to the formation of a glial scar. In layman's terms, that means my boy suffered damage to the neurons in his brain, particularly to the axonal fibers which make up most of the white matter. As a reaction to such damage, the surrounding neuron support cells (called glial cells) have proliferated in certain areas, a sign of the body working hard to attempt damage control. Such traumatic damage to the deeply situated white matter of the brain is only possible during birth, when the head is subjected to high contraction forces – as in Pitocin induced labor. This is the "remote white matter insult" that the report is referring to.

Lost Memories Rekindled

Once I saw this MRI report, I started remembering things that had happened during the delivery of the boys. A feeling of guilt of having let this damage happen to our babies started taking up most of my waking hours and led to many sleepless nights. When my wife was induced for our first baby boy, about 5 to 6 hours into the process, the nurse had come into the delivery room carrying a phone handset, saying the doctor wanted to talk to us. On the other end of the line was the doctor who had demonized the C-section all along suddenly recommending that we consider one. She began by saying "At this point you can decide to proceed with the current course or have a C-section if you want," later adding that a "C-section is not that bad, let's do a C-section." She even had a giggle in her voice as she said it. She knew I was totally confused by her about-face as would have been expected going by her long-held view against C-section. I was pretty surprised by her sudden turnaround. I asked why and she simply said "in some cases it's not a bad choice." To this day, I wish she had given better reasoning, unfortunately, she did not offer anything further by way of explanation. Not convinced by her reasoning (or lack thereof), I responded that having waited this long could we continue for a couple of more hours and check back on progress. Her response was with a question "How is the mother doing? Is she tired? Can she go on for some more time?" My wife was doing perfectly fine as far as I could see and I told her so. Dr. S. then agreed to proceed with the current course. All in all, it was a 5-minute conversation that changed our lives and that of our child forever.

I was totally naïve to what was happening, but in reality, the nurse had warned the ignorant doctor about the risks of proceeding, but it ended up that the doctor had failed to explain her reasoning and ended up giving in to my request to continue for a couple of hours. The nurse couldn't believe the doctor gave in to my request. She simply couldn't hold back and as she was hooking my wife up to the next dose of Pitocin she made a prophetic remark: "Did you know this can cause brain damage?" At that moment I didn't even know if she meant brain damage to my wife or child, especially since the doctor had talked so much about the state of the mother a couple of minutes earlier. My wife looked fine to me and in my mind, I wrote off her comment as potentially some kind of adverse chemical reaction she was warning about. I told the nurse that the doctor didn't say anything like that, and dismissed the concern with a dismissive wave of my hand and a comment that would come back to haunt me: "Don't they write those warnings on every drug out there?" That was the end of the conversation.

I did tell her we had agreed to a couple of more hours, but the nurse and assistant nurse were upset at that time and I couldn't understand why. The older assistant nurse made a sad pout when she heard the decision. But this was pre-Affordable Care Act (Obamacare) times and nurses were not allowed to offer medical advice. I guess that was the reason they didn't pursue the matter any further. But the fresh attempt at induction, which I now know used a higher dose of Pitocin, brought on the dilation. A couple of hours later the nurse came back and sounded surprised when she reported that there had been progress. Eventually the baby was ready to be delivered after reaching 10-cm dilation around 8:30 pm in the night, a full 12 hours from the original start time, and he was born after an additional half hour of pushing.

Shortly after the baby was born, another incident happened. It was when the very experienced Pediatrician Dr. Joe examined the baby for the first time within an hour or two after he was born. Dr. Joe was visibly frustrated with what had happened. He was just done examining the baby at the when the nurse brought me over to him. He actually started yelling at the nurse that had brought me into the nursery room where he was examining our baby.

"I DON'T UNDERSTAND WHY THEY STILL KEEP DOING THIS, HE SHOULD HAVE BEEN C-SECTIONED OUT, WHO WAS THE OBSTETRICIAN?"

He then turned around to me and his exact words were

"His reflexes are poor, He should have been C-sectioned out, C-section is the best in these cases."

He continued with his reading to me on his assessments.

"The baby is fine, he is healthy overall, but his reflexes are weak, that's because he was induced for so long."

At this point I asked him, so when will his reflexes improve? Will he be ok in a few days? To that, Dr. Joe. did not answer but just gave me a helpless look and cast a helpless smile at my naiveté, and just shook his head and said, "I hope so, but it will take a long time." That was the end of our conversation. He didn't quite say how long that time was going to be and I didn't think much about it. Everything I had heard until that point in my life was that babies rapidly recover from most everything because they grow very, very rapidly.

The truth didn't register until I read the MRI results from my second son years later: my first baby had suffered brain damage as well, exactly as the nurse had warned. Dr. Joe's words and frustration now made perfect sense to me. The pediatrician was rightfully upset with the way events had turned out. He knew there were going to be issues down the line, which corroborates with what we are finding out years later. He had obviously not wanted to break the bad news that the baby had suffered permanent brain damage and ruin our happy 'new baby' moments. But because of what happened next, I wish I had deciphered the full extent of what he meant.

The Big Squeeze – The Scar Erasing Effect of Pushing

After getting the MRI back on my second boy and the flood of revelations it triggered, I had an MRI performed on my first son. I wanted confirmation of what had happened so long ago to help me make sense of everything. There was just one hitch: when the result of his MRI scan was returned, it did not show any abnormalities in brain shape or size at 10 years of age. So, no brain damage from a prolonged Pitocin induced delivery?

Not so fast.

It turns out that there's a good explanation for why there's no visible brain damage on my first son's MRI. Recall that he was a big boy, weighing in at about 8.5 pounds, and had to be pushed out after the 10cm dilation of the cervix had been achieved by the 12 hours of Pitocin induction.

Now brain trauma would typically show up on an MRI for you or me if our brains were exposed to this trauma outside the womb. But for my sons – and for the thousands of babies that are born with autism – the trauma happens *inside* the womb as a result of Pitocin induced delivery. And there's one more thing that has to happen before a baby enters the world. It has to travel down the birth canal.

Now a baby's skull is a disjointed set of 5 bones designed for exactly this. It freely takes on a conical shape due to the massage of the even pressure from the mother's pelvic muscles in the birth canal. The brain is the consistency of butter at this stage, and so it is technically pretty fluid and is be able to take shape deformation without too much trouble at this early stage of life. And indeed, we would be poorly evolved creatures if the normal process of birth somehow caused brain damage. Unlike my second son, who as you'll see quickly popped out once dilation was achieved without any pushing whatsoever, there was just over half hour of pushing in the case of my first son before he was born. Unsurprisingly, due to the pushing his head was crowned and he came out with a conical elongation.

But when it comes to identifying the presence of damage, what has the most significant impact is the scar re-distribution of white matter damage. The effect of subsequent skull/brain deformation from pushing means that any localized damaged tissue in the fluid brain is actually distributed over larger areas, thus erasing it from MRI scans (an MRI can only see any scarring or damage that is larger than 1 millimeter in size). In my older boy the pressure and deformation from the pushing had the effect of 'erasing' the scar tissue from being detected in an MRI scan by redistributing any damaged cells over larger areas of the brain.

Key Take Away: Diagnostic evidence in the form of MRI scan images fails to present itself as scarring in the brain in most cases because the pushing stage of labor tends to erase any scarring that has happened in the cervix dilation stage of labor by re-distributing the scar tissue such that it becomes invisible from MRI scan images. The first-born child and sometimes even subsequent children of a mother typically will not have scar tissue showing up in an MRI scan, if pushing is involved. This has allowed traumatic brain injury at birth to remain hidden for decades.

CHAPTER 7

OB-GYNs, Pitocin and the Abuse

Two years down the road we were pregnant with our second child. We went again to Dr. S.; after all, we weren't quite aware of any issues with our first kid, and for all we knew, Dr. S was an expert OB/GYN. But this time we already knew about induced labor. Dr. S. declared that since our first was induced, chances are the second would have to be too. And she was right. This time again, my wife was scheduled for induction on the due date. But unlike last time we didn't go back home; it was one long bout of 18 hours of Pitocin and Cytotec (misoprostol) combined induction.

Delivery #2

Sometime during the induction process, I heard a couple of nurses talking outside the ward. "That Dr. S. is at it again; she has been inducing this poor couple for over 7 hours," said one nurse, with the other nurse replying "oh my goodness."

Moments later the head nurse suddenly rushed into the room and asked in a very declarative tone:

"DO YOU KNOW WHY SHE IS INDUCING YOU FOR SO LONG?"

We responded by saying we had our first boy who was induced born and so we were expecting this one to be the same. The nurse frowned and said "Is he OK?" to which I answered he was. The truth was our first son was hyperactive and not verbal at close to age 2, but we didn't think of it as an issue then. She replied with a "really? ... hmm" and left the room with a frown and a confused look. This time there was no call from the doctor and no other interruption from the nurses.

I didn't quite know what to make of what the nurse was trying to say at that time. After 2 years I had completely forgotten the episode I had with the nurses and Dr. Joe with our first boy. Our induced labor continued on for a total 18 hours until our second baby boy came out. Being a smaller baby by a full pound, he did not have to be pushed but slid right out, after tearing through moms cervix. He had a well-rounded head due to the lack of pushing. This lack of the pushing stage is also the reason his TBI and scarring is visible on his MRI scan.

His MRI scan shows scar tissue and foci of white matter damage distributed all over the brain where he was pressure damaged by the induction process. Due to the lack of pushing and the lack of pressure and crowning of the head, the damage to his brain remained intact, allowing it to show up as scar tissue in the MRI scan. The location of the scar tissue within the brain is also critical in the developmental delays. He has a large scar in the language area of the brain and directly correlates with his lack of ability to pick up language.

Pitocin Contra-indications

Brain damage at birth can happen even without induced labor, due to other reasons like hypoxia, infection, meconium, placenta conditions and so on. But when such complications do not exist and induced labor is pursued beyond the point of contra-indication, then it has a 100% certainty of brain damage. The reason I say this is 100% is because this is traumatic brain injury caused by the mechanical means of uterine contractions and not some kind of subjective chemical effect like in other drugs where the extent of an individual's adverse reaction to the drug might vary. Don't just take my word for it – that's exactly what it says could happen on the Pitocin label.

Reading through the warnings and contra-indications was an eye-opener and ended up giving me a clearer picture of what had happened to my kids and what has been happening across the US in general, causing the autism epidemic.

A contra-indication is defined as something (such as a symptom or condition) that makes a particular treatment or procedure inadvisable. The Pitocin package insert describes the following as contra-indications:

CONTRAINDICATIONS

Antepartum use of Pitocin is contraindicated in any of the following circumstances:

1. Where there is significant cephalopelvic disproportion;
2. In unfavorable fetal positions or presentations, such as transverse lies, which are undeliverable without conversion prior to delivery;
3. In obstetrical emergencies where the benefit-to-risk ratio for either the fetus or the mother favors surgical intervention;
4. In fetal distress where delivery is not imminent;
5. Where adequate uterine activity fails to achieve satisfactory progress;
6. Where the uterus is already hyperactive or hypertonic;
7. In cases where vaginal delivery is contraindicated, such as invasive cervical carcinoma, active herpes genitalis, total placenta previa, vasa previa, and cord presentation or prolapse of the cord;
8. In patients with hypersensitivity to the drug.

OB/GYN's not understanding or paying heed to this single line has been the cause of almost all autism in America and the world !!!

Fig. 7.1: Pitocin Label – Contra-indications section.

While most of the contraindications mentioned on the label are pretty much self explanatory the contraindication # 5 is not very self evident. It warns against using contractions indefinitely to achieve dilation of the cervix. The manufacturers of Pitocin clearly know that the use of excessive contractions can cause adverse reactions. This means when you don't achieve complete dilation of the cervix in spite of 4-6 hours of continuous contractions at the optimal frequency interval, further pursuit of induction is contraindicated and needs to be discontinued. At this point a C-section is the only option. Why? Because of the adverse reactions that could ensue. These too are plainly listed on the adverse reactions section of the Pitocin label captured in Fig 7.2. The complete Pitocin label is included in the Appendix section of this book. This label is also downloadable from the FDA website and is one of the last remaining publicly available evidence of the brain damage Pitocin abuse is capable of, in a world where evidence against obstetric malpractice tends to disappear surreptitiously.

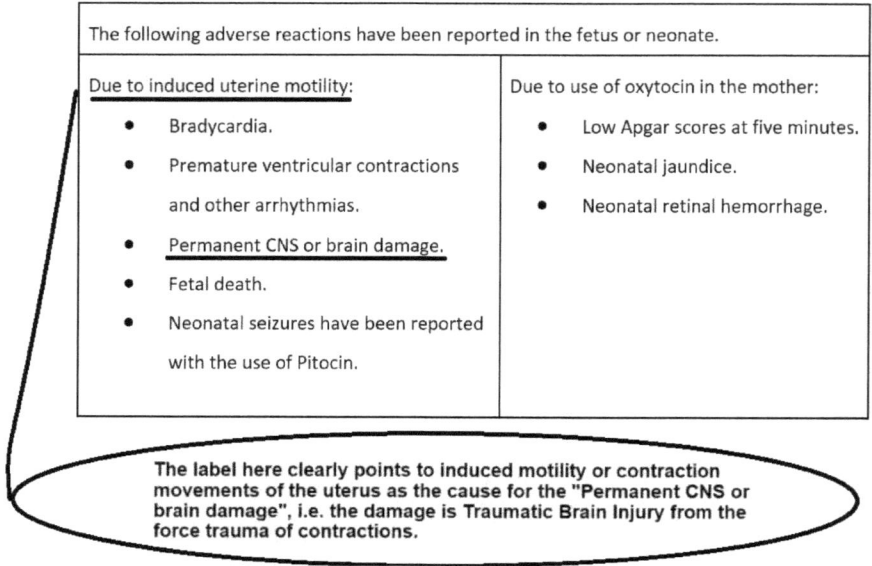

Fig. 7.2: Pitocin Label – Adverse effects section.

Every one of the uterine motility adverse reactions is actually a manifestation of brain damage. Bradycardia is abnormally slow heartbeats of less than 110 beats per minute, which in turn is indicative of fetal distress and leads to insufficient oxygen supply to the brain causing hypoxia. The point about premature ventricular contractions also causes low blood supply from the heart. Permanent CNS or brain damage is the traumatic brain injury – traumatic because it is caused by the movements of the uterus and the consequent forces on the fetal head and the brain inside, that every subjected to prolonged induction has suffered, causing the autism epidemic. Seizures again happen due to traumatic brain damage and result in autism after birth. The Apgar score at birth is indicative of low reflexes and brain damage as was pointed out by Dr. Joe in our case.

ACOG & the "Failure to Progress" Diagnosis Point

The American College of Obstetricians & Gynecologists (ACOG) is the authoritative body in the obstetrics world that provides directives to practicing obstetricians and maternity wards of Hospitals regarding obstetric practices.

To address the contraindication #5 on the Pitocin label, which says further use of Pitocin is contraindicated when adequate contractions fail to bring satisfactory progress, the ACOG clarifies and defines this "failure to progress diagnosis point" as a total of 72 continuous contractions, over a period of 4-6 hours depending on the contraction frequency achieved of 2 or 3 contractions every 10 minutes. If delivery is not achieved or imminent within that numerical limit of 72 contractions, labor induction is to be deemed to have failed and a C-section needs to be performed. This is designed to avoid the brain damage adverse outcome on the Pitocin label. This being traumatic brain damage, it happens to every unlucky fetus that gets induced beyond this limit with the extent of damage directly proportional to the number of additional contractions the unfortunate fetus was subjected to.

While the warning on Pitocin is pretty clear and Pitocin contra-indication is laid out in the instructions for the drug, many OB/GYN's have been in the practice of continuing labor induction, in spite of this contraindicated situation time and time again to this day. The American College of Obstetricians & Gynecologists (ACOG) should have come out strongly against this Pitocin abuse as strongly as they seem to condemn the abuse of C-sections, but instead seems to have remained silent. They were actually warning their ob-gyns to focus on cervical dilation and pursue induction only after proper cervical dilation was assured, in their internal website which was open to institutional access prior to 2018. Even at that time there was no explicit warning on the institutional website about the brain damage consequences while such a consequence is clear on the Pitocin labeling. It's possible they are trying to protect their OB/GYNs from what they might see as unnecessary lawsuits for past deeds. While it is understandable that they might not want to scare people away from a treatment course that is non-invasive and beneficial to some, not highlighting the risks enough and not publicly stating the conditions of failed induction has resulted in malpractice that destroys the lives of victims, their families and impacts society at large.

Unfortunately, the reality seems to be more than just doctors protecting other doctors. Since the early 1980s the ACOG has been actively involved alongside the manufacturers of Pitocin in the development of the practice of inducing labor.

The Pitocin label itself cites a study by the ACOG OB/GYNs, but the paper makes no mention of contra-indication, fetal brain damage possibilities and Pitocin warnings in that study or in their many publications. The closest they seem to come to Pitocin contra-indication is to talk about the adverse outcome of C-section if Pitocin induction fails to result in delivery. The conditions that constitute that failure of induction are never discussed in public. As a result, most obstetricians interpret adverse outcomes as fetal distress requiring C-section while ignoring the contra-indication contraction count and time limit, resulting in the ever-increasing autism numbers. More details on this ACOG behavior follow in the next chapter.

Readiness of the Cervix for Induction

The Bishop score is a system used to assess the readiness of the cervix for labor induction. It helps healthcare providers determine how favorable the cervix is for induction and the likelihood of successful vaginal delivery. The score ranges from 0 to 13 and is based on five factors:

1. Cervical Dilatation :
- 0 cm: 0 points
- 1-2 cm: 1 point
- 3-4 cm: 2 points
- ≥ 5 cm: 3 points

2. Cervical Effacement (thinning):
- 0%:   0 points
- 1-29%:   1 point
- 30-49%:   2 points
- ≥ 50%:   3 points

3. Cervical Consistency:
- Firm: 0 points
- Medium: 1 point
- Soft: 2 points

4. Cervical Position:
- Posterior: 0 points
- Mid-position: 1 point
- Anterior: 2 points

5. Fetal Station:

(the position of the fetus in relation to the ischial spines):

- -3:   0 points
- -2:   1 point
- -1/0:   2 points
- +1:   3 points
- +2 or more: 4 points

Interpretation of the Score:

- Score of 0-4: Unfavorable for induction; vaginal delivery unlikely.

- Score of 5-7: Moderate likelihood of a successful induction.

- Score of 8 or higher: Favorable for induction; higher likelihood of vaginal delivery.

Notice how successful induction requires a high score on multiple fronts with a score of 8/14 needed for the cervix to be considered favorable for induction. This Bishop score helps guide decisions about labor induction, allowing for a more personalized approach to each patient's situation. This score and its interpretation shown above is a measure of the readiness of the cervix for induction and is very critical to successful labor induction. When labor induction is undertaken when the cervix is not ready it results in a failed induction and the appropriate action to be taken if labor induction fails is to resort to a C-section. Further induction beyond the point of induction failure causes traumatic brain injury in the fetus and the child ends up being diagnosed with neurodevelopmental disorder or autism 2-3 years later.

Pitocin abuse begins when labor induction is undertaken by OB-Gyns more as a matter of convenience or as a weeks of pregnancy time limit, without consideration of the readiness of the mother's cervix for induction. Our story described as it transpired in Chapter 5 is a classic example of how Pitocin abuse happens in maternity wards across the US and around the world. It begins with a healthy mother of high bone density that can carry a pregnancy for 46-47 weeks, but is declared to be post-dated by an obstetrician and subjects the mother to labor induction without any consideration of the condition of the mother's cervix. To make matters worse these obstetricians do not engage in any cervix preparation but directly hook up these moms to Pitocin and / or administer misoprostol and expect it to result in a vaginal delivery. Such induction can result in a vaginal delivery, particularly if there's no fetal distress, but only after induction for longer than the "failure to progress diagnosis point" by leaps and bounds, both in terms of the number of contractions and the duration of induction. Such prolonged induction always results in traumatic brain injury to the baby, by way of severed neuronal tracts, which will be years later diagnosed as autism.

Unripe Cervix - no Dilation, no Effacement - only Stretch and Tear

As I have mentioned before, some pregnancies can last longer than others. Longer pregnancies tend to happen to very healthy moms with high bone density as borne out by experience and the research community agrees to this as well, with research papers recognizing a role for the Calcium ion cycle in the labor induction process. (Ref 7.2 – Vanessa M Barnabei et al - Autism and induced labor: is calcium a potential mechanistic link?)

When such a mother with a cervix that is not ready to dilate, at least not at 40 weeks of pregnancy or even as determined by the bishop score mentioned previously, gets subjected to induction, nothing happens, there is no dilation, no change whatsoever. In these cases, the supposed positive feedback loop of cervical stretching causing more natural oxytocin release leading to further natural contractions fails to take hold. This is because the mother's body instinctively knows that the cervix is not ready and bringing on contractions at this point will cause brain damage to the baby. But when an OB Gyn continues to induce contractions, the cervical wall stretches and stretches thereby putting tremendous pressure on the baby's head and brain inside. Eventually after prolonged hours of induction, the cervix eventually tears apart releasing the baby into the birth canal. The point to note here is if tearing is what happens to the cervix, what would be the damage sustained by the head and brain of the baby that caused the tear.

Fig. 7.3: The cervix stretch & tear pathway of abusive labor induction

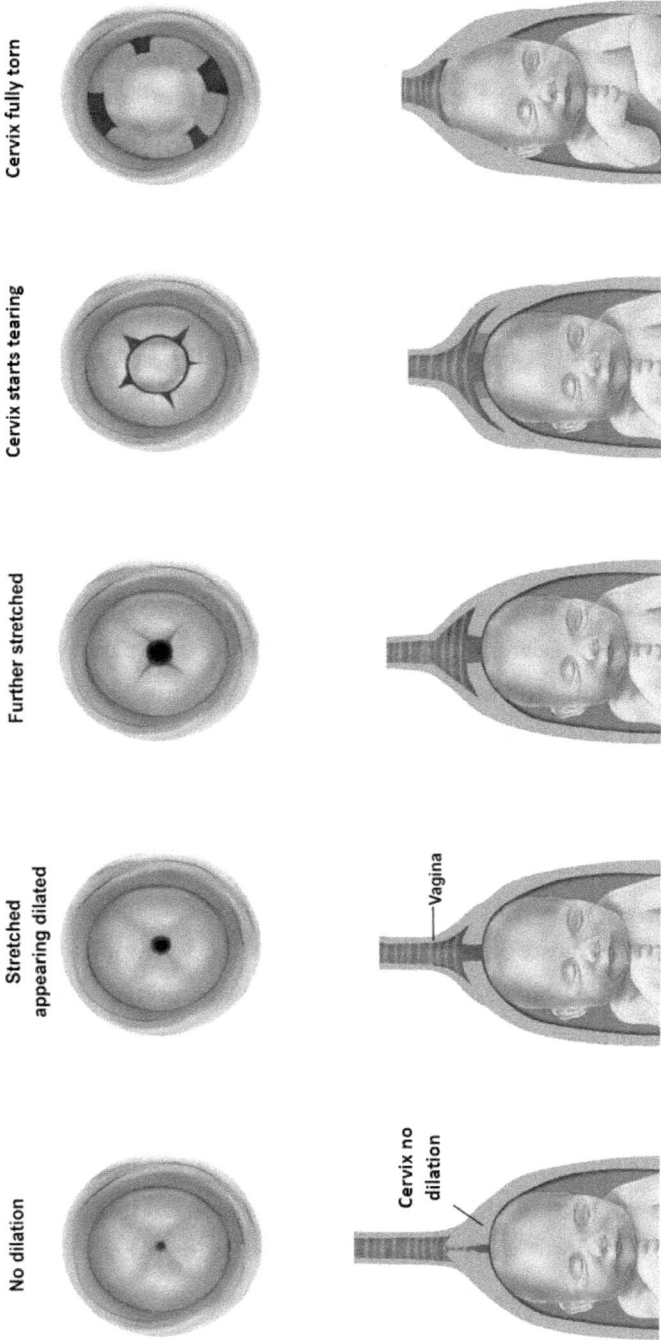

No dilation

Stretched appearing dilated

Further stretched

Cervix starts tearing

Cervix fully torn

Cervix no dilation

Vagina

The Mechanism of Brain Damage

Simply put, the human brain is the crown jewel of our biological existence. The brain is also a paradox of incredible power and profound fragility. While it orchestrates complex thoughts, emotions, and actions, its delicate structure is susceptible to a myriad of insults, both internal and external. Its intricate network of neurons, connected by delicate axons makes it the most fragile, yet the most consequential organ for the functioning of the human body. Even Steve Silberman, the now deceased author of bestselling book – "Neurotribes" and an autism epidemic denier, after watching a video about the soft and squishy brain, published by the University of Utah Neuroscience initiative titled "The Unfixed Brain" on YouTube, famously commented that, watching that video would make some people want to "put on a football helmet and never leave the house again.".

The brain's fragility is particularly evident in cases of traumatic brain injury (TBI). A sudden impact, as seen in concussions, can disrupt neural pathways, leading to cognitive impairment, memory loss, and long-term neurological disorders. The rapid acceleration and deceleration forces associated with head trauma can cause shearing and tearing of axons, leading to diffuse axonal injury (DAI). The impact can also cause contusions, lacerations, and hemorrhages, disrupting the brain's delicate circuitry. The consequences of TBI can range from mild cognitive impairments to severe disabilities and even death.

In spite of our understanding of the fragility of the human brain, until now traumatic brain damage from prolonged induced contractions during birth remains hidden as the predominant cause of neurodevelopmental disorders. The excessive contractions, both the number of contractions and the force of them acting on the baby's head for longer time durations can pulverize the fragile neuronal networks in unimaginable ways. Autism is known to many as a disorder of neuronal disconnects. To make matters worse there does not exist a way of accurately measuring the contraction forces even in modern times, due to the complexity of even modeling intrauterine pressure and intracranial pressure inside the baby's head. While the intrauterine pressure catheter (IUPC) offers the most precise measurement of intrauterine pressure, its invasive nature, requiring transcervical insertion, carries inherent risks of infection and, though rare, uterine perforation. Moreover, despite its perceived accuracy, IUPC readings can be influenced by various factors, including catheter placement, cervical condition, maternal position, and tissue elasticity, potentially compromising data reliability. Furthermore, as the IUPC necessitates amniotic rupture for placement, its use is limited, and it is not routinely employed in most deliveries. Instead, cardiotocographs (Fig 5.4) use another device called the tocodynamometer (toco). This is a non-invasive external monitoring device that consists of a pressure-sensitive transducer attached to a belt wrapped around the mother's abdomen. It detects changes in the tension of the uterine wall as contractions occur. Unlike internal monitors, which are designed to measure actual intrauterine pressure, a toco records relative pressure changes rather than exact contraction strength. As a result of this, there is never any monitoring of the absolute intra uterine pressure. This might be ok, as the toco might still capture the extremely forceful hypertonic contractions which might show up as a serious departure from limits.

Additionally, as the cervix stretches the forces acting on the head also become uneven with the annular ring of force on the head becoming increasingly higher. This is because the forces are acting on a smaller and smaller annular area, the pressure differential on the various parts of the head and brain becomes increasingly intense eventually ripping apart the long-range neuronal connections inside the baby's brain. Figure 7.4 shows the forces acting on the brain as the head gets pushed against the cervix wall during contractions.

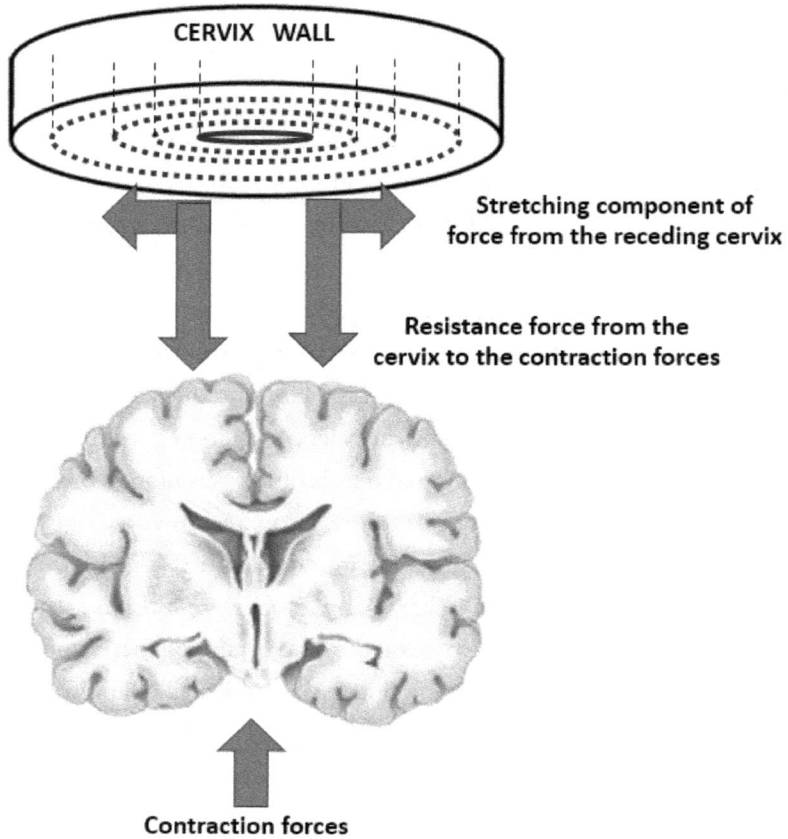

Fig 7.4: Diagram showing the compression forces acting on the brain as the cervix slowly stretches out with every contraction.

Damage is proportional to how long the cervix spends dilating at each station or how many contractions blows the brain takes at each station as the cervix dilates from 0 to 10 cm. Naysayers would say, "oh don't you know the brain is floating in cerebrospinal fluid and this kind of damage cannot happen". To them, all I have to say is please go re-read the Pitocin label, it does say Pitocin can damage the entire CNS, i.e. everything that the cerebrospinal fluid encloses. The truth is, this kind of prolonged induction injury pretty much pulverizes the neuronal cabling in the brain and it is the reason kids never recover from this kind of injury, while those that suffer hypoxic injury actually have a possibility to recover.

Understanding the diagrams presented here requires some imagination on the part of the reader. Consider that the non-dilating cervix is a strong piece of muscle tissue and belonging to the same make up as the uterus which is the strongest muscle in the female body. The head of the baby is being forced through this strong annulus by contractions. Numerous researchers particularly those looking at advanced DTI MRI scans find that children with autism seem to show neuronal disconnects at the corpus callosum. I present this schematic diagram in Figure 7.5 as an illustration of how the severing of neurons along the corpus callosum might happen as has been noticed in MRI scans of kids with autism. This explanation might help researchers avoid the indignity of having to research the genetic reasons as to why such severed neuron connections might occur!

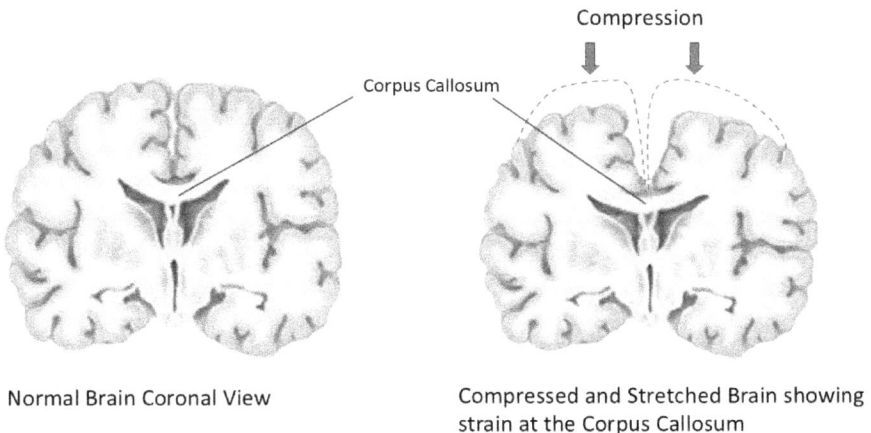

Normal Brain Coronal View   Compressed and Stretched Brain showing strain at the Corpus Callosum

Fig 7.5: Schematic comparison of normal brain with one under compression from strong induced contraction.

We'll continue this discussion in the chapter on MRI scans including the research performed, the research papers and their conclusions. The effects of contraction abuse not only end with the traumatic brain injury, there's other equally harmful consequences from some other mechanisms. Sometimes, the entire uterus could tear, from the forces of contraction, which puts the mother in serious danger of bleeding to death unless immediate surgical intervention is undertaken to do an emergency hysterectomy along with the C-section to remove the uterus or if tear is minor other corrective surgery is performed. Thus, labor induction comes with risks for both the mother and the baby particularly when undertaken while the cervix is not ready to dilate. Labor induction can also accentuate other risks such as development of fetal distress, tachycardia, bradycardia, meconium aspiration, placental abruption, all of which are implicated in additional hypoxic trauma and neurodevelopment issues in the baby down the line.

Key Take Away: Details of delivery of our second boy and the attempted intervention by nurses at the "Failure to Progress" diagnosis point, and the Pitocin label warnings have been discussed. Complete evidence of the cause of traumatic brain injury at birth with abusive labor induction has been provided. The cause of the neuronal disconnects so common in subjects with autism is clearly identified. The exact mechanism of the damage has been described.

CHAPTER 8

Pitocin Abuse – ACOG's "Failure to Progress" 72 Contractions Limit

I n the United States, no single agency is exclusively responsible for obstetric medical practices. Instead, like in every other field of medicine, several agencies and organizations influence and regulate these practices:

1. American College of Obstetricians and Gynecologists (ACOG): While not a government agency, ACOG sets practice guidelines and standards for obstetric care that are widely followed by healthcare providers.

2. Centers for Disease Control and Prevention (CDC): Provides guidelines on infection control, prenatal care, and public health issues relevant to obstetrics.

3. U.S. Food and Drug Administration (FDA): Regulates pharmaceuticals, medical devices, and products used in obstetric care to ensure their safety and efficacy.

4. State Medical Boards: Each state regulates the practice of medicine within its jurisdiction, including obstetric care, through licensing and adherence to state-specific medical laws.

There are other organizations like the American Board of Obstetrics and Gynecology (ABOG), an organization that tests knowledge of the subject and provides board certification, but OB/GYNs do not need to be board certified to practice. These entities collectively shape and oversee the standards and practices for obstetric care in the U.S. while also influencing care internationally. The American Journal of Obstetrics and Gynecology (AJOG) puts out the latest studies and scientific papers and advancement in the field of Obstetrics in the US. Many of these papers (as is common in this field) point to 'unknown' origins of autism. There are other international organizations like the International Federation of Obstetrics and Gynecology (FIGO) who provide resources to educate doctors and nurses, at the international level but sometimes suggestions coming from international organizations tend to get written off in the US apparently due to superior practices of their own.

The American College of Obstetricians and Gynecologists

The ACOG is a professional non-profit organization of Obstetricians and Gynecologists. Like other self-governing professional organizations in other fields of knowledge, they provide centralized practice guidance and standards for obstetric care. These are the people that are distinctly aware of the central role Pitocin has come to play in modern obstetrics, by providing obstetricians the ability to control the uterus. They are also the people fully aware of the dangers of the unbridled obstetric control of the uterus, the contra-indication conditions and adverse outcomes Pitocin is capable of.

Prior to the advent of Pitocin in 1980, the only intervention Obstetricians were able to offer during the birth process, were pain alleviation and mechanical interventions like forceps and vacuum extractions and C-section delivery. Hence it is understandable if they feel strongly about the usefulness of contraction control afforded by labor and delivery drugs. But when such drugs start becoming so commonplace that their dangers are getting forgotten and caution is replaced by complacency, it leads to disastrous consequences for the patients involved. Unfortunately, this has become reality for thousands of kids suffering from autism, who have permanently been brain damaged as a consequence of abusive labor induction damaging their brains at birth and changing their lives forever.

When Pitocin first delivered the ability to fully control the uterus after its approval in 1980, the responsibility for explaining the conditions of usage of this all-powerful new tool must have fallen squarely in the hands of the ACOG. Given the rather vague definition of the contraindication #5 of the Pitocin labelling, which states "where adequate uterine activity fails to achieve satisfactory progress", chances are mistakes were made on that front early on before the brain damage consequences became obvious.

The problem with contractions is they are literally hammering the baby head-first against the mother's cervix. These contractions cannot be too feeble such that they will never get the baby out. If they're too strong as in some women that are hypersensitive to Pitocin it leads to contractions that are so strong that they could damage the baby's brain with a few blows. Contraction strength has to be just right, strong enough to push the baby out of the cervix yet not too strong to damage the baby's brain in the process. Even then, if such contractions still don't bring about any significant dilation of the cervix wall, how long can you keep hammering that head before it starts to sustain brain damage? Inside the baby's head is a fragile network of neuronal tracts connecting the different parts of that growing fetal brain. It almost comes down to a strength of materials type of engineering question.

Somewhere along the line, a few years after 1980 it looks like the ACOG working with the manufacturers had eventually figured out the safety threshold. An exact number of safe continuous contractions allowable for safe induction was defined to be 72 at the maximum. Any contractions beyond this point would be making the damage being caused to the fetal brain from the force of contractions to start becoming irreversible. Such damage to the fragile neuron tract network that forms the fundamental networks on top of which all future development of the baby depends on, would be disastrous to any baby subjected to such trauma. Thus, they seem to have come up with this "failure to progress diagnosis point" of 72 continuous contractions beyond which the only safe alternative to avoid brain damage in the baby is a C-section.

They then advertised it within obstetric circles, gave directives to hospitals who then established labor induction protocols to deal with the situation. This was the reason the nurses in our case tried to intervene at this failure to progress diagnosis point in each of our 2 deliveries. But by the time ACOG realized what was happening, quite a few babies had already been brain damaged with this reason unknown to their parents. Given that there's no external indication of this trauma damage to the brain, no fetal distress, no NICU stay, there's no way these parents or anyone else were going to question obstetricians about their child's neurodevelopmental issues. These children would have been moved into pediatric care anyway out of the purview of obstetrics anyway.

The exact dates as to when the ACOG gave these hospital directives and had them establish these protocols is unknown to me and any experts I have had the privilege of discussing it with. The best guesses put the actual dates sometime in the 90's. All I know is, quite a significant number of years had passed between 1980 and the time ACOG came up with this 72-contraction limit and over which time numerous babies had been induced beyond this subsequently established 72 contraction limit. This makes it obvious that obstetricians have been sitting on some serious liability issues in terms of the babies that were previously damaged.

The ACOG might have done better had they come out clean on these mistakes of the past, instead they seem to have chosen to keep it hidden. They seem to continue to be trying to keep the exact contraindication conditions hidden from the general public even after a full 45 years have passed by as of 2025. While their intention for their keeping their flock of practitioners safe from malpractice suits is fathomable, their attempts at keeping it hidden has also meant, not all obstetricians are getting the message loud and clear about the dangers of inducing beyond their "failure to progress" diagnosis point. And it's probably not just them. Obstetric mistakes and liabilities are covered by malpractice insurers and hospitals are not given an easy pass in lawsuits, when it comes to obstetrics mistakes on their premises either. So, in this age of managed healthcare and hospital and insurance conglomerates, the ACOG have probably been under pressure from these entities also, to keep mistakes under wraps for financial liability reasons.

This means, for over four decades since 1980, the autism epidemic of supposed unknown causes has been unleashed on healthy mothers and babies unlucky enough to be induced by their obstetrician when the mom's cervix is not ready. If they picked an obstetrician who didn't get that mid 90's memo on the failure to progress contraindication situation and its brain damage consequences or fully understand the hospital protocols instituted since then, they would be induced all the way to a vaginal delivery, disregarding this brain damage consequence. These unfortunate babies would suffer silent traumatic damage to their fundamental neuronal networks. These babies then experience neurodevelopmental delays growing up, and a vaccine double whammy that I will talk about in subsequent chapters and end up with autism of supposedly unknown causes a few years later. Obstetricians who do not understand the seriousness of the Pitocin brain damage consequences, end up extolling the benefits of Pitocin induction, as a safe and natural method, like our OB-GYN did, while demonizing the C-section. To parents with healthy pregnancies, a surgical intervention like a C-section is obviously a last resort. In cases where the cervix is not ready for delivery, as in most post-dated women and where the obstetrician does not engage in cervix preparation prior to induction, it invariably results in a failed induction and when induction is pursued further the contractions begin to cause irreversible traumatic brain damage.

Uniqueness of Labor Induction Drugs

Most medicines work at the cellular chemical level by binding to a molecular target, usually proteins like receptors or enzymes, thereby either blocking or supporting its activity, which results in their therapeutic effects. Receptors are proteins on a cell's surface that can trigger a variety of responses inside the cell when activated. The effect of the drug brings about a better chemical balance in the body, helps get rid of invading antigens, brings about pain mitigation or alleviates other symptoms.

Labor induction drugs are very unique in that they bring about contractions of the uterus, physical movements of an organ inside the body. The adverse reaction and traumatic brain injury as a result of such a different type of drug action are unfathomable to many. But the details on the adverse reactions on the Pitocin label are pretty clear and clearly warn about the possibility of brain damage to the baby as a result of the contraction movements.

The Contra-indication Directive Concealed from Public View

The ACOG have useful information on obstetrics including labor induction on their website acog.org. After my realization of what caused my boys' condition, I got busy researching the ACOG directives on labor induction. I was able to login to the then protected parts of the site using my educational institution access back in 2017, which is where I learnt about the 72-contraction limit. It was corroborated by the times at which the nurses tried to intervene to stop induction during the deliveries of my 2 boys. I have personally come across documents outlining the 72 continuous contractions limit for labor induction and the ACOG directives warning their flock against attempting induction without achieving proper cervical dilation. But the directives on inducing labor are not available to the public, it was probably never public. In their public site they speak of a C-section as the undesirable outcome of failed induction although the criteria for failed induction are never mentioned. Looking at the public information makes one conclude that a C-section is to be done only in the case of fetal distress.

The ACOG site as seen in 2024 has been split into three parts, one for public view, one for paid members and one other part reserved exclusively for practitioner only access. It is believed they removed institutional access completely in 2021, replacing it with the paid member view which is a $200+ paywall per individual member. Their directives on Pitocin even in the public site has been constantly changing. It is really hard to imagine why their documentation on a drug and process in use for 45 years needs to keep changing. They even claim it will change, based on emerging clinical and scientific advances in spite of the process of uterine contractions and birth having stayed the same. Have they been playing a game of trial and error all this time, with a drug that carries a slew of brain damage and loss of life warnings?

Notice how things seem to be changing in the ACOG language over the years. Any clues of the Pitocin contraindication seem to have quietly disappeared.

Fig 8.1: Screenshot from the ACOG website in 2020.

Comparing figure 8.1 with figure 8.2 you will notice the reference to C-section delivery and fetal death as adverse effects of labor induction have conveniently disappeared in the 4 years between 2020 and 2024. That is because the ACOG have withdrawn the "failure to progress diagnosis" point which required the C-section upon lack of progress with labor induction. It was a safety precaution against brain damage from excessive contractions. But this critical safeguard was dropped after the conclusion of the "ARRIVE" trial in 2018 and ACOG's acceptance of the recommendations of the Society for Maternal Fetal Medicine, another obstetric organization that came up with totally contrary recommendations on labor induction upon completion of their "Arrive" trial. More details about this flawed trial which did not take into consideration the contraindication warning #5 in the Pitocin label are in the upcoming paragraphs.

https://www.acog.org/womens-health/faqs/labor-induction

What are the risks of labor induction?

One risk is that when oxytocin is used, the uterus may be overstimulated. This may cause the uterus to contract too often. Too many contractions may lead to changes in the fetal heart rate. If there are problems with the fetal heart rate, oxytocin may be reduced or stopped. Other treatments may be needed to steady the fetal heart rate.

Other risks of labor induction may include

- chorioamnionitis, an infection of the amniotic fluid, placenta, or membranes
- infection of the baby
- rupture of the uterus (this is rare)

Medical problems that were present before pregnancy or occurred during pregnancy may contribute to these complications. To help prevent these complications, the fetal heart rate and force of contractions may be electronically monitored during labor induction.

What if labor induction does not work?

Sometimes labor induction doesn't work. If you and your pregnancy are doing well and the amniotic sac has not ruptured, you may be given the option to go home. You can schedule another appointment to try induction again. If your labor starts, you should go back to the hospital.

If you or your baby are not doing well during or after attempting induction, a cesarean birth may be needed. Although most cesarean births are safe, there may be additional risks for you, including

- infection
- hemorrhage (heavy bleeding)
- complications from anesthesia

The recovery time after a cesarean birth is usually longer than for a vaginal birth.

There are also considerations for future pregnancies. With each cesarean birth, the risk of serious placenta problems in future pregnancies goes up. In addition, the number of cesarean births you have had is a major factor in how you will give birth to any future babies.

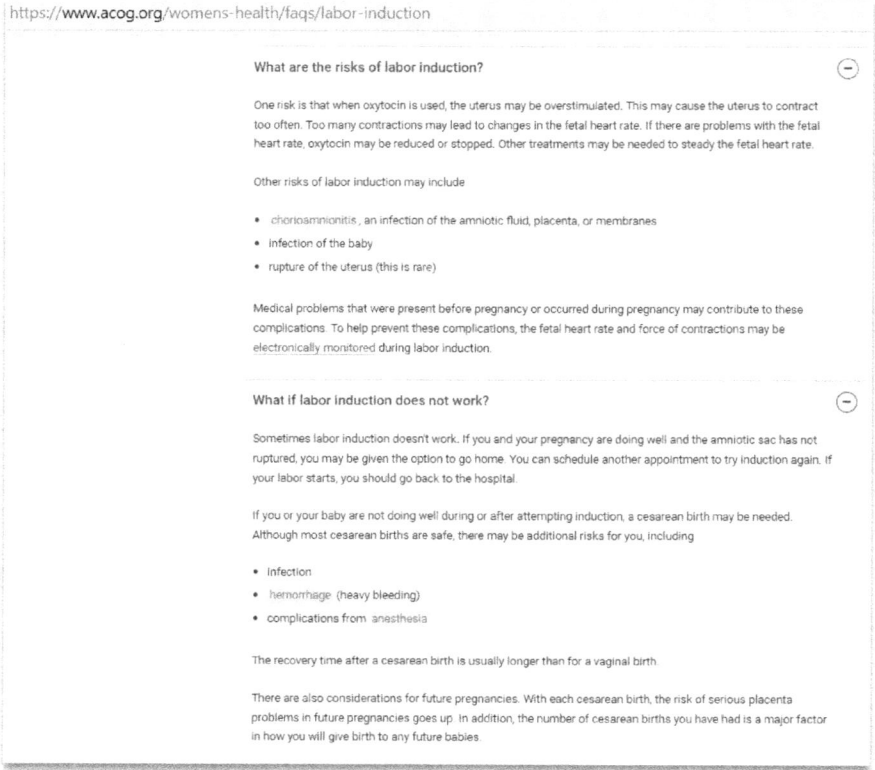

Fig 8.2: Screenshot from the ACOG website in 2024

The ACOG should have been the first people to link neurodevelopmental disorders to birth injury and the word autism, but they seem to have avoided the topic altogether, leading one to think it's an obvious conflict of interest and they are trying to protect their practitioners from legal exposure and lawsuits for mistakes from their past. Most of their experts seem to be busy diverting attention, (using their committee opinion page described later) postulating about the chemical effects of externally administered oxytocin on the fetus, faulty oxytocin signaling pathways, alteration of fetal oxytocin receptors, etc., as the purported cause of autism and then going on to cite evidence to the contrary, thereby claiming Pitocin doesn't cause autism. All this while fully aware that the actual cause is physical trauma to the brain from forceful Pitocin contractions against an un-ripe cervix. This brain damage outcome from excessive contractions is something the ACOG are very much aware of and very obvious on the Pitocin label. But instead, they seem to be moving to bury all their recommendations from the past with regard to the safety of labor induction.

Notice the login requirement to read more about induction of labor in the next screenshot Figure 8.3.

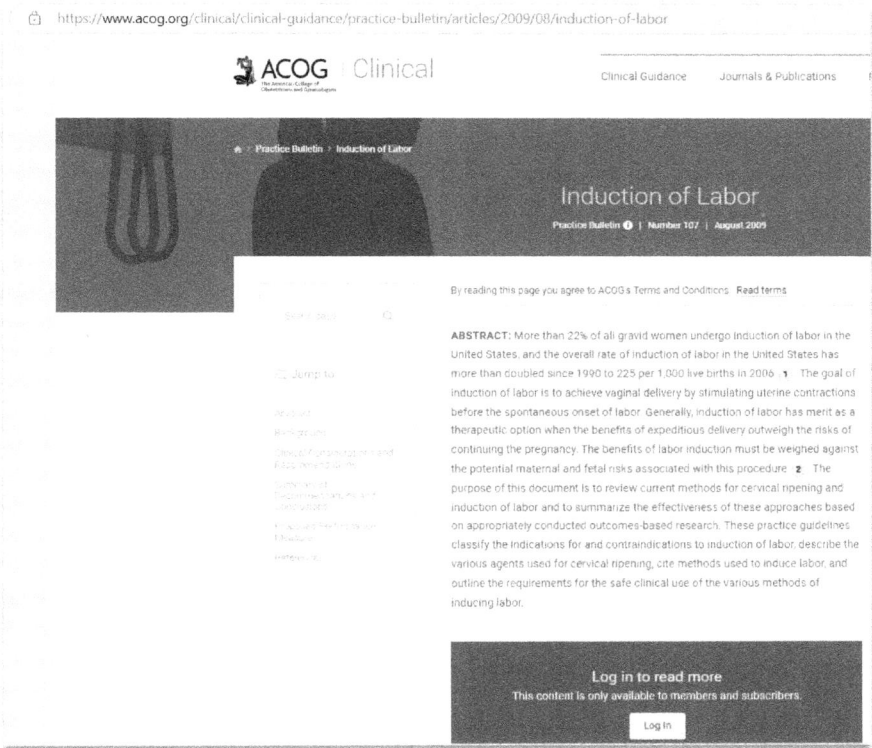

Fig 8.3: Screenshot from the ACOG website in 2025

Gaming the Headlines with False Sciences

When it comes to the labor induction autism link the ACOG has strategically published a paper on their website titled "Labor induction or augmentation and autism - a committee opinion" originally from the year 2014 and consistently reaffirmed it every couple of years up to the present. This page consistently ranks in the top couple of results on google when the term "Pitocin autism" is searched. In this paper they divert the entire topic of the Pitocin autism causation mechanism to a chemical effect. They have conveniently taken a flawed hypothesis that presumes the cause of autism is due to faulty Oxytocin signaling pathways due to impacts from fetal exposure to exogenous Oxytocin during labor induction. It is a play on oxytocin's alternate role in the brain as a neurotransmitter. The ACOG committee then go on to argue that this alternate mechanism cannot cause autism and cite studies to back them up. The only problem is everybody and their brother knows that Autism is not as simple as faulty Oxytocin signaling, it comes with speech, cognitive, fine motor and other development issues at every level and not just a social disability from faulty Oxytocin signaling or scarcity. As I have mentioned before, Oxytocin acts as both a hormone and a neurotransmitter on the 2 sides of the Blood Brain Barrier (BBB). It is a hormone on the body side, that causes uterine contractions and on the brain side of the BBB it is considered a love neurotransmitter enabling social interactions. The committee opinion seems to be citing only the brain side effects and claims there is no down-regulation of oxytocin receptors in the fetal brain from external oxytocin in the mother and hence does not cause autism while the primary effect of oxytocin causing uterine contractions and causing traumatic injury from the abuse of it, is being surreptitiously left out. The committee seems to be conveniently forgetting that augmented pituitrin (oxytocin sourced from cattle) had a history of brain trauma and fetal death in its past from uncontrolled contractions and its use was banned before being re-approved in 1980 after the advent of synthetic version of oxytocin and electronic fetal monitoring. The link to this committee opinion posted in the figure below has changed since the release of my prior book, (Autism Answers and Action – Dinesh Danny - 2021) and so has the content on the page that has replaced it in 2025. The biggest change is that they have moderated their stance, prioritizing cited research over direct assertions. The first line on their document states "The Society for Maternal Fetal Medicine endorses this document". To me, it sounds like they don't exactly agree with this content completely, but yielding leadership on the subject to this "Society for Maternal-Fetal Medicine". More on this in the upcoming pages.

Labor induction or augmentation and autism. Committee Opinion No. 597. American College of Obstetricians and Gynecologists. Obstet Gynecol 2014;123:1140–2.

Old Link (link defunct in 2025)

The link to it on the ACOG website is as follows

https://www.acog.org/Clinical-Guidance-and-Publications/Committee-Opinions/Committee-on-Obstetric-Practice/Labor-Induction-or-Augmentation-and-Autism.

New Link

https://www.acog.org/clinical/clinical-guidance/committee-opinion/articles/2014/05/labor-induction-or-augmentation-and-autism

In the opinion paper itself the only thing they don't talk about is traumatic brain injury. So, they are walking the same path of defending their stance and hiding the truth in the wake of mounting evidence of their wrongdoing with the increasing autism numbers. They also continue taking that extra step in their defense by suggesting that all autism is genetic. It's not like there's been a dearth of scientific papers citing the risks in active management of labor. There's also been papers highlighting the risk of malpractice when it comes to labor induction. What's been missing is the tagging of what these papers call 'adverse outcomes' with the term 'Autism.' Below is a small sampling of science papers and studies that have talked about malpractice risks from as far back as 1987, within a few years of the official approval of Pitocin for inducing labor in 1980 by the FDA for elective induction:

1. **Perinatal malpractice. Risks and prevention**. Nocon JJ, Coolman DA. J Reprod Med 1987;32:83–90.

2. **The Use and Abuse of Oxytocin**. Oláh KSJ, Steer PJ. The Obstetrician & Gynecologist 2015;17:265–71

3. **Association of autism with induced or augmented childbirth in North Carolina Birth Record (1990–1998) and Education**

Research (1997-2007) databases. Gregory SG, Anthopolos R, Osgood CE, Grotegut CA, Miranda ML. JAMA Pediatr 2013;167:959–66.

4. **Increased Risk of Autism Development in Children Whose Mothers Experienced Birth Complications or Received Labor and Delivery Drugs.** Smallwood M, Sareen A, Baker E, Hannusch R, Kwessi E, Williams T. *ASN Neuro.* 2016 Aug 9;8(4):1759091416659742. Doi: 10.1177/1759091416659742. PMID: 27511908; PMCID: PMC4984315.

Each of these articles cite about 30 other articles each, so there's no scarcity of opinions and studies supporting the argument against Labor induction and highlighting the possibility of malpractice. Unfortunately, people in positions of influence in the OB/GYN community have chosen to ignore these voices and have ended up perpetuating labor drug abuse malpractice and autism.

When a research paper refers to "adverse perinatal outcomes," it is primarily discussing outcomes related to the baby. These adverse outcomes typically include:

▸ **Stillbirth**: Loss of the fetus at or after 20 weeks of gestation.

▸ **Neonatal mortality**: Death of the baby within the first 28 days after birth.

▸ **Neurological issues**: Conditions ranging from cerebral palsy to developmental delays i.e. Autism.

▸ **Birth weight**: Low or high birth weight that can indicate potential health issues.

▸ **Apgar scores**: Low scores at one and five minutes after birth, indicating the baby's physical condition.

While the adverse outcomes of stillbirth and neonatal mortality are easily observed and remain the highest in the United States among the developed world, the other problems like neurological issues, the actual impact of Apgar scores, and such are not immediately visible and take longer times to play out. Too long for most scientific studies to follow and report on it. Even parents tend to forget incidents at birth to be able to correlate their child's neurological issues to their birth circumstances.

Sometimes it is possible to miss the point even after reading some of these papers, even if you agree they all are solid evidence that perinatal obstetric malpractice might play a major role in causing autism. That's because common folks may not make the connection in words used in scientific literature which actually translate to autism in common parlance:

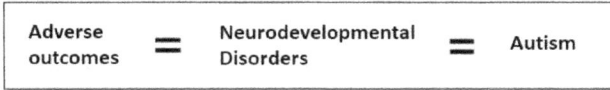

| Adverse outcomes | = | Neurodevelopmental Disorders | = | Autism |

It makes a world of difference reading through the above papers to your understanding of the causes of autism once you make the above connection.

Almost Outed

Out of these the 2013 paper by Dr. Simon G Gregory et al[8,9], of the Duke Center for Autism and their analysis of North Carolina birth records between 1990 - 1998, correlating it with the education research database 1997-2007, created quite a bit of uproar in the parent and medical circles. Labor induction has become the norm in obstetric wards around the globe and here was a paper correctly correlating it to autism. The data used is from the North Carolina Detailed Birth Record (NCDBR) which is known to be very accurate. The school register includes all public schools and is maintained by North Carolina Education Research Data Center (NCERDC). The diagnosis of autism is by school psychologists using criteria universally accepted for the diagnosis of autism and the diagnosis by age 8 which is what the CDC uses to calculate its autism numbers. Of 910,887 births, 678,078 (74.4%) were successfully matched between the birth and education records. Thus, it is the largest study of its kind ever performed. The correlation between autism and labor induction turned out to be exceptionally strong. The study found 23% of induced kids ended up being diagnosed for autism. That is almost one fourth of the induced population. And in male children subjected to induction or augmentation at birth, the odds where even higher at 35% compared to the non-induced/non-augmented population.

Some of the other known causes of autism like twin births, multiple births, congenital anomalies, very premature births < 24 weeks and some where there was missing data on potential confounding factors were excluded from the analysis. This excluded a significant number of autism births. Yet, out of more the 625k births considered, there were over 5500 children with autism or about 0.9% autism occurrence in this dataset of births in the 90's. The birth data in the North Carolina records is so rich, the researchers were even able to see there were more cases of placental abruption and meconium staining in cases where there was induction/augmentation vs the natural non-intervention group. They had the cause of autism pretty much nailed down to labor induction / augmentation. There was no way anybody could say this data was lying. Or so you would think.

Unfortunately, the Duke/Chicago research group fell prey to prior research that had previously discovered the social bonding aspect of Oxytocin, which is its neurotransmitter function. These researchers postulated that the chemical effect of external Oxytocin on the infant brain might somehow be responsible for causing autism. They failed to track down the autism causation mechanism to the traumatic brain damage outcome mentioned in the adverse reaction section of the Pitocin labelling, or the failure to progress contraindication found in the labelling and ACOG directives and hospital protocols not being followed. I guess it might have been assumed that doctors are following protocols or the details about Pitocin and contraindications might not have been known to these researchers as the failure to progress diagnosis condition seems to be a closely guarded secret of the ACOG. These researchers instead picked the plausible explanation as the impact of exogenous oxytocin on the oxytocin signaling pathways that play a critical role in social behavior and cognition development as the possible cause of their findings.

This research paper with undeniably strong evidence pointing at Pitocin use for autism causation, perhaps put the entire Pitocin abuse malpractice defense and misinformation complex made up of malpractice insurance companies, hospitals and ACOG on high alert. They immediately set into action their research wings to create studies that could contradict this claim. And a counter study came, just a couple of years later in the form of another analysis of data. This time a look at the Swedish birth records between 1992 and 2005 which was a much larger dataset at 1.36 million births by a group of Academic researchers and practitioners with impressive credentials.

"Association of Labor Induction with Offspring Risk of Autism Spectrum Disorders" Sarah Oberg et al.
https://jamanetwork.com/journals/jamapediatrics/fullarticle/2534479

Interestingly Sweden had a much lower labor induction rate of about 10.5% This set of researchers actually found the same correlation between labor induction and autism occurrence thus confirming the findings of the North Carolina research group. But given that their research set out to prove the opposite, they came up with further ways to eliminate data to remove this relationship. To accomplish this, they had to return to the flawed genetic basis theory (flaws explained in chapter 9). They restricted the data to only siblings that were discordant with respect to labor induction, i.e. they restricted the dataset to cases of siblings where one sibling was induced and others were not. This way they claimed that when born to the same mother and one child was induced and other not induced, the occurrence of autism in the induced child was no higher than in the non-induced child.

To me the reasoning for this finding is pretty clear but different from what the researchers had to say. When a mom has multiple children and one of them is induced and the others are not, it is mostly the first child of the mother that has difficulty coming out and is induced. Experience shows that subsequent children are susceptible to other forms of hypoxic injury that can happen without induction. It was probably really hard to find samples where the first child was not induced and subsequent ones were induced. So, they potentially whittled down the autism occurrence data sets in the data to a really small fraction of the original. The study did not report how many autism cases fell in the sibling cohort where they found close to equal amounts of autism diagnosis amongst siblings that were induced and non-induced. Thus, they claimed labor induction had no effect on autism occurrence by fudging the data by building an unproven genetic theory into it to make it fit the expected outcome.

But the bottom line is this. While the North Carolina data was actually richer than the Swedish data in terms of the medical outcomes like meconium staining and placental abruption, neither the Swedish data or the North Carolina data actually contained the real causal information. They both had only check boxes marked or procedure codes for labor induction and not the duration of induction, which is the factor that can establish the causal relationship to autism. Thus, this study of the large Swedish data accomplished nothing above what was said in the North Carolina study except use a flawed genetic comparison of siblings to prove lack of correlation of autism to induction without disclosing detail on the actual autism numbers in the restricted group. They were using Statistical Analysis Software (SAS) typically used in clinical trial data analysis, and given that it came from reputed institutions and had a slightly larger data set, this study met the requirements of the people managing the narrative on the safety of labor induction and hiding Pitocin abuse. They were able to go to town with this false study and reclaim the safety of labor induction. Another interesting point to note is that the studies that point fingers at Pitocin are typically not sponsored by the NIH, but the ones supporting Pitocin always are. While it might be pure coincidence it does indicate that obstetrics researchers coming up with papers in defense of Pitocin are pretty influential and able to obtain NIH funding at will.

The detail that is being lost in all this research is the fact that these papers seem to be looking at induction from a chemical exposure to Oxytocin standpoint vs the risk from actual direct effect of Oxytocin which is the uterine contractions and the potential for head trauma. That particular point cannot be proven with population studies but only proven by MRI scans of children with autism that show neuron tract disconnects. We'll look at this in a subsequent chapter on MRI scans. However, all the attention given by these papers to the chemical effects, to some hypothetical downregulation of oxytocin receptors in brain damaged individuals serves only one purpose and that is to game the headlines to say Pitocin doesn't cause autism by simply switching the underlying mechanism of damage to something that doesn't exist.

Adding Insult to Injury – The ARRIVE Trial (2015-2018)

Acronym for – "A Randomized Trial of Induction Versus Expectant" Management, a catchy name for a trial supposedly undertaken in response to concerns raised regarding the risks and benefits of elective induction of labor.

Unfortunately, this ARRIVE trial has been the source of a lot of newfangled nonsense coming through in the obstetric community.

The trial was initiated by the National Institutes of Health (NIH), specifically through the National Institute of Child Health and Human Development (NICHD). This large, multicenter, randomized controlled trial aimed to examine the effects of elective induction of labor at 39 weeks of gestation compared to expectant management (waiting for spontaneous labor) in low-risk women with a singleton pregnancy.

The study, which began in the mid-2010s, enrolled nearly 6,000 women and aimed to determine whether inducing labor at 39 weeks could reduce the risk of adverse outcomes such as cesarean delivery, fetal distress, and neonatal complications, while also considering the impact on maternal health.

The findings of the study are published in
https://www.nejm.org/doi/10.1056/NEJMoa1800566
WA Grobman, et al. Labor Induction versus Expectant Management in Low-Risk Nulliparous Women.
The key findings from the ARRIVE trial were:

▶ Induction at 39 weeks was associated with a slightly lower rate of cesarean delivery compared to expectant management.

▶ There was no significant difference in neonatal outcomes between the two groups, such as neonatal intensive care unit (NICU) admissions or Apgar scores.

▶ Inducing labor at 39 weeks did not lead to better overall outcomes for mother or baby in most cases but could reduce the risks related to complications of prolonged pregnancy.

As benign and inconsequential as this sounds, the study actually contradicted everything about the brain damage risks of labor induction that had been learnt over the years by the ACOG. Rather than stick with the study objectives of measuring outcomes from labor induction at 39 weeks, using established labor induction protocols they strayed into suggesting new labor induction protocols exposing that they were unaware of the existing ones. They suggested it was ok to induce labor for about 20 hours! The ACOG had been so secretive of their protocols to handle labor induction that the newbie obstetricians involved in the Arrive trial were obviously not familiar with them or the reasons for their existence. This is clear from their paper about their key findings I mentioned previously. The paper references another paper by the same set of authors that displays their total lack of knowledge of the warnings on the Pitocin label, the reason for the ACOG and hospital labor induction protocols. They have probably never seen the Pitocin label as hospitals switched to inducing with off label use of misoprostol since 2010 a prostaglandin approved only for abortions and not live births and hence does not carry the brain damage warnings that the Pitocin label does. (More on this in the next section).

Prior to the Arrive trial there was a paper published by its principal investigator William A Grobman in the AJOG, which should have served as a warning shot to the obstetric community of things to come.

"Defining failed induction of labor" W A Grobman et al
https://pmc.ncbi.nlm.nih.gov/articles/PMC5819749/

This paper was published in the American Journal of Obstetrics and Gynecology 2017 Nov 11; Everything about this paper is wrong and subpar, it should never have been accepted for publication in any professional journal of any standing. They made it about the hours of induction, a step back from the precise contraction count that the ACOG had arrived at. The paper doesn't display any understanding of the Pitocin labeling or the ACOG "failure to progress diagnosis point" and the reason for its existence and any understanding of the possible brain damage consequences of abusing uterine contractions. These studies only followed near term neonatal outcomes such as still birth or neonatal death within 7 days of birth and complications like neonatal encephalopathy, respiratory distress syndrome, and meconium aspiration. The study never followed the subjects once they leave the hospital.

But to make matters worse for the ACOG, another obstetric organization the "Society for Maternal Fetal Management" (SMFM.org) ended up buying into the arrive trial. (The trial was conducted by Members of the SMFM) They apparently specialize in high-risk pregnancies. To me that means they don't know much about labor induction as labor induction is only attempted in low-risk pregnancies. The idea of the arrive trial was to induce labor in women ahead of the pregnancy turning into high risk with the development of pre-eclampsia (mother developing a sustained high blood pressure with related kidney, liver damage problems) and related complications in mothers mostly at the tail end of pregnancy. So, to them, inducing ahead of time, without a full understanding of the complications caused by induction itself sounded like a great idea and they embraced it fully. This obviously put the ACOG in a tough spot.

As unlikely as it seems, a bunch of newbie obstetricians armed only with the audacity of the clueless, seem to have run roughshod over years of wisdom accumulated by the ACOG. A closer scrutiny of the Arrive trial and its papers reveals something quite extra-ordinary. The principal investigator of the arrive trial, William A Grobman seems to have pretty much done it singlehandedly. With an MD from Harvard University and MBA from Northwestern, and a fellowship in Maternal Fetal medicine from Northwestern, he seems to have attempted to disrupt the obstetrics practice and revolutionize it in ways older wiser, more experienced obstetricians seem to have been wary to try. Obstetrics in the US is highly interventionist and Grobman's efforts seem to be aimed at making it even more interventionist at a time when people are casting doubts about the safety and prudence of these interventions. He appears to have leveraged his academic achievements to advance his career within the obstetrics community and assume positions of unparalleled influence. He was chosen to become editor of American Journal of Obstetrics and Gynecology (AJOG) in 2010, which explains his foray into labor induction with his subpar paper, "Defining failed induction of labor" in 2011, which exposes his total lack of knowledge of the known dangers of labor induction and the protocols in place in hospitals at that time. His paper would never have been published, if not for he himself being the basic science editor of the AJOG. He had also been made President of the SMFM organization for a while, which explains why the SMFM seem to have readily accepted the outcome of the flawed ARRIVE trial he spearheaded. Thus, an academically accomplished doctor with a "smarter than thee" attitude seems to have broken down obstetric safety limits with his flawed research. This way, an obstetrician educated and specializing in high-risk pregnancies seems to have influenced the course of obstetric practices for low-risk pregnancies completely unaware of the long-term neurological consequences of the interventions he seems to have injected into the obstetric community. Being a large trial of over 6000 cases, there were further papers analyzing the arrive trial data, coming up with further conclusions about the safety of induction. The trial itself did not track patients after they left the hospital, so it's very probable that there will be a significant amount of autism diagnosis among the babies of mothers subjected to the 20 hours or more of induction, who will be told autism is genetic.

Unfortunately, even the ACOG seem to have given in to recommendations of Grobman about prolonged induction and abandoned their definition of the "failure to progress" diagnosis point in labor induction.

Let me try to explain the reasons behind it next.

ACOG's Fools Exposure Paradox

The fool's exposure paradox is this paradoxical situation, where wise or experienced individuals cover up a mistake to maintain their reputation, control, or perceived authority. However, when an outsider (the fool) unknowingly escalates the mistake, the wise people find themselves trapped. Correcting the fool would risk exposing their own earlier missteps. Thus, they are forced to watch as the mistake grows, unable to intervene without revealing the truth.

When a group of newbie obstetricians secured NICHD funding to conduct the arrive clinical trial, they appeared to proceed without fully integrating established insights from the ACOG. This emerging cohort, often trained with the notion that labor induction was "safe and natural", obviously overlooked or dismissed potential traumatic brain damage outcomes associated with induction and without any regard to the traumatic brain damage outcome warning by the Pitocin label. Meanwhile, ACOG remained unresponsive, possibly because the trial aligned, either by design or chance, with a strategic shift away from its historical association with the dangers laid out in the Pitocin labelling. Whether this was a planned alignment or an unexpected opportunity, ACOG seemed willing to adapt and leverage the situation. They decided to bury the years of legal liability that was building up against their flock, who were anyway not all abiding by their directives. They dropped the "failure to progress" diagnosis recommendations and decided to cede leadership of labor induction to their new found fall guys at the Society for Maternal Fetal Medicine, the SMFM in 2018.

The Sinister Coverup

In the last couple of decades, a new drug has come into being as the primary drug used for induction of labor. Misoprostol was originally approved for preventing NSAID induced ulcers in 1988. However, in 2000 its use in combination with mifepristone (a progesterone blocker) for medical abortion was approved by the FDA. Misoprostol also causes uterine contractions similar to Pitocin and causes the abortion by expelling the fetus with its uterine contraction effects. Misoprostol is also reputed to aid in cervical dilation. Although not proven or approved for its cervical dilation abilities, this additional capability if true, makes it an even superior drug to Pitocin for labor induction. Thus, beginning in the year 2000 misoprostol (Cytotec) has started replacing Pitocin as the main labor induction drug. But there is a major issue with this new off-label role of misoprostol.

Misoprostol is not approved for use in live births, it is only approved for abortions. As a result, it's label doesn't carry the warnings, precautions, contraindications and safeguards included for protection of a live baby as with the Pitocin label.

In short, use of misoprostol off-label for live birth labor induction might be outright illegal. Misoprostol is a cheaper drug than Pitocin, which might be one reason for its popularity in hospitals, and it is used alongside Pitocin for both cervical dilation and to stimulate contractions in labor induction. This is because misoprostol lasts longer in the body than Pitocin which has a shorter half life and only lasts in the body for about 6 minutes and thus allows for better control of contractions than just misoprostol. Unlike Pitocin, misoprostol is administered through tablets via oral, vaginal or sublingual routes and in small doses due to this lack of ability to control contractions very closely.

Remember the warnings on the Pitocin label is about traumatic brain injury.

The key Pitocin warning is about the count of the contractions safely allowed, before the traumatic injury caused by these contractions, becomes irreversible... Thus, any medication that is used for controlling contractions in a live birth should be subjected to the same guidelines as Pitocin.

The fact that misoprostol marketed as Cytotec is used for labor induction but doesn't carry the warnings necessary in a live birth, means that newbie OB-GYN's reading the warning labels are going to assume it cannot cause any brain damage. To them it would be ok to pursue labor induction indefinitely, without regard to the contraction count or the time taken, eventually hammering the baby out vaginally in the absence of fetal distress. They will continue to cause autism at unprecedented levels either blissfully unaware of the issue or continue with total impunity, knowing that they could always get away blaming it on genetics.

My second boy was induced for 18 hours using Cytotec and he is the one with the traumatic brain damage showing up on his MRI scan. The problem is with traumatic brain damage from excessive contractions; it does not matter which drug is used to induce those contractions. As mentioned in the previous paragraph in a strategic shift following years of trying to rein in their flock secretly and failing, the ACOG have now given in to the flawed findings of the arrive trial blaming it on the SMFM's embrace of it. I am not sure if all hospitals have given up on the failure to progress diagnosis, but quite a few of the younger obstetricians I have talked to, seem to believe the new recommendations allow for inducing all the way until vaginal delivery is achieved and the failure to progress diagnosis point doesn't matter anymore. Thus, the sinister cover up of one of the most rampant malpractices has come full circle with all that is left of it is the Pitocin label and the contraindication condition on it. But the Duke paper also discovered some other conditions of brain damage that become more frequent occurrences with labor induction, like placental abruption and meconium staining which are responsible for hypoxic brain damage and other complications as seen in the figure 8.4 which lists the various ways abusive induction damages the fetal brain.

Mechanisms of Brain Injury in Abusive Labor Induction

Hypoxic Brain Damage:

Tachysystole from high frequency contractions

Placental abruption caused by high force contractions

Meconium aspiration from the stress of contractions.

Unaddressed fetal distress during induction.

Traumatic Brain Damage:

Axonal shearing from numerous contractions beyond allowed 72-contraction contraindication limit.

Fig 8.4 – Brain damage pathways of Abusive Labor Induction

Pitocin Abuse: Pathways to Brain Damage

Abuse of contractions by Pitocin augmentation carries a whole variety of risks falling under both hypoxic and traumatic injury realms.

Tachysystole: This is a condition from contractions that are too frequent allowing little or no time between consecutive contractions. With every contraction, the placenta gets squished between the baby and the uterine wall, particularly in contractions of active labor after the amniotic fluid has been lost. The blood in the placenta also gets squished out in this process. The placenta needs time to recover between contractions so it can be refilled with a fresh blood supply. If the next contraction comes before the placenta and baby have recovered from the previous one, then the baby can become oxygen deprived resulting in brain hypoxia. This could lead to hypoxic fetal distress and needs to be avoided.

Placental Abruption: This is a serious pregnancy and delivery complication where the placenta detaches from the uterus before delivery, which can lead to heavy bleeding and deprive the baby of oxygen and nutrients. While rare, during pregnancy, it is known to occur most commonly in the third trimester and can cause significant risks for both the mother and baby. But contractions from Pitocin abuse are known to increase incidence of this during the delivery process. When it happens, it is an obstetric emergency and there is a need for hospital staff to identify the signs and intervene immediately. Any time delay in identifying and performing immediate C-section in such cases can cause adverse outcomes from hemorrhage for the mother and hypoxic brain damage or even death of the baby.

Meconium Staining and Aspiration: Meconium aspiration syndrome (MAS) is a serious condition that arises when a baby passes meconium, their first stool, either in utero or during labor and subsequently inhales this mixture with amniotic fluid into their lungs. Risk factors for meconium passage before birth include post-term gestation and intrauterine growth restriction. However, when meconium passage occurs during labor, it often signals fetal distress, potentially stemming from prolonged labor and resulting in hypoxic or traumatic brain injury, which leads to increased intestinal motility and loss of anal sphincter control. While many astute obstetricians opt for a Cesarean section at this point, others unfortunately continue with induction, causing further harm. The presence of meconium in the lungs can trigger a cascade of problems, including partial or complete airway obstruction, chemical pneumonitis (inflammation due to meconium's irritant properties), surfactant dysfunction (impairing lung expansion), and persistent pulmonary hypertension of the newborn (PPHN), a dangerous failure of the normal circulatory transition after birth. The severity of MAS is variable, but it can cause significant breathing difficulties requiring respiratory support and, in severe instances, lead to long-term lung damage or even be life-threatening. Critically, the initial brain damage and the subsequent respiratory distress can compound, resulting in further hypoxic brain injury, contributing to neurodevelopmental disorder, which gets diagnosed as autism.

Unaddressed Fetal Distress: Fetal distress on a fetal heart rate (FHR) monitor is indicated by several concerning patterns. These include a persistently high (tachycardia) or low (bradycardia) baseline heart rate, and abnormal variability such as absent, minimal, marked, or a smooth sinusoidal pattern. Decelerations, which are drops in heart rate, are also significant; late decelerations often suggest placental insufficiency, variable decelerations typically point to cord compression, and prolonged decelerations are particularly concerning. The absence of accelerations, which are reassuring increases in heart rate, can also be a sign of potential issues. Interpreting these patterns requires expert evaluation in the context of the entire labor and maternal history to determine the need for timely interventions to ensure fetal well-being. There are many cases where fetal distress is missed by hospital staff and it results in NICU admissions and immediately visible life threatening or adverse neurological consequences. These are the only instances where if the parents are made aware of the obstetric mistakes, there is legal consequences and this is the only case where Pitocin abuse in spite of FHR readings indicating fetal distress results in court victories and compensation. The impacted kids typically fall into the autism spectrum if not quadriplegic and falling into the cerebral palsy category.

Traumatic Brain Damage: This is a situation which happens to the healthiest of fetuses, where excessive contractions are needed to dilate the mother's cervix as labor induction is undertaken at a point when the mother's cervix is not ready to dilate. Under such circumstances every contraction can be stressful to the brain as it is being pounded in place being compressed by every contraction against a rigid cervix. Unfortunately, since the brain does not feel pain upon physical trauma to itself, this does not register as fetal distress except in the most extreme circumstances. Here, the only protection is the failure to progress diagnosis point limit on contractions as required by the Pitocin label and previously defined by the ACOG as 72 contractions. Any contraction beyond this is considered excessive and results in damage happening at the corpus callosum and other long-distance connections in the brain. This causes the disconnected brain which is a very common description of autism. Unfortunately, this damage gets hidden from basic MRI scans if there is longitudinal deformation of the head during the pushing phase in a vaginal delivery. This damage however is visible in the more powerful DTI MRI scans which can locate the areas of neuronal disconnects or fractional anisotropy which shows white matter alterations from this kind of damage.

An Urgent Call for Action

The ACOG stepping away from their "Failure to progress diagnosis point" during labor induction in the wake of the flawed Arrive trial, which did not take into account the long-term effects of prolonged induction, and the warnings on the Pitocin label, represents a crisis in maternity wards across the world. The newbie trial researchers have recommended continuous induction all the way to vaginal delivery, going completely against the warnings on the Pitocin label. The ACOG seem to have walked away from "failure to progress" contraction count to define the failure of labor inductions in an attempt to hide their mistakes from the past. In fact, they don't say anything at all, (and if they do, it's probably locked up behind their exclusive professionals only parts of their site). They seem to have shifted focus more to the importance of cervical dilation and cervical readiness for successful induction. But leaving a gap in their recommendations for failure of labor induction has meant that the only reason for failure of induction, is fetal distress, and nothing else, which goes completely against the contraindication #5 of the Pitocin label. The ACOG potentially felt emboldened by the fact that their flock have not seen any legal repercussions from not following their guidelines. But the truth is parent awareness has been kept under check with the online disinformation and tort reforms that have made lawyers unwilling to take on cases outside of established hypoxic injury cases. Thus, in cases where mothers are post-dated and labor induction is attempted and runs long, the child is mostly condemned to traumatic brain damage and autism. It's about time this is stopped.

Thus, the ACOG keeping the failure to progress diagnosis point in labor induction a relative secret, has resulted in a wide-ranging abuse of the obstetric control of the uterus afforded by Pitocin and prostaglandins. This is resulting in hidden traumatic brain injury at birth in cases where mothers are induced when the cervix is not ready, which is causing the autism epidemic.

Key Take Away: The failure of the ACOG to come out clean, publicly on mistakes of the past has meant that numerous new ob-gyns are not getting the message on the traumatic brain injury caused by Pitocin and similar uterine control drugs when abused past labeled contraindication limits. The fact that traumatic brain injury is not detected in the fetal monitors, has meant there is no external indication of damage. Add to that the molding of the head during the pushing stage of birth has meant normal MRI doesn't detect evidence of traumatic damage.

CHAPTER 9

The Genetic Basis – A Flawed Speculation

T he genetic origin theory of autism is based on studies of twin births by renowned child psychiatrist Dr. Michael Rutter(1933-2021) back in the 1970's. He is credited with transforming child psychiatry from a disjointed collection of theories and practices into a disciplined and compassionate field of study. His 1972 book, Maternal Deprivation Reassessed, countered prevailing views that inadequate mothering was the principal cause of psychiatric problems in children. The 1950's and 60's were the age of the "refrigerator mother" hypothesis, as one of Autism's first researchers Leo Kanner, a physician from Johns Hopkins, had gotten the cause and effect backwards and blamed the mother's behavior for the child's psychiatric problems. It was also times when mentally ill patients were institutionalized and subjected to what was seen as inhumane electric shocks called electroconvulsive therapy (ECT). Thus, Dr Rutter's work was a breath of fresh air and provided a more scientific alternative to the pseudo-science that ruled the field of psychiatry in those times. This exoneration from maternal fault, also effectively liberated the future generations of working mothers.

Rutter proposed investigating autism in twins to better understand the influence of genetic and environmental factors. To gather data, Susan Folstein, a trainee psychiatrist in the US at the time, visited 21 pairs of twins across the United Kingdom, where at least one twin had been diagnosed with autism. The study revealed an impressive level of concordance (82%) in the symptoms of autism and cognitive abilities among identical(monozygotic) twins, a finding that was not observed in non-identical(dizygotic) twins, at least not to the same extent (30%)

as the identical ones (Infantile autism: a genetic study of 21 twin pairs. S. Folstein and M. Rutter, J. Child Psychol. Psychiatry 18, 297–321; 1977).

His unexpected discovery made Rutter hopeful that he could identify the few genes he believed might be linked to autism. However, ever open to correction, he soon realized that the involvement of hundreds of genes was likely, and that the connections between genes, brain function, mind, and behavior were too complex to yield a single, clear explanation. But his supposed discovery of a genetic basis for autism, published in the 1977 paper mentioned above, transformed understanding and launched a new era of research. His 1977 paper has been cited 1000+ times, which points to the extent of influence this paper had on subsequent autism studies including diversion of a lot of autism research towards genetics. Taking a closer look at this paper reveals that Dr Rutter did consider the possibility of what he calls "biohazards" including kernicterus, perinatal apnea, neonatal convulsions, multiple congenital anomalies. Kernicterus is severe jaundice with high bilirubin count capable of causing brain damage if left untreated and perinatal apnea is where premature infants stop breathing for 20 seconds or more causing bradycardia (slow heart rate). Considering the high correlation of autism with these factors he even widened the scope of anomalies to include lower birth weight by 1 lb. between twins and pathologically smaller umbilical cord diameter and this covered 12 of 17 twins under consideration where one twin was autistic, where the autistic twin had suffered these "biohazards". Hence, he has a second conclusion on his paper that autism is associated with these "biohazards" and establishes the important role of these "environmental factors" in the causation of autism. I still wonder why this wasn't his primary finding and why he still went on to conclude genetic influence in autism causation only based on zygosity in spite of all his "biohazard" evidence suggesting the opposite.

In the forty-five plus years since the publication of Rutters paper, the field of genetics has seen a quantum leap in our understanding of the science and our abilities to uncover the secrets buried within the 3 billion base pairs of encodings in the DNA double helix. The human genome project (HGP) was a collaboration of government entities and research organizations from multiple countries that began in 1990. The first draft of the fully sequenced human genome was published in 2001. A further updated genome sequence was published at the end of the project in 2003. Thus, the initial sequencing took a good 11 years and enormous effort and collaboration and data sharing among multiple nations to complete. The HGP was a monumental scientific endeavor, significantly advancing our understanding of genetics and paving the way for future research in genomics and medicine.

Since then, the time taken to sequence an individual's genome has been significantly reduced. sequencing an individual's genome typically takes about 1 to 2 days using advanced technologies, particularly next-generation sequencing (NGS). As of 2024 there are multiple companies online offering whole genome sequencing as a service with reports that help doctors look at deviations from the norm to diagnose certain conditions.

The Autism Genome Project (AGP) was launched in 2005 by an autism organization called National Association for Autism Research (NAAR, later merged with Autism speaks), along with the National Institute of Health with the goal of identifying genetic factors associated with autism spectrum disorders (ASD). This large-scale collaborative research initiative involved other institutions with an interest in autism, like the Simons foundation (SFARI) and aimed to better understand the genetic underpinnings of autism by analyzing the genomes of individuals with ASD and their families. The key goals and objectives, included genetic mapping: to identify chromosomal regions linked to autism and pinpoint specific genes involved. They intended to explore the genetic diversity among individuals with autism. The project also considered how genetic factors might interact with environmental influences in the development of autism. The project utilized advanced genetic techniques, including, Genome-wide association studies (GWAS) to find genetic variants associated with autism. There was also linkage analysis to examine genetic markers in families with multiple cases of autism. Whole-exome and whole-genome sequencing were used to identify rare mutations. The AGP identified numerous "potential" genes and genetic variations associated with an increased risk of autism. Some notable genes identified to be linked to ASD include CHD8, SCN2A, and ASD-associated de novo mutations. However, none of these could be definitely identified to be causative factors in autism, so studies have been inconclusive. understanding how identified genetic variations contribute to autism symptoms is also an ongoing challenge

The AGP continues to influence ongoing research efforts, including initiatives focused on understanding the relationship between genetics and environmental factors in autism. But there are numerous other known genetic syndromes that cause neurodevelopmental deficits and unlike autism their incidence has remained constant through time.

Disorder /Syndrome	Genetic Cause	Occurrence Rate
Autism Spectrum Disorder (ASD)	Unknown with a few genes implicated by research.	1 in 31
Down Syndrome	Caused by an extra copy of chromosome 21 (trisomy 21), it results in intellectual disability and developmental delays.	1 in 700 to 1 in 1,000 live births
Neurofibromatosis Type 1 (NF1)	Caused by mutations in the NF1 gene, it can lead to cognitive impairments and learning disabilities along with characteristic skin changes.	1 in 3,000 live births.
Fragile X Syndrome	Caused by mutations in the FMR1 gene, it leads to intellectual disabilities, behavioral challenges, and developmental delays.	Males 1 in 4000, Females 1 in 8000
Tuberous Sclerosis Complex (TSC)	Caused by mutations in the TSC1 or TSC2 genes, it can lead to seizures, intellectual disability, and autism.	1 in 6,000 to 10,000 live births
Williams Syndrome	Caused by a deletion of genetic material from chromosome 7, it is associated with developmental delays, intellectual disability, and distinct facial features.	1 in 7,500 to 1 in 20,000 live births
Rett Syndrome	Primarily affects females and is caused by mutations in the MECP2 gene, leading to severe cognitive and physical impairments.	1 in 10,000 to 15,000 female births. 1 in 40,000 to 100,000. of male births
Angelman Syndrome	Caused by a deletion or mutation of the UBE3A gene, it leads to severe developmental delays, speech impairment, and movement disorders.	1 in 15,000 to 20,000 live births
Prader-Willi Syndrome	Caused by the loss of function of genes on chromosome 15, it leads to cognitive disabilities, behavioral issues, and obesity.	1 in 10,000 to 30,000 live births
Smith-Magenis Syndrome	Caused by a deletion of chromosome 17p11.2, it is associated with intellectual disability, behavioral problems, and distinctive physical features.	1 in 15,000 to 25,000 live births
Sotos Syndrome	Caused by mutations in the NSD1 gene, it leads to overgrowth, learning disabilities, and behavioral challenges.	1 in 10,000 to 14,000 live births
Cornelia de Lange Syndrome	Caused by mutations in several genes (including NIPBL), it leads to developmental delays, growth deficiencies, and characteristic facial features.	1 in 10,000 to 30,000 live births

It's very striking to see this data in such tabular format. The autism numbers are at a minimum 2 to 4 orders of magnitude higher or a hundred to ten thousand times more prevalent than any of the known and most prevalent genetic diseases known to cause neurodevelopment issues. To the trained geneticist and genetic theory enthusiasts this might mean there's at least hundreds of genetic disorders hidden out there waiting to be discovered. This was the response of Dr Rutter for example. To the rest of us, looking at this data, the answer is even more obvious. The real cause of autism must lie elsewhere, outside of genetics!

Wikipedia lists over 230 different genetic disorders discovered so far that could impair brain development. Some of them as rare as one in 10 million or more. While such rare cases can be traced back to genetics, autism is far more common, occurring with every 1 in 31 births. Researchers trying to find genetic roots for autism always come up empty-handed and point to the 'complexity' of the problem to explain their failure to find a genetic cause. And I can tell you they fail simply because they are looking for a genetic problem that doesn't exist. It's been these modern birth interventions causing hypoxic and traumatic brain injuries at an ever-increasing rate as the obstetrics community gets more and more complacent with their practices, as they continue to get away with their very avoidable and easily corrected malpractices with impunity.

Another point to note with this data is the fact that every one of these genetic syndromes comes with various other effects distinct and unrelated to the brain, such as distinct facial features, skin changes, physical growth deficiencies or excesses, distinctive physical features and so on. These traits are not found in autism, another pointer to the fact that these are genetically normal kids suffering brain damage at birth from modern obstetric practices. Hypoxic injury is even accepted in courts as the cause of neurodevelopment delays but none of the genetic research seems to even take into account the birth conditions of the participants leading to flawed research results finding genetic inconsistencies that do not amount to anything and certainly not causative to autism.

Twins are a Divergence from the Norm Already

Dr Rutter revisited his twins research in 1995 again confirming his earlier findings in twins this time with an even larger data set. He still found that identical twins with autism meant both twins had autism, while that was not the case with most non-identical dizygotic twins. Thus, he confirmed his earlier findings from about 20years prior that autism was all in the genes. However, similar to the first study he failed to look into the chorionicity i.e. possibility of a shared placenta in identical twins being a factor.

Twins represent a fascinating divergence from the typical pattern of human reproduction. According to data from the CDC's National Center for Health Statistics, the twin birth rate in the United States reached 31.2 per 1,000 live births in 2022. This statistic translates to approximately 3% of all births, which is significant considering that it reflects about 1.5% of total pregnancies. The occurrence of twin pregnancies is influenced by a variety of factors, which have been the subject of extensive research. These factors include maternal age, genetic predisposition, and the use of fertility treatments, all of which contribute to the likelihood of conceiving twins. Understanding these influences can provide deeper insights into the complexities of human reproduction and the increasing prevalence of multiple births in contemporary society.

The factors that cause twin pregnancies have been previously investigated. A research study in 1997 by the imperial cancer research institute and oxford university indicated that mothers of twins typically had a 49% higher concentration of Follicle stimulating hormone and certain binding globulins during their menstrual cycles, while during pregnancy, the mothers carrying twins had 58% higher geometric mean estradiol (a form of estrogen) concentration ($p = 0.02$) and a 50% higher testosterone concentration ($p = 0.03$) than women carrying singletons. The increased concentration of follicle stimulating hormone during the menstrual cycle of mothers of twins, which was also reported in two other previous studies, lead the researchers to conclude follicle stimulating hormone level may be an important determinant of dizygotic twinning.

A sizeable percentage of twinning is also known to come from the use of fertility treatments. Clomiphene citrate commonly known as Clomid is a drug that stimulates ovulation in women and was approved as a fertility treatment by the FDA in 1967. Clomid and similar drugs have been implicated by multiple studies as causing autism in kids, with the autism occurrence risk directly depending on how long the mother was exposed to the drug. These drugs are also known to increase the twinning rate. Thus, use of fertility drugs seems to have a direct correlation to both twinning and autism.

The Inherent Complexity of Twin Pregnancies

Twin pregnancies add an extra layer of complexity to an already intricate process. Twins can arise in various ways, each with distinct configurations of placenta, chorion, amnion, and amniotic sac, depending on how conception and splitting occurs. The amnion and chorion are two membranes that begin separately in the first trimester. The amnion is the inner fluid-filled sac surrounding the embryo, while the chorion is the outer membrane enclosing the amnion, placenta and two early artifacts, yolk sac and allantois. In singleton pregnancies, the amnion and chorionic membranes fuse after the first trimester, becoming indistinguishable as the amniotic sac. However, in twin pregnancies, the chorion and amnion may remain distinct in certain cases.

Dizygotic, or fraternal, twins - the most common kind of twins, develop from two separate eggs which are fertilized by two different sperm. Each twin has its own placenta and amniotic sac. The twins can be two girls, two boys, or a boy and a girl. In contrast, monozygotic or identical twins form when a single egg splits a few days after conception. Identical twins might share a placenta and an amniotic sac or the twins might share a placenta and each have separate amniotic sacs. Genetically, the two babies are identical. They'll be the same sex and share physical traits and characteristics.

Depending on the status of the placenta and amniotic sac the different types of identical twins are:

▸ **Monochorionic Twins (70%)** - Identical twins with a single shared placenta are known as monochorionic twins. This occurs in around 70 percent of identical twin pregnancies.

- **Monochorionic-Monoamniotic (MoMo) Twins (1-2%)** - They are twins who share the same placenta as well as the amniotic sac.
- **Monochorionic-Diamniotic (MoDi) Twins (70-75%)** — Identical twins that do not share an amniotic sac but do share a placenta are known as monochorionic-diamniotic twins.

▶ **Dichorionic Twins (DiDi) (25-30%)** - They have separate placentas and amniotic sacs. This occurs in approximately thirty percent of identical twin pregnancies.

All fraternal twins are also Dichorionic twins. Monochorionic twins, given the shared placenta are inherently high-risk pregnancies, at higher risk for in-utero hypoxia among others. Of this the MoMo twins that share both the placenta and amniotic sac are the highest risk for complications such as cord entanglement and cord compression, which are linked to hypoxic brain injury and autism. Thankfully they represent only 1% of all twins, but even the identical twins with shared placenta (70%) puts them at a higher risk for autism from the factors listed in the subsequent paragraph. Among all twins, the dichorionic twins, the ones with their own placenta and amniotic sac in which are 30% of monozygotic and 100% of dizygotic (fraternal) twins are the ones at lowest risk for the complications of twin pregnancy. Chorionicity and amnionicity are crucial factors in pregnancy risk assessment in a multiple pregnancy. Thus, in the realm of twins the subtype of twins plays an important role in the risk for autism with 70% of identical twins at higher risk due to the shared placenta. This differentiation was lost in the work of Dr Rutter, as it only considered zygosity and none of the other true risk factors in twins. The incidence of shared placenta in 70% of identical twins puts them at higher risk for autism, vs the 0% sharing of placenta and amnion for non identical twins, lowers their autism risk significantly.

Combinations of Chorion and Amnion in Twin Pregnancy

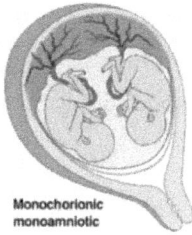

Monochorionic
monoamniotic

Monochorionic Monoamniotic (Mo/Mo) Twins

- Twins share a placenta/chorion and amnion.
- Extremely high risk pregnancy
- 1-2% of all identical(monozygotic) twins.

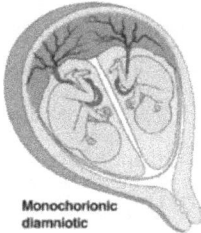

Monochorionic
diamniotic

Monochorionic Diamniotic (Mo/Di) Twins

- Twins share a placenta/chorion and have own amnion.
- High risk pregnancy
- 70-75% of all identical(monozygotic) twins.

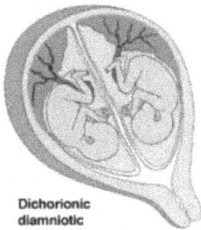

Dichorionic
diamniotic

Dichorionic Diamniotic (Di/Di) Twins

- Twins have their own placenta and amnion.
- Lowest risk of all twin pregnancies
- 25-30% of all identical(monozygotic) twins
- 100% of non-identical(dizygotic) twins

Fig. 9.2 – High risk pregnancy of Mo/Mo and Mo/Di Twins. Figures adapted from https://icombo.org/chorionicity/. Twin chorionicity occurrence rates from Judith Hall (Lancet 2003 - Volume 362, Issue 9385 Pages 673-752)

The major risk factors for autism in twins in general, is from brain hypoxia arising from hypoxic ischemia in-utero, the causes of which include

1. In utero hypoxic ischemia from shared placenta, unable to support both babies fully well.
2. Maternal insufficiency to keep 2 babies oxygenated and supplied in late pregnancy.
3. Twins are mostly delivered premature with undeveloped lungs and are at risk for postpartum hypoxia.

4. Twin pregnancy from use of fertility drugs known to be an autism risk factor.

5. Occurrence of twin pregnancy is itself due to maternal hormone imbalances, namely higher follicle stimulating hormone levels.

6. Twin to twin transfusion syndrome - imbalance of blood supply between the 2 twins.

Thus, by not taking into account the high-risk pregnancy with increased risk of hypoxic injury from the unique condition of a predominantly shared placenta associated with identical twins, Dr Rutters research has erroneously implicated genetics as the sole cause of Autism. His research took into consideration only zygosity of twins with no consideration of chorionicity and amniocity of twins and the associated higher risk of autism in twins from these factors through increased risk in utero hypoxia or hypoxic ischemia, both perinatally and after premature delivery. His plausible but flawed research has had most of the research community and autism community misled into believing genetics as the cause of autism while the real cause has been perinatal brain damage from hypoxia, trauma or both.

Of course, I am not the first person to point out that Dr Rutters theory is flawed. Papers have been published in the past implicating the twinning process itself as the source of autism in twins. Two studies (Greenberg et al. 2001 [9.1]; Betancur et al. 2002 [9.2]) suggested that the twinning process itself is an important risk factor in the development of autism. Even the original co-author of Dr Rutter, Susan Folstein authored a paper in 2001[9.3] that showed a 70% concordance of autism in monozygotic twins and 0% concordance in dizygotic twins, which is the exact number that can be expected based on the occurrence rate of shared placenta in monozygotic vs dizygotic twins. However, every time a paper questions the genetic basis theory of autism, other studies appear out of the woodworks defending the theory with flawed and mostly absurd arguments of their own. The interesting point to note is, these counter studies are sponsored by integrated care management consortiums of hospital systems and insurance companies. These parties have a vested interest in keeping the source of autism from being traced back to the hypoxic or traumatic birth injury causes, for fear of legal ramifications. The defense of the genetic basis theory is taking the same lines as the deceptive defense of the sanctity of labor induction in spite of the warnings in the drug label saying the opposite.

Twin Autism Rates are not Rising but Overall Rates Are!

Finally, the study of autism in twins might actually end up providing counter-productive evidence that results in disproving the genetic basis theory of autism that it supposedly provides solid evidence for. A study of the Swedish twin births revealed that the autism rate in twins of 1 in 44 has remained fairly constant over the years. What does that tell us. Are twins not being affected by whatever is impacting the rest of the population. So, what is that?

The answer is actually pretty straight forward, twins are mostly born prematurely and they are never subjected to labor induction. Twins are not good candidates for labor induction even in the hypothetical case of being postdated twins, as they are considered a high-risk pregnancy. The only mothers subjected to labor induction are healthy mothers with healthy low risk singleton pregnancies and they are the ones that pay the ultimate price in terms of brain damage in their kids when they are induced when their cervix is not ready. This also clarifies why the autism rate is increasing only in the rest of the population and the 1 in 31 autism rate in US children as of 2022 data, even surpasses the traditional twin autism rates. Originally it started out that twin autism rates were an order of magnitude higher than the rest of the population. Thus, the constant autism rate among twins vs the increasing autism rates in the rest of the population is a clear indication that obstetric control of the uterus in the non-twin healthy mother population and the resulting abuse have turned the tables on the autism rates in twins vs the rest of the population on such a vast scale.

Birth Hypoxia as the Historical Cause of Autism

In modern times just before the meteoric increase in autism numbers started in 1980 the primary cause of mental retardation (now intellectual disability in DSM 5) was known to be birth hypoxia. The categorizations of mental retardation vs autism were still unclear and subject to individual physicians' interpretation. Hospital births while popular were still not the only game in town. Midwifery and home births were still a possibility, with people only rushing to hospitals to seek medical attention in case of complications i.e. childbirth was not a fully medical event yet. The one major intervention hospitals could offer was the C-section delivery alongside better post-delivery maternal and neonatal care. A lot of the modern gadgetry, portable ultrasound, fetal monitoring, scopes and probes of today, were not yet available to obstetricians. Labor induction was not approved until 1980 and the practice of Obstetrics was still in its infancy compared to what it is now.

All this meant one thing, the avenues for hypoxic brain injuries were abundant in the times before 1980. The brain is the first organ to get damaged when oxygen supply is cut out. Hypoxic brain damage happens very quickly. For an adult human between 30-180 seconds of oxygen deprivation, causes loss of consciousness. At the one-minute mark, brain cells begin dying. At three minutes, neurons suffer more extensive damage, and lasting brain damage becomes more likely. At five minutes, death becomes imminent. While babies might do slightly better, hypoxic injury at birth is widely accepted as a cause of neurodevelopmental delays and disorders including everything that falls into the current autism spectrum definition. This acceptance is universal including in courts of law and causing hypoxic injury has been the only basis for obstetricians being sued in current times.

But with the introduction of labor induction in 1980 the additional traumatic brain injury component has been added to the mix although it has potentially not been litigated or litigated correctly in court in the past.

In Summary, Autism incidence can be traced to 2 main pregnancy/birth causes.

- Hypoxic brain injury in utero, at birth or first weeks after birth.
- Traumatic brain injury from Pitocin abuse.

In fact, more than 90% of cases labelled as 'Autism', 'ADD', 'ADHD', 'Learning disabled,' etc., can really be traced back to brain damage at birth.

Hypoxic brain injury can be caused by a whole slew of conditions that modern medicine is fully aware of, including but not limited to the following conditions.

1. Premature delivery where the lungs are not fully developed.

2. Meconium aspiration causing undetected respiratory distress in the first 2-3 weeks after birth,

3. C-section after fetal distress during labor.

4. Scheduled C-section with undetected respiratory distress after birth.

5. Sickness/fever in the first few days after birth causing undetected respiratory distress.

6. Umbilical cord tight around the neck (nuchal cord) during delivery.

7. Kinked cord or cord compression during delivery.

8. Placental abruption (characterized by bleeding during pregnancy or delivery).

9. Hypoxia in-utero from a variety of factors including severe long-term maternal diseases (including heart, lung and kidney diseases), pregnancy with anemia, hemoglobinopathy, placental insufficiency, maternal infection, umbilical cord compression, alcohol consumption, maternal smoking, preeclampsia, and administration of glucocorticoids [8.1] (to help lung development) to name a few.

The second main cause, i.e. Traumatic Brain Injury is known to many within the obstetric and pediatric circles although not widely publicized within the general population, including researchers, due to the fact that it mainly started happening with abusive labor induction in 1980, any prior research would only have looked at cases of hypoxic injury causing autism, except a few cases of possible traumatic damage by forceps, skull fracture from craniosynostosis etc.

The Convenience of Blaming Genetics

Turns out genetics is the most convenient and easiest scapegoat of all possible reasons autism causation can be blamed on. There are no counter parties that would be upset, no financial interests impacted. It's the ideal place to cast blame for anything without an easily established cause. The advantages are simply overwhelming.

1. Too complex for common people to understand.

2. Blames the parents and their genes for their kids' condition.

3. Causes social stigma for the kids' family.

4. Pushes people into a shell such that they don't ask questions.
5. Creates the "it happens to other people" attitude among the public.
6. Easy to say we don't know, as genetic science is still evolving.
7. Provides for better control of the narrative on social media.

In short, the best way to keep birth injury unknown to parents is to blame something that goes back to conception itself and pointing to genetics fits the bill quite nicely. However, genetic diseases are historically known and proven to be the result of inbreeding. Most cultures are aware of the dangers of marriage among first cousins for example and explicitly forbid such unions In the US, 25 of the 50 states forbid marriages among first cousins. These genetic symptoms and diseases have also typically been described since historical times, while autism is a relatively new phenomenon, conflicting with it having a genetic cause. Modern genetics also confirms, that autosomal recessive inheritance caused by inbreeding as the cause of multiple genetic diseases

In the United States there exist communities of Amish people totaling about 250,000 who live their lives in the countryside in a very traditional way, away from the thrills and frills of modern living. In their rural communities, they grow their own foods and livestock, avoiding fertilizers, pesticides and other modern agriculture techniques. The Amish do not go to hospitals to have their babies and they don't vaccinate, and in these communities the incidence of autism is close to zero (as no scientific studies exist these estimates are based on people receiving services). Additionally, being a small closed community that descended from families of Swiss immigrants, they are susceptible to inbreeding and consequently have higher incidence of genetic diseases that are mostly unheard of in the general population – and there are many Amish receiving services for these genetic diseases. This is another glaring example of how we can draw a common-sense conclusion that genetics has nothing to do with autism as much as hospital birth interventions and injuries and possibly vaccinations might have.

The human genome contains approximately 20,000 genes, with this estimate down from the original 30,000-60,000 genes estimated in the 1980's and 90's. Less than about 10% (around 1,500 genes) are implicated in neurodevelopment with a far fewer number about 22 estimated to influence neuron growth, causing brain structural malformations and intellectual disorder. Considering that the prevalence of known genetic diseases is roughly 1 in 10,000, and many of these have been identified, it seems unlikely that rare genetic variations within these neurodevelopmental genes alone could account for the rising prevalence of ASD, which currently affects approximately 1 in 31 children as of the 2022 count by the CDC.

This concept of de-novo mutations and copy number variations (CNV's) that geneticists have come to blame autism on, have not proven that they have anything to do with significant neurological development impacts and probably never will. The presence of CNVs in one's genome is not necessarily indicative of a 'breakdown' of the genetic makeup. Many genetic variations are neutral or even beneficial. These copy number variations have probably existed for millions of years and odds are it is all part of the overall genetic evolution process. Genetic evolution happens slowly over multiple generations while autism, happens to normal parents and there is simply no genetic process that could explain it.

The canary in the coalmine when it comes to autism and genetic causation is the fact that the current ASD incidence of 1 in 31 in normal births even exceeds the 1 in 44 autism rate for twins with the twin rate remaining static through history. This development clearly points to autism causation by hospital interventions that are not targeted at high-risk twin pregnancies but only at low-risk singleton pregnancies like in induction of labor.

Pivoting Genetic Research to Look at Recovery Treatments

Genetic sciences and gene technologies have come a long way after the human genome project. Genetics research continues to attract top talent in colleges and people involved in research are some of the very best we have. They choose to be in sciences to try and solve the toughest problems for mankind. When it comes to Autism genetic researchers would serve themselves and the autism community better if they pivot their research to look at the kind of genetic changes if any, hypoxia and trauma bring about in the immune privileged areas of the brain, the effects live vaccine viruses have on the neurons of the brain if they get past the blood brain barrier, the causes of neuro inflammation that is so typical in autism and many other mental health conditions. Knowledge of these conditions help device better treatments for those impacted by autism.

Current autism research in genetics has now been reduced to causing mutations in the suspected genes responsible for neuro development in mice and confirming that the mice end up with neurodevelopmental issues. While this can be useful to identify the genes involved in neurodevelopment, there has not been any confirmation of these mutations occurring in individuals with autism in any of the genetic studies. Such studies have only been useful to the 'autism is genetic' crowd simply because they make for headlines that carry the words 'Autism' and 'Genetic' in the same sentence. Further, for DNA damage to be passed on to a subsequent generation, damage needs to occur in the haploid gamete cells (eggs and sperm) which is unlikely to happen in these fortified, immune privileged organs; the testicles and ovaries. Even if this had this been the case, it would have been detected very easily, instead of years of research turning up nothing.

Gene technologies are advanced enough, they can identify genetic disease conditions with the rarest of rare rates of occurrence but have come up empty handed when it comes to autism, so much that most genetic researchers have given up trying to explain autism as a genetic condition.

The only people screaming "autism is genetic" on top of their lungs are internet trolls working on behalf of special interests wanting the truth about the birth injury causes of autism to stay under wraps. There is a powerful segment of the medical intellect who want this to remain hidden backed by malpractice insurance, hospital conglomerates and other powerful special interests trying to protect their own economic interests from what they see as menacing lawsuits that could prove to be an existential threat. Years of enormously restrictive tort reform in most states have meant victims of medical wrongdoing stand no chance of even being heard, leave alone seek justice. The lack of this crucial feedback loop has meant obstetric interventions responsible for the autism epidemic continue unchecked to this day.

Key Take Away:

To summarize we've looked into the flaws of Dr Rutters approach which is regarded as the gold standard study that provided proof of autism being genetic.

▶ Twinning inherently comes with high autism risk from hypoxic brain damage.

▶ The rate of autism in twins has remained constant through time, while the rest of the population is seeing an increase.

▶ Concordance of autism in twins is correlated to hypoxic risks and effects of a shared placenta in a certain subtype of twins and not to genes.

Genetic research has come up empty handed, although it solved numerous rare genetic disorders simply because the cause of autism lies outside of genetics.

CHAPTER 10

The Autism Epidemic - Beyond the Blame Game to the True Cause

T his book is based on the observed fact that in more than 90% of cases labelled as 'autism', 'ADD', 'ADHD', 'learning disabled,' etc., is really infant brain damage at birth. Autism really comes down to 2 main causes.

1. Hypoxic brain injury in utero, at birth or first weeks after birth.
2. Traumatic brain injury from labor abuse by excessive contractions.

As mentioned in the previous chapter hypoxia in-utero can be caused by a variety of factors including severe long-term maternal diseases (including heart, lung and kidney diseases), pregnancy with anemia, hemoglobinopathy, placental insufficiency, maternal infection, umbilical cord compression, nuchal cords, knotted cords, alcohol consumption, maternal smoking, preeclampsia, and administration of glucocorticoids to help with lung development among some others.

A lot of these risks have existed throughout human history and have contributed to a small fraction of the total autism numbers. In current times with expecting mothers taking pre-natal vitamins and other pregnancy precautions, some of these risks have been significantly reduced while not completely ruled out. In such cases where development is impacted right during pregnancy there tends to be a few other impacts outside of brain abilities. There are usually visible features. Case in point - Fetal Alcohol Syndrome or FASD, which is one of the more studied impacts. It causes visible features like small eyes, thin upper lip, smooth philtrum and it could include growth deficits, low height, low weight, microcephaly, and numerous other visible symptoms inconsistently. I believe intrauterine hypoxia from any of the many causes previously listed could be responsible for visible features like hypodontia, microcephaly etc. found in a tiny fraction of children diagnosed with autism. The point to notice here is everything involving changes in the intrauterine growth environment causes changes in multiple parts of the body, not just the brain. The same is true of all genetic abnormalities. The symptoms of genetic abnormalities are more far reaching than just the brain damage effects of autism. Genetic abnormalities involving neurodevelopment also manifest themselves as groups of structural abnormalities visible in brain MRI scans.

Given this background, let us look at some of these arguments and reasons being cited as a potential cause for autism. Many of them are valid possibilities. But could they be happening at the scale of being responsible for the autism epidemic.

Medications During Pregnancy

The Thalidomide scandal of the 1950's and 60's exemplified everything that could go wrong during pregnancy with the use of an untested novel new drug in pregnant mothers. Thalidomide, a drug originally introduced as a tranquilizer was later approved and prescribed for anxiety, trouble sleeping, tension, and morning sickness during pregnancy. Prescribed to pregnant women in over 46 countries for morning sickness, thalidomide caused severe birth defects, most notably phocomelia (abnormally short limbs), in thousands of children and led to numerous miscarriages. Originally introduced in the mid 1950's in West Germany, in this instance again it took a while before the connection to thalidomide was established. Some researchers argued that the increasing cases of dysmelia were caused by nuclear testing, others tried to promote other teratological theories implicating improper nutrition and maternal behavior. Finally, by the time the drug was banned in 1962 in West Germany, about 2500 German babies had been born with birth defects, impacted by thalidomide. The US apparently circumvented this disaster thanks to denial of approval by the FDA citing insufficient testing, but many other countries which had approved the drug, suffered the consequences of congenital birth defects in their children impacted by thalidomide.

This event is considered one of the most significant medical disasters of the 20th century, highlighting the critical importance of rigorous drug safety testing and monitoring during pregnancy. This prompted adoption of more rigorous standards for the approval of drugs for use in pregnant mothers and safe drugs lists were established that were acceptable for use in pregnancy. Even in current times there are mass torts in progress against established drugs like Tylenol (named acetaminophen in US, called paracetamol elsewhere) for allegedly causing Autism, ADD and ADHD symptoms after being taken continuously for 28 days or more in early pregnancy. While not proven in court, it goes to show why drugs in pregnancy need to be avoided and even the safe ones, be used only when necessary, where the benefits of using it outweigh risks of avoiding it pretty significantly.

Environmental Toxins

There are numerous chemicals in our environment that are toxic with the potential to cause brain damage. The predominant ones are heavy metals including mercury, lead, arsenic, cadmium, chromium and the whole host of other chemical derivatives found in pesticides, building material, furniture, plastics, and so on. While their effects are true and they are undeniably dangerous, they have become the default scapegoats for everything that ails our modern society. They are now being implicated in numerous health issues including autism.

These chemical toxins can affect various parts of the body. They can be allergen, carcinogenic, cardiotoxic, genotoxin, hepatotoxic, nephrotoxic, neurotoxin, sensitizer, or teratogenic. From the autism standpoint we need to consider the effects of neurotoxins, which affect the brain and nervous system, and teratogenic agents, which cause birth defects.

With respect to teratogenic agents, birth defects tend to be severe, causing effects in many parts of the body, and typically more devastating than just cerebral shortcomings such as seen in autism. More broadly, the reason why damage from chemicals tends to be severe is because the human body is capable of repairing minor DNA damage; consequently, damage from the chemical needs to be really severe for birth defects to occur. It's important to note that the human body can tolerate trace amounts of various toxins pretty well and in many cases excrete them effectively. Any other exposure like the trace amounts someone may get from casual contact with furniture or building materials have to be accumulated without being excreted over long periods of time – possibly decades – for any negative impacts to show up. Even then the effects would show up later in the lives of individuals rather than the first few years. These also mostly end up causing cancers than neurologic defects.

People are right to be concerned about chemicals in the environment; but there are some telltale signs that are missing, in case chemicals are the cause of autism. For example, impact of environmental chemicals tend to show up first in smaller living animals with a shorter life span before its impact shows up in humans. No such major impact to the entire ecosystem across multiple species is being seen due to any of the chemicals currently being studied as possible cause of autism. Chemical contamination of the water supply, food sources or air also happens in clusters and the symptoms are universal and more obvious than just 1 or 2 in a 100 being affected by it. And if autism was caused by chemicals, accumulated over long periods of time and passed on by way of de-novo mutations, the kids of people growing up in less industrialized countries with very little incidence of autism like me would not be impacted in the subsequent generation. But I know numerous people who immigrated from practically every nation under the sun that have been affected because their kids were born in the United States. Autism is apparently neutral to parents' nationality.

Perhaps most damning to the chemical causation thesis is just how widespread autism is. Newborn children are diagnosed within the first 2 to 3 years of their life with an affliction that only seems to impact their brain functioning. No impacts are found anywhere else in the body. But chemical effects (if congenital) would be more severe than involving just the brain. And when it comes to autism, the environment being talked about is really the uterine environment. If it was chemicals other organ systems like the liver and kidney that are involved in the process of keeping the body free of chemicals would be the first ones impacted. However, no such effects are seen in kids with Autism, ADD and other attention deficiency and hyperactivity disorders. It's time to reject the chemical explanation of autism as not fitting the facts.

Ultrasound Scans in Pregnancy

While not given very serious attention, another purported culprit in autism causation is ultrasound scans. Some recent discoveries have led to casting doubt on the safety of ultrasound scans during pregnancy as a possible factor in fetal brain damage and autism. Ultrasound monitors for medical imaging were invented in the 1960s and have been used in fetal ultrasound scanning in the US since the mid-1970s. They work by the principle of the echo reflection of ultrasonic sound waves by objects. The ultrasound probe transmits sound pulses which then travel into the tissues of the body. Some of the pulse is reflected at tissue boundaries while some of it passes through, only to have other tissue boundaries reflect it. By accurately measuring the reflections and the time it takes to be reflected (to the millionths of a second), the ultrasound machine creates a depth and density image of tissues and organs in the body on the screen. Millions of pulses and echoes are sent and received each second.

It's important to note that ultrasound waves are not electromagnetic radiation and do not cause any ionizing effects on tissues at an atomic/molecular level. There are two ways the acoustic pulses might perturb the target tissue. They can bring about a temperature increase in the target area or can cause mechanical movement of the tissue in a phenomenon called acoustic cavitation (defined as the growth and collapse of pre-existing microbubbles in liquids under the influence of an ultrasonic field). Safety limits have been established in terms of a Temperature Index (TI) and a Mechanical Index (MI). Commercial ultrasound scanners are required to display these safety indexes on the screen at all times so the operators can stay under prescribed limits. And in fact, the guidance given operators is to use the lowest possible probe output for the shortest possible time compatible with obtaining diagnostic information.

Experiments in pregnant mice have shown that ultrasound directed at the mice fetus during typical neuron migration times in development for prolonged durations results in irregular distribution of neurons in the brain after birth.

However, the mice in these experiments were subjected to hours of ultrasound and such irregular brain development is easily identified in scans. Needless to say, human fetuses are not subjected to these levels of ultrasound, nor is this kind of irregular brain development characteristic of autism. We can reasonably conclude autism is not caused by the limited exposure to ultrasound that is the norm in human births.

Mysterious Bacterial or Viral Infections

Autism sometimes gets blamed on bacteria and viruses. There could be some truth to this, but it's not the obvious. We know autism is not some communicable disease. However, maternal infections during critical stages of pregnancy are known to impact the development of the child. Viruses like Zika have made headlines for causing mental retardation in unborn babies, so viruses could certainly impact brain development during pregnancy. But the point to note is viruses like Zika that impact the brain typically influence the growth of the fetal brain, resulting in a condition called microcephaly where there is a noticeable reduction in the size of the head due to reduced or stopped brain growth in-utero. Viral impacts to the brain are easily identified in an MRI scan as continuous lesions in the brain – again something not seen in the MRI scans of children with autism.

Historically we have seen many diseases that impact the brain like polio, smallpox, rubella, and scarlet fever. These have left numerous children paralyzed, deaf, blind, etc. Many of these diseases have been eradicated by vaccinations and so it's highly unlikely that some undetected disease lurks out there secretly causing autism. And as seen in most of these cases, the manifestation of these diseases is much more severe than the predominantly brain damage related speech and social development impacts of autism.

But that said maternal infections during pregnancy, particularly pelvic floor infections which could result in inflammation of the chorion can impact the development of the baby, cause intra uterine growth restriction etc. These are known to cause cerebral palsy and autism in some cases. But these are cases where abnormal MRI scans can readily point to the potential cause of the condition.

C-section

When it comes to the autism blame game, lifesaving C-sections have also become the target of blame as the source of autism. When a child is C-sectioned out because of fetal distress, then there is always the chance that the child had already suffered brain damage before being saved by the C-section. But then, there are instances where the mom went in for a planned C-section and the child was diagnosed with autism years later. How do we explain something like that. Here again there are multiple explanations, and the fairly naïve explanation is that the lack of vaginal delivery means the child did not somehow get a dose of gut bacteria from the mother's birth canal. This however can't be further from the truth. But the notion that C-sections are causing autism is a dangerous one and it has somehow been popularized among obstetricians of all people. I have met multiple obstetricians that have told me that! The true reason for it might be the fact that uterine contractions trigger the release of fetal hormones regulating lung fluid clearance during transition from the uterine to an air-breathing environment. With planned C-sections babies end up making that transition going from being inside the liquid filled amnion to air without the stress of birth and it leaves their lungs ill-prepared to take on the stress of the transition to air. This is borne out by evidence that shows elective C-sectioned babies have a much higher incidence of respiratory distress and NICU admissions in the first weeks of life. The following table lists a select few research papers on the subject.

Table – 10.1. Select research papers on C-section and respiratory distress

Elective Cesarean Section: It's Impact on Neonatal Respiratory Outcome - Ashwin Ramachandrappa, Lucky Jain https://pmc.ncbi.nlm.nih.gov/articles/PMC2453515/
Improving Neonatal and Maternal Outcome by Inducing Mild Labor before Elective Cesarean Section: The Lacarus Randomized Controlled Trial Sven Wellmann; Gwendolin Manegold-Brauer ; Tina Fischer; Leonhard Schäffer; Vincent D. Gaertner; Sara Fill Malfertheiner; Tilo Burkhardt Neonatology (2021) 118 (1): 116–121. https://doi.org/10.1159/000512752
Caesarean section and severe upper and lower respiratory tract infections during infancy: Evidence from two UK cohorts Neora Alterman ,Jennifer J. Kurinczuk,Maria A. Quigley Published: February 16, 2021 https://doi.org/10.1371/journal.pone.0246832

I believe such respiratory distress happening unnoticed at a subclinical level might be the cause of mild autism in these cases. Or it might be that the hypoxia suffered during that early phase is forgotten or goes unnoticed by parents and not considered serious enough to cause brain damage for it to be traced back as the cause of the autism years later.

They typically have milder autism and are mostly verbal but might have some social deficits. And in some cases, this is also the reason we have geniuses on the autism spectrum where the brain's repair mechanisms have gone on an overdrive resulting in higher memory, cognition and other aspects of intelligence. But the point is most kids diagnosed with autism were not C-sectioned out, so this explanation doesn't cover the more serious non-verbal autism out there.

Denying the Epidemic Altogether

Despite the reasons covered thus far, the most convenient diversion for explaining rising autism numbers is to simply deny an autism epidemic exists. It has become fashionable to attribute the increase solely to changes in diagnostic criteria, evolving categorizations, and improved record-keeping due to advances in information technology. While these factors play a role, the meteoric rise in numbers is undeniable; one would have to be living under a rock not to notice it. Everyone now knows someone impacted by autism, and that number continues to grow. This trend is most evident in the increasing sizes of special education classes in schools and the proliferation of small businesses offering ABA therapy, occupational therapy, and other brain treatments for children. This rise is contained within the scientific data collected by the Autism and Developmental Disabilities Monitoring (ADDM) Network a program instituted by the CDC. The ADDM began collecting data on children receiving services in school at age 8 in the year 2000. They chose age 8 as it would be enough time for these children to have been through the medical system and school system to have received a diagnosis from the medical system or school psychologists. While early diagnosis is critical, autism diagnoses tend to be more stable and reliable at 8 years old than at younger ages. By age 8 children have accumulated adequate health and educational records and having these records aids the ADDM to ascertain cases. While they also collect age 4 and age 16 numbers in certain cases, the age 8 has been their most reliable indicator of the incidence rate of autism in a given age group of the population and its change over time. As mentioned in the initial chapters, the American Psychiatric Association's Diagnostic and Statistical Manual, (DSM) provides standardized criteria to help diagnose ASD. Its most recent version, its fifth edition published in 2013 the DSM consolidated multiple categorizations into the Autism spectrum effectively going back to definitions of Autism in the 70's and 80's. The CDC's autism diagnosis follows the rigorous and stringent criteria set forth in the DSM-versions, a stark contrast to the casual way 'autism' is bandied about on social media.

To meet diagnostic criteria for ASD according to DSM-5, a child must have persistent deficits in each of three areas of social communication and interaction (see A.1. through A.3. in Table 10.2) plus at least two of four types of restricted, repetitive behaviors (see B.1. through B.4. in Table 10.2).

Severity is based on social communication impairments and restricted, repetitive patterns of behavior. For either criterion, severity is described in 3 levels:

- Level 3 – requires very substantial support
- Level 2 – Requires substantial support
- Level 1 – requires support

Table - 10.2. Autism Diagnostic Criteria

A. Persistent deficits in social communication and social interaction across multiple contexts, as manifested by the following, currently or by history (examples are illustrative, not exhaustive; see text):	
A.1	Deficits in social-emotional reciprocity, ranging, for example, from abnormal social approach and failure of normal back-and-forth conversation; to reduced sharing of interests, emotions, or affect; to failure to initiate or respond to social interactions
A.2	Deficits in nonverbal communicative behaviors used for social interaction, ranging, for example, from poorly integrated verbal and nonverbal communication; to abnormalities in eye contact and body language or deficits in understanding and use of gestures; to a total lack of facial expressions and nonverbal communication
A.3	Deficits in developing, maintaining, and understanding relationships, ranging, for example, from difficulties adjusting behavior to suit various social contexts; to difficulties in sharing imaginative play or in making friends; to absence of interest in peers
B. Restricted, repetitive patterns of behavior, interests, or activities, as manifested by at least two of the following, currently or by history (examples are illustrative, not exhaustive; see text):	
B.1	Stereotyped or repetitive motor movements, use of objects, or speech (e.g., simple motor stereotypes, lining up toys or flipping objects, echolalia, idiosyncratic phrases).
B.2	Insistence on sameness, inflexible adherence to routines, or ritualized patterns of verbal or nonverbal behavior (e.g., extreme distress at small changes, difficulties with transitions, rigid thinking patterns, greeting rituals, need to take same route or eat same food every day).
B.3	Highly restricted, fixated interests that are abnormal in intensity or focus (e.g., strong attachment to or preoccupation with unusual objects, excessively circumscribed or perseverative interests).
B.4	Hyper- or hypo reactivity to sensory input or unusual interest in sensory aspects of the environment (e.g. apparent indifference to pain/temperature, adverse response to specific sounds or textures, excessive smelling or touching of objects, visual fascination with lights or movement).
C. Symptoms must be present in the early developmental period (but may not become fully manifest until social demands exceed limited capacities, or may be masked by learned strategies in later life).	
D. Symptoms cause clinically significant impairment in social, occupational, or other important areas of current functioning.	
E. These disturbances are not better explained by intellectual disability (intellectual developmental disorder - previously called mental retardation) or global developmental delay. Intellectual disability and autism spectrum disorder frequently co-occur; to make comorbid diagnoses of autism spectrum disorder and intellectual disability, social communication should be below that expected for general developmental level.	

The scientific data meticulously compiled by ADDM every 2 years between the year 2000 and current is presented alongside some of the older data in this table.

Table – 10.3. Autism Rates From 1970's to 2014.

Survey Year	Birth Year	Number of ADDM Sites Reporting	Combined Prevalence per 1,000 Children (Range Across ADDM Sites)	This is about 1 in X - children
2022	2014	16	32.2 (9.7 - 53.1)	1 in 31
2020	2012	11	27.6 (23.1-44.9)	1 in 36
2018	2010	11	23.0 (16.5-38.9)	1 in 44
2016	2008	11	18.5 (18.0-19.1)	1 in 54
2014	2006	11	16.8 (13.1-29.3)	1 in 59
2012	2004	11	14.5 (8.2-24.6)	1 in 69
2010	2002	11	14.7 (5.7-21.9)	1 in 68
2008	2000	14	11.3 (4.8-21.2)	1 in 88
2006	1998	11	9.0 (4.2-12.1)	1 in 110
2004	1996	8	8.0 (4.6-9.8)	1 in 125
2002	1994	14	6.6 (3.3-10.6)	1 in 150
2000	1992	6	6.7 (4.5-9.9)	1 in 150
Mid-1990's			~20 per 10,000	~1 in 500
80's – 90's			~4-10 per 10,000	~1 in 1,000 - 2,500
70's – 80's			~2-4 per 10,000	~1 in 2,500 - 5,000

The earliest and largest epidemiological study on autism was conducted on close to 900,000 children aged 2-12 years in Wisconsin in 1970 by Darold A. Treffert, published in "Epidemiology of Infantile Autism." While the diagnostic criteria for autism at that time considered it a form of childhood schizophrenia, the listed symptoms—including detachment from reality, preoccupation with inner thoughts, unevenness and inadequacy of development, and gross immaturity—remain pertinent today. These historical descriptions corroborate with, and are arguably even broader than, current autism definitions. In this study, the incidence of autism was between 1 in 2,500 and 1 in 5,000 (2-4 per 10,000). Later studies from the late 1980s and early 1990s, incorporating DSM-III and DSM-IV definitions, consistently identified autism as a neurodevelopmental disorder beginning in early childhood, characterized by social, behavioral, language, and cognitive deficits. In each case, there are some serious criteria for some serious behavioral and social and developmental deficits that are not easily misdiagnosed or missed.

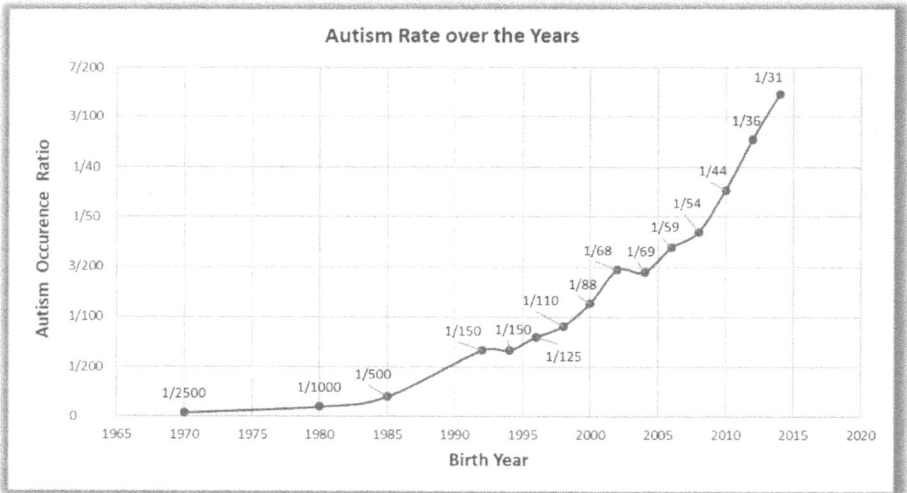

Fig 10.1 - Graph of current CDC data and prior data showing the meteoric rise in autism rates.

Therefore, the ongoing arguments by "epidemic deniers" that the rise in autism is merely due to increased identification are not logical reasoning, but an argument of facetious reasoning with an agenda. Here again, the perspective of impacted parents should carry significant weight. If you still have doubts, ask a parent with both an autistic child and a neurotypical one, and they will tell you why the world of difference between the two is simply impossible to miss.

In recent times, the neurodiversity movement, which has championed acceptance and inclusion for a now grown-up generation of autistic individuals (primarily those at the highest-functioning end of the spectrum), has also been at the forefront of autism epidemic denial. This denial stems from its dissonance with their theory of genetic diversity as the cause of autism. Genetic evolution, however, unfolds over significantly longer timescales and cannot account for changes of epidemic proportion within any given period. Proponents of the neurodiversity theory of autism consider the inherent genetic diversity of people as the cause of what they term an 'alternate developmental style' in autistic individuals. They are, however, conspicuously oblivious to the fact that this rapidly increasing neurodiversity, evident since 1980, is not attributable to genetics. Instead, it arises from the forced rewiring of brains following hypoxic or traumatic birth injury, particularly from the abuse of obstetric control over the uterus through excessive contractions during labor by a new breed of obstetricians empowered by these new uterus control drugs and egged on by insurance companies to achieve 'natural' vaginal delivery.

The neurodiversity perspective has gained traction because it's narrative aligns conveniently with birth injury cover-up narratives pushed by the truth suppression squads on social media (I will elaborate more about this in upcoming chapters). It is further amplified by conventional media and research groups that persist with their flawed approach of using twin studies to bolster claims of autism's heritability. At no point in the natural history of the world has genetic evolution exploded to such high rates, corresponding to the explosive growth of autism within such a short period, as to support the neurodiversity theory or the genetic causation theory of autism.

According to the ADDM, approximately 85% of parents of autistic individuals in their surveillance counts reported a developmental concern to their doctors by age 3, and virtually all (100%) had received a diagnosis by just under 4.5 years. The bottom line is, it is hard for parents to not notice the abnormalities in their children when a child only has a 5-8 second attention span, who won't stand in one place for more than that time, whose mind is constantly switching context and thoughts at that frequency. It's impossible to miss it, no matter what era we live in, be it the 70's, 80's, 90's or beyond the 2000's.

The Definitive Cause of the Autism Epidemic

What then is the cause of autism? The nurses at the large Midwest hospital where our boys were born were aware that inducing labor beyond a certain point would result in brain injury from excessive contractions. The hospital had developed its own protocol as per ACOG guidelines to avoid it. But our OB/GYN went against the hospital's established norms and failed to advise us correctly. She ended up inducing when the mom's cervix was not ready and without adequate cervical preparation. Once induction proceeded to the point of contra-indication, we were pretty much trapped with C-section being the only option out. Our Ob/Gyn believed C-sections are evil and we know because she had told us so multiple times before. The nurses tried to stop her in case of our first child and again questioned her strategy in the case of our second child but unfortunately were unsuccessful in a pre-ACA world where nurses were not allowed to give medical advice. I mistook the nurses' comment about brain damage as one of a chemical adverse effect, and failed to connect the dots, where the action of this unique drug was physical brain trauma and would cause traumatic brain injury (TBI). An injury that would stay silent and would only manifest itself as neurodevelopmental disorder years later. And as a result, our boys suffered TBI with the fundamental networks of their brains severed by the force trauma of contractions. That – and that alone – was the cause of their autism and they are not alone.

I arrived at this conclusion regarding my own sons only in early 2017. This revelation came quite accidentally, in late 2016 when our neurologist's office requested me to pick up a copy of my second son's MRI scan report directly from the hospital's radiology department, as they hadn't received it. The report in very clear terms pointed to a traumatic insult, resulting in multiple areas of scarring and gliosis in the white matter. This discovery immediately triggered recollections of incidents during both their deliveries, prompting me to wonder if my boys' experiences were unique or part of a wider pattern causing autism. As I began talking to other parents, most shared similar stories of prolonged labor induction. The only other notable observations were nuchal cord complications or C-sections necessitated by fetal distress in some cases.

Years earlier, I had encountered a research study that established a correlation between autism and labor induction. This was not some obscure scientific research paper, but a large epidemiological study by Dr. Simon Gregory et al. from Duke University. In fact, it received significant media attention, particularly since it concerned the emotionally charged topic of autism coming two years after the highly publicized vaccine omnibus trials, where impacted parents lost the case about autism causation from vaccines. Media outlets were abuzz with the labor induction-autism correlation study; all major news networks covered it in their primetime segments. Both Reuters and the Associated Press carried the news of the study, and numerous local newspapers picked up on it as well (media snippets in the next page). However, the study's authors didn't confirm causation, only affirmed an association. I did not know it at that time, but prevailing thought at that time focused on potential chemical effects of the drug Pitocin on the fetal brain, as drug effects are almost always perceived as chemical. I was concerned, but failed to dig deeper, as I recalled that some of my friends had children with typical development after induced labor. Consequently, I didn't closely follow the story, assuming that if it amounted to anything substantial, I would eventually find out. Like other short news cycles, the story faded, and I, like everyone else, forgot about it.

The eye-opener for me, however, came with my son's MRI report showing traumatic brain damage. That realization triggered the sleepless nights I discussed in an earlier chapter and brought vivid recollections of incidents in the delivery ward: nurses upset with the induction, and the pediatrician outraged that my boy had been induced for so long. It all suddenly coalesced. I researched the label of the Pitocin drug and found that it's warning explicitly pointed to permanent brain damage from excessive uterine motility—in essence, it was traumatic brain injury rather than an adverse chemical reaction.

Reuters
World ∨   Business ∨   Markets ∨   Sustainability ∨   Legal ∨   Commentary ∨   Technology ∨   Investigations   More ∨

Inducing, augmenting labor
to autism

By Andre...

NBC NEWS

Autism Linked with Induced Labor

Autism Linked with Induced Labor

Babies born to women whose labor was induced, or whose contractions were strengthened, with medical procedures such as hormone treatments, face an increased risk of autism, a new study suggests.

By Bahar Gholipour, Staff Writer

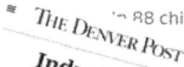

...of induction or augmen...
maternal and fetal health," Simon Gr...

THE DENVER POST

...n 88 children has an autism spec...

Inducing labor may be tied to autism, study fin...

By THE ASSOCIATED PRESS | The Associated Press
PUBLISHED: August 12, 2013 at 1:18 PM MDT

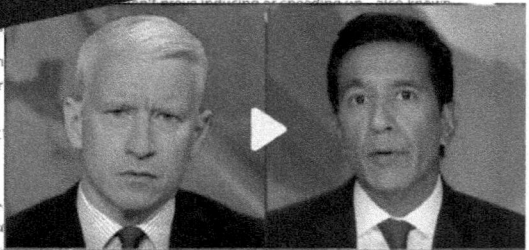

April 2...

STUDY: INDUCING, SPEEDING UP LABOR MAY BE TIED TO AUTISM
Researchers report male infants seem to be most vulnerable   **CNN**

FOX 8   Watch ▾   News ▾   Weather ▾   Sports ▾   PPR ▾   Seen On   Contests ▾   Lifestyle ▾   More ▾   Q Sea

HEALTH

Study links autism to
induced labor

by: Bob Ponting
Posted: Aug 13, 2013 / 11:34 AM PDT
Updated: Aug 13, 2013 / 11:34 AM PDT

Doctors typically use drugs to induce l...
due date. For augmentation, doctors a...

When medically indicated, induction h...
infant death.

Th...   ...formation on b...
e...

Q...

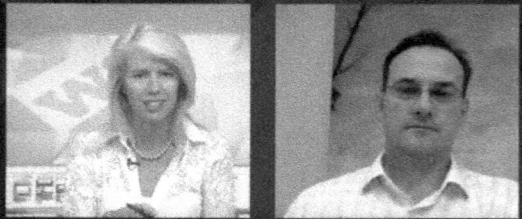

Induced Labor May Lead to Greater Risk of Autism for Child

▶ ◀ 1:13/4:32

The Risks Surrounding Induced Labor

Pregnant women whose labors are induced appear to have a greater risk of bearing children with autism, especially if the baby is m... study from Duke University found. The study takes into account factors such as the mother's age. Lindsay Gellman and Dr. Simon ...

Photo: AP

By Wall Street Journal

August 12, 2013 ⏱ 4:32

Of boys...

percent were delivered after augmenta...
were born after induction and 14 percent after augmentation.

My research extended to the ACOG.org website, where I found articles limiting labor induction to 68–72 contractions. I also learned about an ACOG directive to hospitals that led to the establishment of hospital labor induction protocols. The ACOG site was somewhat less restricted in early to mid-2017, allowing institutional access. But then, I also discovered what had happened to this 2013 Duke University paper. I saw how it had been successfully countered by bogus research that used the flawed genetic origin theory to manipulate the Swedish dataset—a dataset that had also confirmed the association of induced labor with autism, despite Sweden's typically low labor induction rates. I further uncovered how ACOG was twisting the narrative of labor induction and autism causation into one of impact to oxytocin signaling pathways, while fully aware of the traumatic brain injury their members were causing by not following their own protocols. They were seemingly unable to stop this practice without risking exposure for previous mistakes if they spoke too loudly.

Thus, this 2013 Duke University study (and the counter-study based on Swedish data) established a population-level association between labor induction and autism. Critically, my son's MRI scan, showing traumatic brain injury, provided proof of the underlying mechanism of causation. While such MRI findings are unique because the injury is often obscured by the birth process itself, numerous studies discuss compromise to white matter integrity and disconnects to fundamental neuronal networks in autistic individuals which I will elaborate on in the next chapter. Therefore, I can demonstrate that the cause of the autism epidemic beginning with the approval of elective labor induction in 1980 is hidden traumatic brain injury from abuse of labor induction. This is a direct consequence of obstetricians failing to adhere to protocols, which were later abandoned in 2018 for reasons of vested interests. This failure has led to an ever-increasing, hidden birth injury-based epidemic, one that is being actively covered up by parties facing legal consequences and enormous monetary losses should the truth about these birth injuries be exposed. Worse still, restrictive tort reforms have completely closed avenues for legal remediation allowing this type of birth injury to grow unchecked, worsening the epidemic.

The Alarming Escalation of Labor Induction Rates.

In the United States, the National Center for Health Statistics (NCHS), a component of the CDC, has collected labor induction data as part of its birth statistics since 1989. Following the 2018 revision of labor induction protocols and the recommendation to induce labor at 39 weeks, the labor induction rate in the U.S. has notably increased, as identified in government data from U.S. birth certificates. Even these numbers, compiled by the NCHS (2022a, 2022b), are not expected to fully capture all cases, suggesting the true rate could be higher.

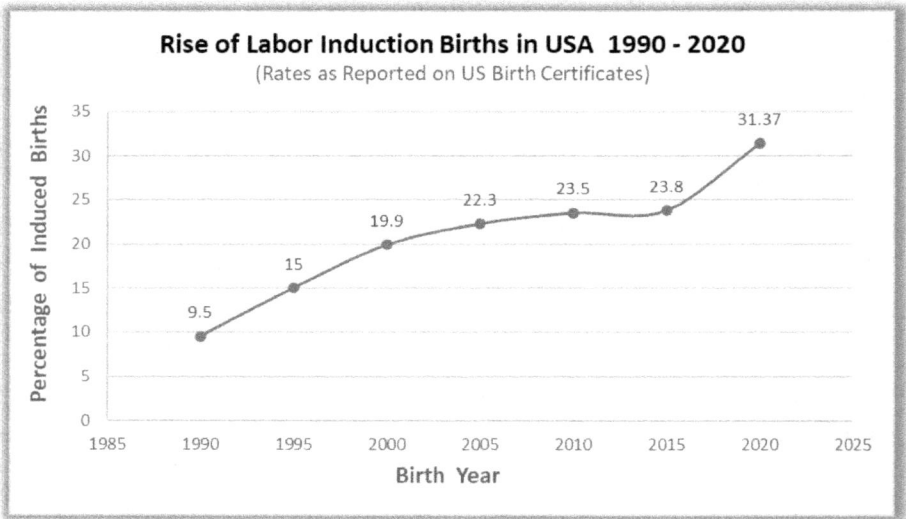

Fig 10.2 Labor induction as a fraction of total births in the US.

This NCHS data was elegantly compiled by Kathleen Rice Simpson, PhD, in her paper titled 'Trends in Labor Induction in the United States, 1989 to 2020.' Simpson's work[10.1] visually highlights the gravity of the situation. It demonstrates how labor induction rates, which stabilized in the low 20th percentile between 2005 and 2015, suddenly surged to over 31% after the ARRIVE trial recommendations by ACOG and SMFM to induce labor at 39 weeks, ostensibly to avoid complications in late pregnancy.

The current U.S. autism prevalence rate of over 3% of births (1 in 31), as per 2022 data, reflects diagnoses in children born approximately eight years prior (i.e., in 2014). This is because the CDC measures autism numbers using school data from 8-year-olds diagnosed by school psychologists and receiving services. Critically, these figures still reflect a period when labor induction protocols were generally in place in hospitals, and only negligent obstetricians were likely engaging in labor drug abuse beyond those limits. These reported numbers could be significantly higher once we receive post-2018 data, following the removal of established induction protocols and the shift towards targeting induction at 39 weeks of pregnancy. Of course, not all induced mothers will exceed labor drug contraindication limits; many may deliver well before, particularly if their obstetrician performed adequate pre-induction cervical readiness checks and preparation techniques.

The 2013 paper by Stephen Gregory et al. found an incidence rate for autism ranging from 13% (in some models) to 28% (in others) among induced births. Given the U.S. birth rate of approximately 3.5 million, a 20% labor induction rate would translate to 700,000 induced births. If we apply an autism incidence rate of approximately 15% to these induced births, this yields 105,000 autism diagnoses. This means 105,000 individuals are brain damaged by labor induction resulting in autism, out of 3.5 million total births, which is precisely 3%, roughly matching the prevailing autism rate of 1 in 31.

Extrapolating this to the future, given the current 30% labor induction rate, would lead to a total autism prevalence rate of 4.5%. However, with the removal of safety protocols and obstetricians seemingly given a 'free pass' to aggressively induce vaginal deliveries, the brain damage rate from labor induction could potentially rise from 15% towards 20-25%. This would effectively double the autism rate from 3% to 6%, or approximately 1 in 16 births. Considering the significant gender gap of 3.4:1 in autism diagnoses, this could mean the incidence in boys might double to 1 in 10, while girls could reach 1 in 35 in the near future.

I openly acknowledge that this argument is based on the presumption that labor induction abuse is the primary factor contributing to the rise in autism. While other static factors contribute to a baseline autism rate—which I will explain in upcoming chapters—the undeniable bottom line is that escalating abusive labor induction is the cause of the escalating autism rate. The situation has become dire since 2018, demanding urgent action, as in 'yesterday.' Otherwise, we risk suffering generational societal damage, with 10% of our male population and 3% of our female population permanently brain-damaged by what is a very avoidable consequence of systemic obstetric malpractice.

What about Vaccines?

I would be remiss in covering autism causation without addressing the elephant in the room: the vaccine question. This subject is so vast that I have dedicated an entire section of this book to it, yet even there, I will only be scratching the surface. Whole books have been written on the topic, including many by Robert F. Kennedy Jr., who serves as the current U.S. Secretary of Health in 2025. Physicians like Joseph Mercola, Sherri Tenpenny, and Kelly Brogan have been prominent in their opposition to vaccines, citing various adverse effects. These include neurological impacts, autism, common respiratory and food allergies, life-threatening food allergies, and autoimmune disorders affecting multiple organs like Lupus or specific organs, such as Type 1 diabetes.

The theory linking vaccines to autism first emerged with the publication of a 1998 study by British gastroenterologist Andrew Wakefield in The Lancet, a globally recognized medical journal. In this paper, the author suggested a connection between the MMR vaccine and autism. The paper was subsequently retracted, and Andrew Wakefield was severely censured, stripped of his medical license, and widely dubbed a fraud. It's a common misconception that the paper focused on the thimerosal adjuvant and its mercury content (this was the focus of the vaccine omnibus trials). Instead, the paper specifically addressed the live virus variants within the injection itself and proposed how they might persist in the gut, causing dysbiosis that later resulted in autism. And he was potentially correct. However, the heavy-handed response this idea elicited from the health establishment, which essentially annihilated Dr. Wakefield and made him an example of what could happen, effectively dissuaded any further independent research on the subject.

It is a common observation among parents of autistic children to notice a regression of skills in their children after certain vaccinations, particularly live vaccines. When so many individuals, including parents and physicians, observe this, it suggests a basis in truth. In fact, similar skill regression is observed by parents of children with prior labor-induction brain damage after contracting most viral illnesses. I believe Dr. Wakefield's research was indeed correct, but it needed to be examined in conjunction with pre-existing traumatic brain damage in his research subjects resulting from birth trauma. We will explore this angle in the next section of this book, including the impact of live vaccines on pre-existing brain damage, the brain immune deviation known as the ACAID phenomenon and its effect on gut dysbiosis, and how live vaccines could be responsible for inhibiting recovery from brain damage, potentially serving as a secondary cause of the autism epidemic. For now, let's continue focusing on the primary cause of the epidemic: traumatic brain injury, as revealed by MRI imaging.

Key Take Away: While various theories and causative pathways have been proposed for the etiology of autism, none of them can account for the increasing incidence of autism among children by age 8 as per the CDC accounting. The only argument that holds any water is brain damage occurring from hospital birth interventions particularly labor drug abuse, by way of excessive contractions in labor induction. This is exactly as it happened in the case of my two sons and this practice is getting more abusive and more rampant in hospitals, causing the Autism Epidemic.

CHAPTER 11

The Clarity Brought on by MRI Scans

Imagine trying to solve a mystery, without any clues, that would have been the situation of medical practitioners before the advent of modern imaging tools. Doctors would have had to fly blind in a whole host of situations, involving surgeries, injuries, cancers and so on. Diagnostic imaging tools are such an integral part of modern medicine, there's this whole field called radiology dedicated to the study of imaging. Even there, there's multiple specializations aligned with the type of use like ultrasound, CT scans, MRI scans, SPECT scans and so on. The specializations and instrumentation are so vast and diverse that each of these is a separate field of study within medicine.

Magnetic Resonance Imaging (MRI) scans play a crucial role in modern medicine, offering detailed insights into the human body without the use of ionizing radiation, which is a concern with other imaging modalities like X-rays and CT scans. MRI is particularly valuable for its ability to provide high-resolution images of soft tissues, making it an essential tool for diagnosing a variety of medical conditions, especially those related to the brain, spinal cord, and joints. Neurologists rely on MRI to identify abnormalities such as tumors, strokes, multiple sclerosis, and neurodegenerative diseases, allowing for timely intervention and management. In orthopedics, MRI is instrumental in evaluating soft tissue injuries, such as ligament tears and cartilage damage, providing a clearer picture of musculoskeletal disorders. Additionally, MRI is increasingly used in cancer diagnosis and treatment planning, as it can help determine the size and spread of tumors, guiding surgical and therapeutic decisions. Functional MRI (fMRI) adds another dimension by measuring brain activity through changes in blood flow, which is invaluable in research and in understanding various neurological conditions. Furthermore, advancements in MRI technology, such as diffusion tensor imaging and spectroscopy, continue to enhance its applications, enabling clinicians to assess conditions like hydrocephalus and metabolic disorders more effectively. Overall, the non-invasive nature and versatility of MRI make it an indispensable tool in diagnostic imaging, contributing significantly to patient care and outcomes across multiple fields of medicine.

Magnetic resonance imaging obtains images of the various interior organs of the body by utilizing the interaction of the body with magnetism and radio frequencies. It relies on the fact that the human body is composed of 65% water and the ionized hydrogen atoms (protons) in water and fat molecules are specifically targeted by this technique. Putting the hydrogen atoms through a heavy magnetic field causes them to align their random atomic spin directions along with the magnetic field. A radio frequency is then used to perturb this spin alignment, which happens when the frequency is in resonance with the spin. When the radio frequency pulse is turned off, energy is given off by the hydrogen atoms as they return to their previous positions. This energy is measured by a coil to create accurate images of the interior organs. "Sliced" views can be obtained from any angle with the resolution being quite high: on the order of millimeters for magnetic field strengths of 1.5 tesla and as low as 0.5mm for the 3 tesla machines. It is typical to generate the 3 axial imaging planes with a single MRI scan. Trained radiologists reading these images can identify abnormalities including scarring, structural deficiencies, tumors and the like.

Sectional Planes

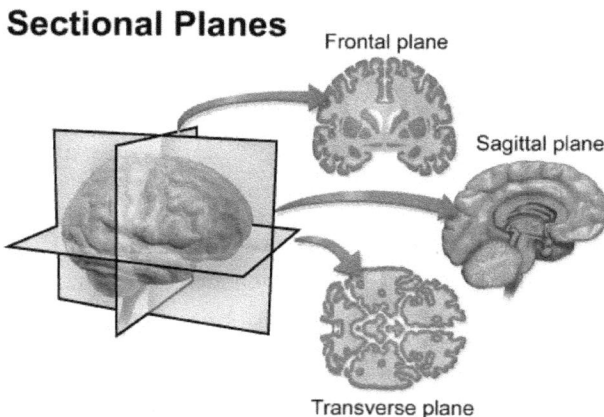

Frontal plane

Sagittal plane

Transverse plane

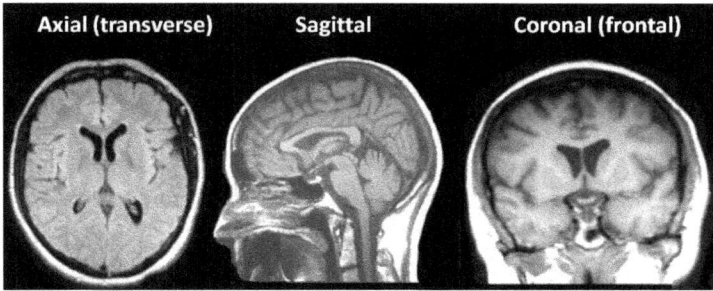

Fig. 11.1a, b: The three different planes in brain imaging with MRI.

Unfortunately, many autism caregiver doctors do not order an MRI scan as they do not anticipate any major treatable findings in an MRI scan. While this is true it mostly results in any trauma or hypoxia related scarring in the brain getting missed. The only doctors who might order an MRI scan are neurologists as they are the only providers that try to ascertain the source of the problem. Autism care pediatricians are mostly impacted parents themselves or impacted in their immediate family or close circle and choose to take up such specialized care. Due to the young age of children and the need to be anesthetized for this procedure, many parents with children experiencing neurodevelopmental disorders have never had an MRI done on their children.

One of the most critical current uses of MRI scans in children is to identify brain structural defects otherwise called brain "cephalies" (abnormalities), known to be caused by genetic disorders. Here's a list of a dozen brain "cephalies" that can be identified in MRI scans: These conditions can vary in severity and implications, and MRI is a crucial tool for diagnosis and assessment.

	Condition	Description
1	Hydrocephalus:	Accumulation of cerebrospinal fluid (CSF) in the ventricles of the brain, leading to increased pressure.
2	Microcephaly	Abnormally small head size, often associated with developmental issues.
3	Macrocephaly	Abnormally large head size, which can indicate underlying conditions such as hydrocephalus or brain tumors.
4	Lissencephaly	A condition characterized by smooth brain surfaces due to abnormal brain development.
5	Porencephaly	The presence of cysts or cavities in the brain tissue, often resulting from injury or malformation

6	Polymicrogyria	An abnormality characterized by an excessive number of small gyri (folds) on the brain's surface
7	Pachygyria	Broadened gyri with simplified sulci (grooves).
8	Schizencephaly	Clefts or slits in the cerebral hemispheres.
9	Chiari Malformation	A structural defect where brain tissue extends into the spinal canal, affecting CSF flow
10	Dandy-Walker Malformation	An abnormality involving the cerebellum and the fourth ventricle, often associated with hydrocephalus.
11	Agenesis of the Corpus Callosum	A condition where the corpus callosum, which connects the two brain hemispheres, is partially or completely absent.
12	Septo-Optic Dysplasia	A condition characterized by the absence of the septum pellucidum, optic nerve hypoplasia, and pituitary abnormalities.
13	Tuberous Sclerosis	A genetic disorder characterized by the growth of noncancerous tumors in various organs, including the brain
12	Encephalomalacia	Softening or loss of brain tissue, often due to injury or lack of blood flow.

Table 11.1 List of brain "cephalies" identifiable in MRI scans.

Most of these conditions except the last one #12 occur as a result of genetic abnormalities and congenital deficiencies which are easily detected by MRI scans and these show up correlated with mental development challenges. Patients with these conditions are also diagnosed with ASD, but the incidence of these conditions is very low as explained in the previous chapter on genetics and the numbers do not add up to explain the incidence rate of autism which is almost at 3 in a 100 and growing. So, as we can see here, genetic abnormalities impacting neurodevelopment occur mostly as groups of malformations in the brain that are easily identified by MRI scans. The last one on the list #12 encephalomalacia is of interest to us, as it is non-genetic and caused by brain injuries that MRI can detect.

Mechanisms of Damage and Death of Neurons

To understand the mechanisms of brain damage and detection of damage by MRI scans we first need to understand the mechanisms by which brain damage can occur at birth. We already know the two possible avenues of damage are hypoxic injury and traumatic injury. We have also seen, in our chapter 2 how the grey matter in the brain is comprised of neuron bodies, while white matter contains the axon tails of the neurons that are responsible for the connectivity of various parts of the brain. This connectivity ranges from local interconnectivity of the various cerebral areas, the intermediate range connectivity between the two cerebral hemispheres of the brain across the corpus callosum and the longer connectivity down the spinal cord into the rest of the nervous system. We also know that the brain consists of various types of neurons and neuron support cells called astrocytes, oligodendrocytes and microglia. Neurons when subjected to hypoxic distress or injured by physical trauma end up dying in different ways depending on the intensity of the trauma suffered. The two possible modes of death of a neuron cell are necrosis and apoptosis.

Necrosis is the kind of neuronal death where, the neuron cell disintegrates spilling the contents of the cell into neighboring environment resulting in inflammation, edema and causes possible secondary damage to neighboring neurons in its environment. This is due to cell damage being seen as danger signals which activate the immune system. This also causes astrocytes and glial cells to migrate to the damage area and also proliferate more by cell division to work on damage control. They remove cellular debris, but contribute to inflammation by signaling the immune system, all of which is good during the initial stages of damage This increase in concentration of glial cells and astrocytes is called gliosis. When larger areas of neuron death by necrosis is involved, it causes glial scars. While gliosis initially works to control the damage these scars then impede any future connectivity across the areas of scarring. Thus, inflammation and glial scarring resulting from necrosis can also cause further damage and it all depends on the extent of neuronal damage and the injury continues to evolve over time

Apoptosis is a form of neuronal cell death where the neuron is marked for atrophy due to loss of cellular function from factors such as oxidative stress, calcium dysregulation and glutamate excitotoxicity. Even in cases of minor trauma, in the hours and days following the initial injury, apoptotic pathways can be activated. During apoptosis, the entire neuron, including both the cell body (soma) and the axon, undergoes a controlled process of self-destruction. The cell body shrinks in size. Chromatin (DNA) within the nucleus condenses and fragments. The cell membrane forms small bulges or blebs which eventually divides the cell into small, membrane-enclosed fragments called apoptotic bodies. The axon also fragments into smaller pieces. The synaptic connections with other neurons are retracted. Apoptotic bodies and cellular debris are efficiently cleared away by microglia in the brain. This process minimizes inflammation and prevents the release of harmful substances that could damage neighboring cells. Thus, glial cells play a role in clearing away cellular debris and participate in the repair process in both necrosis and apoptosis. In fact, when an MRI scan is performed months or years after the original injury, this reactive proliferation of glial cells that occurs in response to neuronal injury called gliosis is what shows up in the scan and its presence is what confirms the neuronal injury from the past.

MRI Sequences and Brain Injury Progression

In both hypoxic and traumatic brain injury the immediate consequences involve death of the neurons either immediately by necrosis or being marked for apoptosis due to cellular dysfunction including energy failure and cellular imbalances. There is evolution of the injury as damage control mechanisms kick in during the initial phases and the healing pathway takes its course. There could also be alternate pathways triggered from continuous festering of the damage, secondary injury from inflammation resulting in longer lasting evolution of the injury, including possible interference from foreign particles like viruses. Hence, in neuro-imaging the time since injury also plays an important role in how the injury presents itself in the images. Understanding the different sequences of MRI imaging is key to reading and understanding MRI reports or even understanding research papers involving studies of MRI scans of subjects on the autism spectrum.

An MRI imaging sequence is essentially a set of instructions that tells the MRI scanner how to acquire images of the body. It's a carefully timed series of radiofrequency (RF) pulses and magnetic field gradients that manipulate the behavior of protons (hydrogen atoms) in the body's tissues. The resulting signals are then processed by a computer to create detailed images.

The sequences most commonly used in MRI of the brain are:

MRI Sequence	Usage
T1 Weighted	Provides excellent anatomical detail and is used broadly for anatomical definition and tissue characterization.
T2 Weighted	Sensitive to water content, it shows oedema and pathology issues such as gliosis as high or 'white' signal.
FLAIR	Fluid-attenuated inversion recovery: suppresses cerebrospinal fluid signal and makes 'white' pathology of lesions and other abnormalities more visible.
Diffusion Weighted Imaging (DWI)	Measures water diffusion within tissue, valuable for detecting acute stroke and other conditions affecting tissue integrity. Areas with restricted diffusion appear bright.
Diffusion Tensor Imaging (DTI)	Measures the diffusion of water molecules in white matter. Diffusion Tensor Imaging is based on DWI and is used to evaluate the integrity of white matter tracts using a key diffusion directionality measurement called Fractional Anisotropy (FA).
Perfusion Weighted Imaging (PWI)	Very useful for blood flow analysis, works by injecting contrast and tracking its flow through the brain tissue.
Susceptibility Weighted Imaging (SWI)	Uses subtle difference in magnetic properties of deoxygenated blood, iron and calcium to detect microbleeds, DAI lesions, stroke, vascular malformations, tumors.

Table 11.2 Important MRI sequences in Neuro radiology.

These different sequences provide clarity in the different phases of progression of brain damage and mostly the progression is similar in cases of both neonatal hypoxic and traumatic injury, with the main difference being that there is more white matter damage in traumatic injury while hypoxic injury involves more grey matter damage at the initial stages. But the progression of secondary damage can be similar in all types of brain injury.

Acute Phase (Days to Weeks): Diffusion-weighted imaging is the most sensitive MRI sequence in the acute phase. It shows areas of restricted diffusion, appearing as areas of high signal intensity. This reflects cytotoxic edema within brain cells, indicating cell injury. T2-weighted and FLAIR images may reveal areas of edema and hemorrhage. Susceptibility-weighted imaging (SWI) is particularly sensitive to detecting hemorrhagic lesions, including microbleeds in cases of trauma. Additionally, MRI can help visualize contusions, lacerations, and any mass effect from hematomas or swelling. The primary focus of MRI in this phase is to assess the extent of initial injury and guide immediate medical management.

Subacute Phase (Weeks to Months): During the subacute phase, MRI scans help monitor the evolution of brain lesions and assess the extent of secondary injury. T2-weighted and FLAIR images may show evolving edema and areas of encephalomalacia (softening of brain tissue). Hemorrhagic lesions may show changes in signal intensity as blood products degrade. Diffusion tensor imaging (DTI) can begin to reveal white matter tract damage, which may not be apparent on conventional MRI sequences. Atrophy may begin to become apparent. The changes seen on MRI during this phase help in planning rehabilitation strategies and predicting potential long-term neurological outcomes.

Chronic Phase (Months to Years): In the chronic phase, MRI scans primarily demonstrate the long-term structural consequences of neuron damage. T1-weighted images may show areas of focal or diffuse brain atrophy, indicating neuronal loss. T2-weighted and FLAIR images can reveal areas of gliosis (scarring) and persistent encephalomalacia (softening and degeneration of brain tissue). DTI can demonstrate chronic white matter tract damage, which correlates with cognitive and motor deficits. MRI is essential for monitoring the progression of long-term complications, such as post-traumatic epilepsy and hydrocephalus. The findings on MRI in this phase help in guiding long-term management and rehabilitation efforts.

Brain Damage from Hypoxic Neuronal Injury

Hypoxic injury is a common birth injury and significant contributor to neuro-development disorders. Since a fetus is not breathing inside the mother's womb, the supply of oxygen and nutrients to the fetus is through the maternal circulation through the placenta and umbilical cord. Any deficits in nutrients during pregnancy results in IUGR (Intrauterine growth restriction). During birth however there exist quite a few additional risks of the oxygen supply to the baby being cut off totally, by complications of birth. The main complications are the umbilical cord wrapped around the neck a few times. The umbilical cord is a fairly long cord, but if a lot of it is wrapped around the baby and the cord gets really tight around the neck during birth, then it could strangle the baby by stopping the blood flow to the brain through the arteries of the neck, causing hypoxic ischemia which is lack of oxygen from lack of blood flowing to the brain. Another cause of hypoxia during birth is when the cord comes out ahead of the baby, causing it to get pinched when the head comes out under tight circumstances. This in-turn stops blood flow through the cord, causing hypoxic ischemia. Another common hypoxic condition is when there's fetal distress from the contractions, mostly as a result of tachysystole contractions or high frequency of contractions as a result of labor drugs causing hypoxia from lack of sufficient time for the placenta to recover between contractions.

Some of the brain areas most vulnerable to hypoxic injury include areas of the brain which contain the largest sized and largest concentrations of neurons. These are also areas of high metabolic demand and include the hippocampus, cerebral cortex (gray matter), cerebellum and some other areas prone to low blood perfusion. These are the areas of interest when hypoxic damage is suspected and hypoxic changes are identifiable in an MRI scan. The hippocampus is crucial for learning and memory. It is particularly sensitive to oxygen deprivation. The cerebral cortex or grey matter of the brain, specifically, layers 3, 5, and 6 of the cerebral cortex are vulnerable to neuronal loss. Different areas of the cortex may be affected depending on the severity and duration of hypoxia. Minor hypoxia over shorter duration might result in loss of some of the pyramidal neurons of the layers 3, 5 and 6 of the cerebral cortex, while prolonged hypoxia can lead to damage to deep brain structures like the hippocampus. Babies can recover from minor hypoxia, and these are the kids born into the spectrum that can eventually get significantly better with genius skills in certain areas.

Brain Damage from Traumatic Neuronal Injury

As mentioned previously abuse of labor drugs to pursue an unlimited number of continuous labor contractions to hammer a baby head first out of the mother's uterus, particularly after amniotic rupture causes traumatic brain injury. This is very similar to brain damage suffered after an accidental concussion by adults.

The axons of the neurons get sheared in the white matter areas, leading to reactive changes like gliosis seen in an MRI scan. This is called Diffuse Axonal Injury (DAI). In DAI, the primary damage occurs to the axons of neurons, which are the long, slender projections that transmit signals between brain cells.

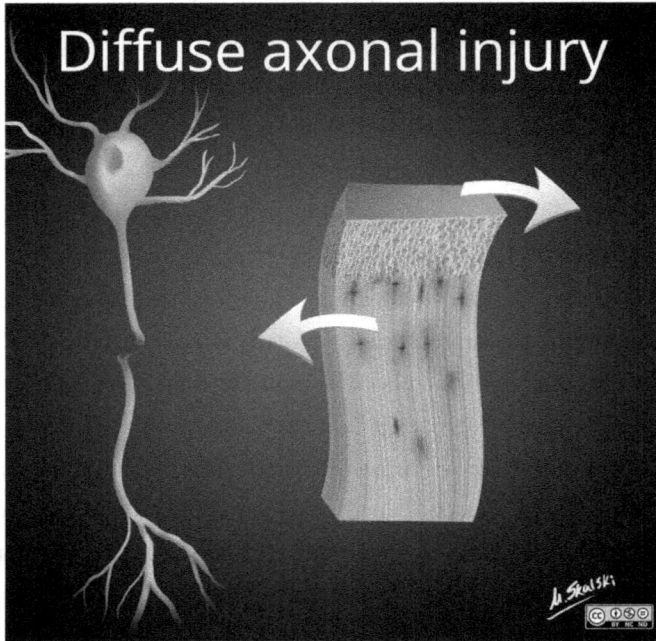

Fig 11.2 showing a schematic diagram of Diffuse Axonal Injury (DAI)
Image source - Case courtesy of Matt Skalski, Radiopaedia.org, rID: 38437

Key consequences of injury from DAI (severe concussion) include.

Axonal Damage:

▶ *Shearing Forces:* The rapid acceleration/deceleration forces associated with DAI cause the brain to move within the skull. This shearing motion stretches and tears axons.

▶ *Disruption of Axonal Transport:* Axons rely on a complex transport system to deliver essential proteins and nutrients from the cell body to the axon terminals. This transport is severely disrupted in DAI, leading to axonal degeneration.

Neuron Death:

▸ Widespread Neuronal Loss - While not all damaged neurons die immediately, significant neuronal death occurs in the days and weeks following DAI.

  o Apoptosis - Many neurons undergo programmed cell death due to
  the disruption of essential cellular functions.

  o Necrosis - In severe cases, neurons may also undergo necrosis,
  from acute injury with inflammation causing secondary damage.

Glial Cell Proliferation:

▸ Inflammation - Glial cells, such as microglia and astrocytes, play a crucial
role in the inflammatory response after DAI.

  o They remove cellular debris and release inflammatory mediators.

  o While initially beneficial, excessive inflammation can contribute to
  further neuronal damage.

▸ Scar Formation - Astrocytes form a glial scar around the injured area,
which can both protect the surrounding tissue and hinder axonal regeneration.

Long-Term Consequences:

▸ Disrupted Brain Connectivity - The widespread axonal damage in DAI
disrupts the intricate network of connections within the brain.

▸ Cognitive and Motor Deficits - This disruption of brain connectivity
leads to a wide range of neurological problems, including:

  o Cognitive impairments (memory problems, difficulty concentrat-
  ing, slowed thinking)

  o Motor difficulties (weakness, balance problems, coordination issues)

  o Behavioral and emotional changes

The extent and location of DAI lesions on MRI are critical for predicting
recovery. Lesions in deep structures like the brainstem and corpus callosum are
associated with poorer outcomes. MRI is a cornerstone in diagnosing DAI and

guiding both prognosis and management decisions. As you might notice most long-term consequences described in DAI are the same as those of autism sufferers. Interestingly the MRI scans of kids with autism also shows similar kinds of damage, just that in their case, damage is even more widespread and in deeper areas like the corpus callosum than in adult DAI from concussions, which is mainly seen close to the grey-matter–white-matter junction areas.

The Unique and Critical Role of Birth as an Agent of Brain Injury

Based on the Diffusion Tensor Imaging MRI scans of kids suffering brain damage and autism from the prolonged forces of contraction in abusive labor induction it is easy to extrapolate how this damage has come about. Damage in these kids is always seen in the white matter areas in MRI scans, which is indicative of traumatic injury along the same lines as DAI. Numerous papers have been published (Table 11.1) on the topic of white matter integrity in autism and it is a known fact that the neuronal tracts are compromised or lack the fiber tract thickness / cross section needed to carry signals fast enough to the various cerebral areas they connect. So how might contraction forces over longer periods of time cause this kind of neuronal white matter damage as in the brain damage warnings of the Pitocin label.

During birth when there is a natural water break or artificial rupture of membranes (AROM) otherwise called amniotomy the natural water bag cushion surrounding the baby is lost. Once this happens, the risk of traumatic and hypoxic injury from interventions increases greatly. The rupture of the membrane naturally brings on contractions, as the mother's body tries to expel the baby quickly through this risky phase of birth. But then the mother's body also knows its limits and understands that unchecked contractions could cause brain damage to the baby particularly when the cervix is not ready. But modern obstetricians promptly jump on this opportunity, apparently to 'help' the natural contractions along with labor induction drugs to induce contractions. These contractions start forcing the baby's head against the cervix wall. The pressure on the baby's head from these contractions is particularly high after loss of amniotic fluid as all pressure is focused on certain parts of the baby's head.

As discussed in chapter 7 in the section on the mechanism of brain damage, prolonged induction causes stretching and tearing of the cervix. If that's what happens to the part of the uterus muscle that's been holding the baby in place inside the mother for the whole pregnancy, we can imagine what might happen to the fragile brain inside the head that is causing the cervix to tear.

Analysis of Forces on a Baby's Head During Birth

During a typical vaginal birth, the fetal head has to endure two distinct forms of compression at the first two stages of birth – the cervical dilation stage, and the pushing stage. During the cervical dilation stage there is vertical compression of the head from uterine contractions that push the head against the cervix attempting to facilitate cervical dilation. In healthy women the cervix has grown stronger during pregnancy as it works to retain a baby and womb that has gotten heavier in the months preceding delivery. The intense vertical pressure from uterine contractions, driving the head against this strong cervix wall, can be very damaging to the baby's brain inside. This is because the baby's brain is not exactly designed to handle this kind of pressure. With such vertical pressure from the top, the brain has nowhere to go except to stay in place and take the pounding. The brain's semi-fluid nature, combined with the rigid confines of the skull, results in the transmission of this force to deeper brain structures. This type of force, for which the fetal head is not optimally designed, may result in vertical compression of the brain as illustrated in fig 11.3. This could result in damage to the neuronal fiber tracts in the cerebral lobes. The long neuron connections that make up the junction between the 2 cerebral lobes called the corpus callosum come under particularly intense stress, causing the long fiber bundles to break, leading to the neuronal disconnects typically seen in those suffering from autism.

COMPRESSED AND SHEARED CEREBRAL LOBES

Stretching cervix wall cross section

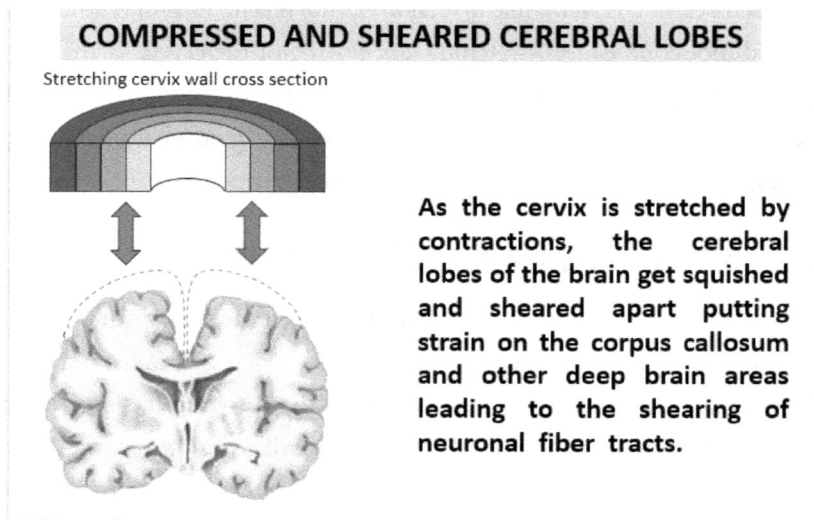

As the cervix is stretched by contractions, the cerebral lobes of the brain get squished and sheared apart putting strain on the corpus callosum and other deep brain areas leading to the shearing of neuronal fiber tracts.

Fig 11.3 Schematic diagram showing how the cerebral lobes might get compressed causing stress and shearing at the corpus callosum.

The white matter alterations being found by researchers in autism brains are the result of traumatic white matter insult sustained from prolonged vertical compression by the contraction forces of excessive or abusive labor induction. This is exactly the kind of brain damage that the Pitocin label talks about. The damage locations in the cerebral white matter marked by gliosis and scarring might for example correlate with the amount of time the cervix spent dilating at that station. Nature understands this and the mother's body does not bring active contractions until the mother's cervix is ready to dilate. This is also the reason why labor gets stuck sometimes, as the mother's body, by design doesn't want to damage the baby's brain. But when obstetricians intervene in these circumstances without adequate reason, and use medication to induce contractions, the result is brain damage to the baby from these forced contractions. This damage shows up as white matter hyperintensities in T2 FLAIR MRI sequences. However, herein lies the catch. The subsequent pushing stage and the lateral compression forces involved there sometimes end up scattering any damage enough that it may not be visible with regular MRI and only DWI / DTI MRI might be able to confirm this white matter damage in the neuronal fibers.

Research Affiliation	Autism – MRI Study
University of Florida, Gainesville, USA	Shin, Y.S., Christensen, D., Wang, J. *et al.* **Transcallosal white matter and cortical gray matter variations in autistic adults aged 30–73 years.** *Molecular Autism* **16**, 16 (2025). https://doi.org/10.1186/s13229-025-00652-6
MIT, Harvard University, Boston, MA, USA.	Hung Y, Dallenbach NT, Green A, Gaillard S, Capella J, Hoskova B, Vater CH, Cooper E, Rudberg N, Takahashi A, Gabrieli JDE, Joshi G. **Distinct and shared white matter abnormalities when ADHD is comorbid with ASD: A preliminary diffusion tensor imaging study.** Psychiatry Res. 2023 Feb;320:115039. doi: 10.1016/j.psychres.2022.115039. Epub 2022 Dec 28. PMID: 36640678.
University of Toronto, CA	Ameis SH, Lerch JP, Taylor MJ, Lee W, Viviano JD, Pipitone J, Nazeri A, Croarkin PE, Voineskos AN, Lai MC, Crosbie J, Brian J, Soreni N, Schachar R, Szatmari P, Arnold PD, Anagnostou E. **A Diffusion Tensor Imaging Study in Children With ADHD, Autism Spectrum Disorder, OCD, and Matched Controls: Distinct and Non-Distinct White Matter Disruption and Dimensional Brain-Behavior Relationships** American Journal of Psychiatry - Volume 173, Number 12 https://doi.org/10.1176/appi.ajp.2016.15111435
National Taiwan University, Taipei, Taiwan	Chiang HL, Chen YJ, Lin HY, Tseng WI, Gau SS. D **Disorder-Specific Alteration in White Matter Structural Property in Adults with Autism Spectrum Disorder Relative to Adults with ADHD and Adult Controls.** Hum Brain Mapp. 2017 Jan;38(1):384-395. doi: 10.1002/hbm.23367. Epub 2016 Sep 15. PMID: 27630075; PMCID: PMC6866870.
Showa University, Tokyo, Japan	Ohta, H., Aoki, Y.Y., Itahashi, T. et al. **White matter alterations in autism spectrum disorder and ADHD in relation to sensory profile.** Molecular Autism 11, 77 (2020). https://doi.org/10.1186/s13229-020-00379-6
University of Tokyo, Japan	Aoki, Y., Abe, O., Nippashi, Y. *et al.* **Comparison of white matter integrity between autism spectrum disorder subjects and typically developing individuals: a meta-analysis of diffusion tensor imaging tractography studies.** *Molecular Autism* 4, 25 (2013). https://doi.org/10.1186/2040-2392-4-25

Table 11.1. Select research papers about investigation of brain white matter with MRI scans in the context of autism.

The second stage of birth in a typical maternity ward involves maternal pushing synchronized with uterine contractions. The mother's abdomen and diaphragm work in concert with the uterus to bear down on the baby, propelling it beyond the pelvis. While this significantly increases pressure on the baby, it's no longer solely vertical pressure on the head as the cervix wall is now out of the way; instead, lateral (sideways) pressure from the walls of the birth canal becomes prominent as the baby moves forward due to the pushing forces. To navigate the pubic arch successfully, the baby typically emerges face down, which may necessitate some rotation during this pushing phase. With the cervix fully dilated and out of the way, this lateral force on the head tends to elongate it. However, the baby's head and its skull plates are generally well-suited to withstand this type of pressure. The fluid nature of the brain allows it to safely deform within the skull, unlike the restricted compression experienced earlier. As long as there are no other complications like hypoxia, this lateral squeeze on the brain may even be beneficial, perhaps analogous to applying pressure to a wound to aid healing. I have often observed that babies born with a conical head without the prior damage from excessive contractions seem to develop into exceptionally intelligent individuals. It's almost as if this second stage of labor serves as a natural mechanism to mitigate potential damage from the first. Of course, the duration of pushing remains critical; if it extends beyond an hour, the risk of hypoxic damage increases. Pushing is typically a problem only in first time mothers. Subsequent pregnancies are much easier from the pushing perspective with the mom's pelvis having been expanded from prior deliveries.

Overall, the effect of the forces acting on the brain from the 2 phases of labor counteract each other, the cervical dilation phase causes the brain to be pounded in place, by vertical pressure on the brain causing neuron tract damage including but not restricted to the corpus callosum, while the pushing phase typically involves lateral pressure which elongates the brain which helps with healing and redistribution of scarring. Thus in MRI scans on autism brains, while scarring may not be found, DTI MRI scans with fractional anisotropy which is a measure of directionality of water diffusion along white matter tracts shows problems with integrity of white matter, mainly due to damage having been caused by excessive contractions being covered up later in the pushing stage.

FORCES ACTING ON A BABY'S HEAD DURING BIRTH

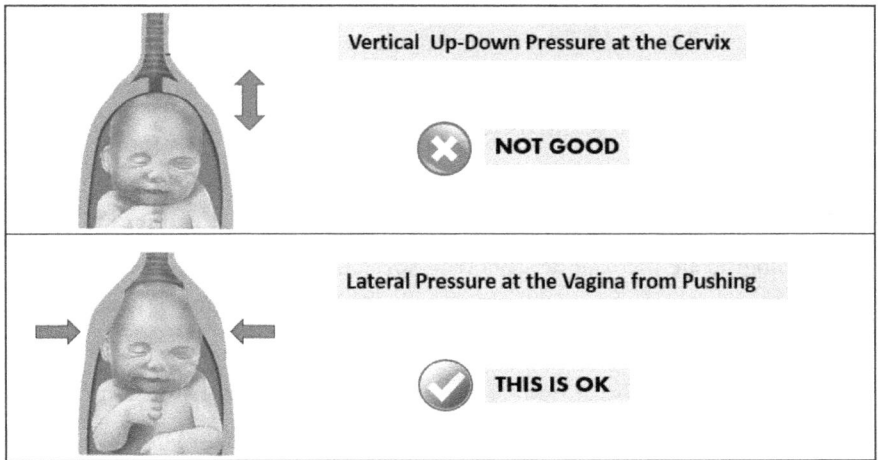

Vertical Up-Down Pressure at the Cervix

NOT GOOD

Lateral Pressure at the Vagina from Pushing

THIS IS OK

Fig 11.4: Schematic diagram showing the effect of the 2 types of pressure in the 2 stages of labor.

Correlating Cause and Effect with MRI Scans

From a forensic MRI perspective, all forces that the brain has been through during birth, needs to be factored in for a full analysis to determine causation. This can be analyzed based on the hospital charts, the contractions the brain was subjected to at birth, the duration of the various stages, the torsion during pushing, the molding of the head, skull fractures any other notations on the records and even from talking to parents involved. For example, if MRI shows gliosis and scarring then it can be deduced that there was not any significant head molding during pushing, or not much pushing was involved.

On the contrary if DTI MRI shows white matter damage, but there is no visible cerebral scarring then it can be verified if prolonged induction was followed by significant pushing it can be reasonably assumed that if the baby had to go through the squeeze of pushing and came out with an elongated head, the MRI scan would typically not find any scarring or gliosis. Any MRI visible scarring or damage in these circumstances might be purely from incidents that occur towards the end of the pushing phase like abuse of forceps or vacuum suction. If the child was subjected to prolonged labor induction and no other scarring is visible, and the DTI MRI shows white matter damage, then it can be determined that the child ended up getting pushed out at birth with a good head squeeze and the damage and scarring sustained from the contraction forces in the cervical dilation stage got dispersed during the pushing stage and thereby invisible to MRI scans.

Radiologists and MRI Interpretation

Radiologists are medical doctors who specialize in interpreting medical images, including those produced by MRI. Radiologists are the detectives in the world of medicine. They play a critical role in unraveling the mysteries of illness and injury within the human body. Just as detectives meticulously examine clues at a crime scene, radiologists scrutinize the intricate details within medical images like X-rays, CT scans, MRIs, and ultrasounds.

Their crucial role involves carefully analyzing the intricate details within MRI scans to identify normal anatomy, detect abnormalities, and ultimately provide a diagnosis or contribute to the overall clinical picture. By recognizing subtle variations in tissue signal intensity, morphology, and contrast enhancement across different MRI sequences, radiologists can differentiate between various pathological conditions, guiding treatment decisions and playing a vital part in patient care. Their expertise allows them to correlate imaging findings with clinical history and other relevant investigations, ensuring a comprehensive and accurate interpretation of the information provided by the MRI examination. Like detectives piecing together fragments of evidence, radiologists correlate imaging findings with the patient's clinical history, symptoms, and other laboratory results to form a comprehensive understanding of the underlying medical issue.

Their expertise allows them to distinguish between various possibilities, rule out certain conditions, and pinpoint the most likely diagnosis. They can identify a tiny fracture invisible to the naked eye, detect the subtle signs of early cancer, trace the path of an infection, or assess the damage caused by trauma. They are the silent witnesses, the expert analysts, and ultimately, the medical detectives who bring clarity to complex clinical cases.

Unfortunately for parents of kids on the autism spectrum, radiologists do not directly consult with patients and the chances of them crossing paths with a neuro radiologist are almost none. Radiologists only analyze the pictures taken by a technician in a radiology lab and provide a written report to the physician that ordered the scan. A head MRI is almost never ordered for newborns unless there were serious complications where neurological impacts are suspected. Of all the medical doctors an autism parent might consult, the only doctors who might order a head MRI scan are neurologists and even they have no way of helping even when brain scarring and damage is detected. The fact that radiologists are also doctors means that the dynamic of doctors protecting other doctors comes into play. Most radiologists are hesitant to come forward and write their findings to the full extent when it might point to malpractice on the part of another physician. Case in point- I went online to a reddit forum of radiology, where I wanted clarification on a few questions, that came to mind as I was writing this chapter and the admin out there refused to post my question. His answer to me was, "this looks like you want these answers so you can sue somebody. Nobody here is going to help you with that". I ultimately was able to find my answers through personal contacts, but this incident opened my eyes to why the cause of autism has remained under wraps for this long. There is resistance from even the detectives that are expected to solve the case for you! Along the same lines I tried to consult with a neuro radiologist who works with trauma and head injury cases from auto and other accidents. There I was told they needed a legal indemnification letter from a lawyer's office and they can't even look at any pictures without a lawyer's office involved. Therein comes a catch 22 situation where lawyers are hesitant to accept a case without evidence and people that can provide the evidence won't do it without a lawyer involved first. This incident again brings to the forefront the hesitancy among radiologists particularly neuro radiologists to come forward with their findings where the stakes are high and legal battles might be involved.

Hence, while neuro radiology is expected to play an important part in identifying autism causation, there exists a systemic resistance to it all from the medical community involved, leading to the perpetuation of the autism epidemic. While the Hospitals wont share patient records particularly if there might be liability involved for them, so unless the patients come forward to directly work with researchers, there could be no solution to this impasse.

Key Take Aways:

1. MRI scans can help differentiate between brain structural variations caused by genetic diseases and changes caused by death of neurons from hypoxic and traumatic brain injuries

2. The types of forces that acted on a baby's head during birth and the damage they might have caused can be correlated based on different sequences of MRI scans and the type of damage that shows up in each.

3. Numerous studies have shown white matter damage in autism but have not gone far enough to correlate these with actual birth records and the birth trauma that caused the white matter damage as laid out in the Pitocin label.

4. Birth involves a complex sequence of events and associated forces acting on the baby's head. Potentially damaging contraction forces during the cervical dilation stage are followed by soothing lateral compression of pushing which works to eliminate scarring from normal MRI visibility. But DTI MRI sequences can detect this type of white matter damage.

5. Radiologists, often considered medical detectives who correlate damage with its cause, frequently hesitate to identify malpractice in their reports, fearing entanglement in legal quagmires, rather than do what is right.

PART III

The Impact of Vaccination on Prior TBI

N umerous parents of children impacted by autism have observed significant retrogression in the skills of their children after vaccinations. If observation is the basis of all science, the scientific community has not been able to provide a satisfactory explanation for this observation. Is it just a case of these observant parents being paranoid or are there other explanations?

CHAPTER 12

How Vaccines Work

In late 2019 – early 2020 when the Covid-19 pandemic hit, it suddenly turned life upside down all over the globe. Almost overnight as a society we suddenly went from one casting doubts on vaccines to one begging for a vaccine to counter a fast-spreading virus. It disrupted life in every part of the world and brought on financial ruin and many unnecessary deaths. It has served as a reminder of how vaccines remain our most potent defense in the fight against viruses.

The knowledge level of common people about vaccines and medical research also hit a new high, making us more aware of the complexities involved in developing a vaccine. Terms like pandemic, herd immunity, zoonotic, immune privilege, immune suppression, etc., that were not common knowledge prior to the pandemic are now more widely understood, making some of my explanations that follow much easier to understand and perhaps even superfluous.

But Covid-19 also brought out varied reactions in people, mostly bringing out the best in people, but it also highlighted the low tolerance some have for the slightest of inconveniences. It has emphasized the desperate need for people to have social interaction for maintaining mental health and sanity. It has also brought to the forefront the varied effects a viral disease can have on different segments of the population. We became aware of the inflammatory syndrome inflicted on children by the Covid-19 virus. We learned of how Covid-19 specifically wiped-out entire Alzheimer wards of senior living facilities while the rest of the facility escaped relatively unscathed.

We also saw bizzare behaviors like Covid-19 parties, proof that the deadly and permanently-debilitating effects of viruses from the past have been completely lost on the current generation. It's a tribute to the success of vaccines while the pandemic has revived memories of the deadly effects of viruses on human life and health.

I see all this as direct evidence of the arguments I am making in the subsequent pages. Viruses continue to play a critical role in shaping human health, as well as mental and physical well-being. They have profoundly influenced human history in both known and potentially unknown ways, a trend that continues today and is expected to persist into the future.

Vaccines and the Immune System

Vaccines have had a checkered past when it comes to safety, and have for a long time been the suspect in the search for the causative factor in autism. Numerous parents have reported massive regression in the development and behaviors of their kids after vaccine doses. There have been many cases where kids that were seemingly developing normally suddenly developed autism symptoms right after their vaccine dose. These occurrences have been the single largest reason why an increasing number of parents refuse to vaccinate their kids. In fact, that is the reason I will dedicate a whole chapter about my observations with vaccinations and their role in the entire autism puzzle. But before we go about looking at causes and effects, it important to know about the immune system and vaccines in general: what vaccines are, what they are made of, and the basic mechanisms used to create these vaccines.

Before looking at vaccines let's review our very simplified representation of the immune system and about how immunity works previously discussed in chapter 3.

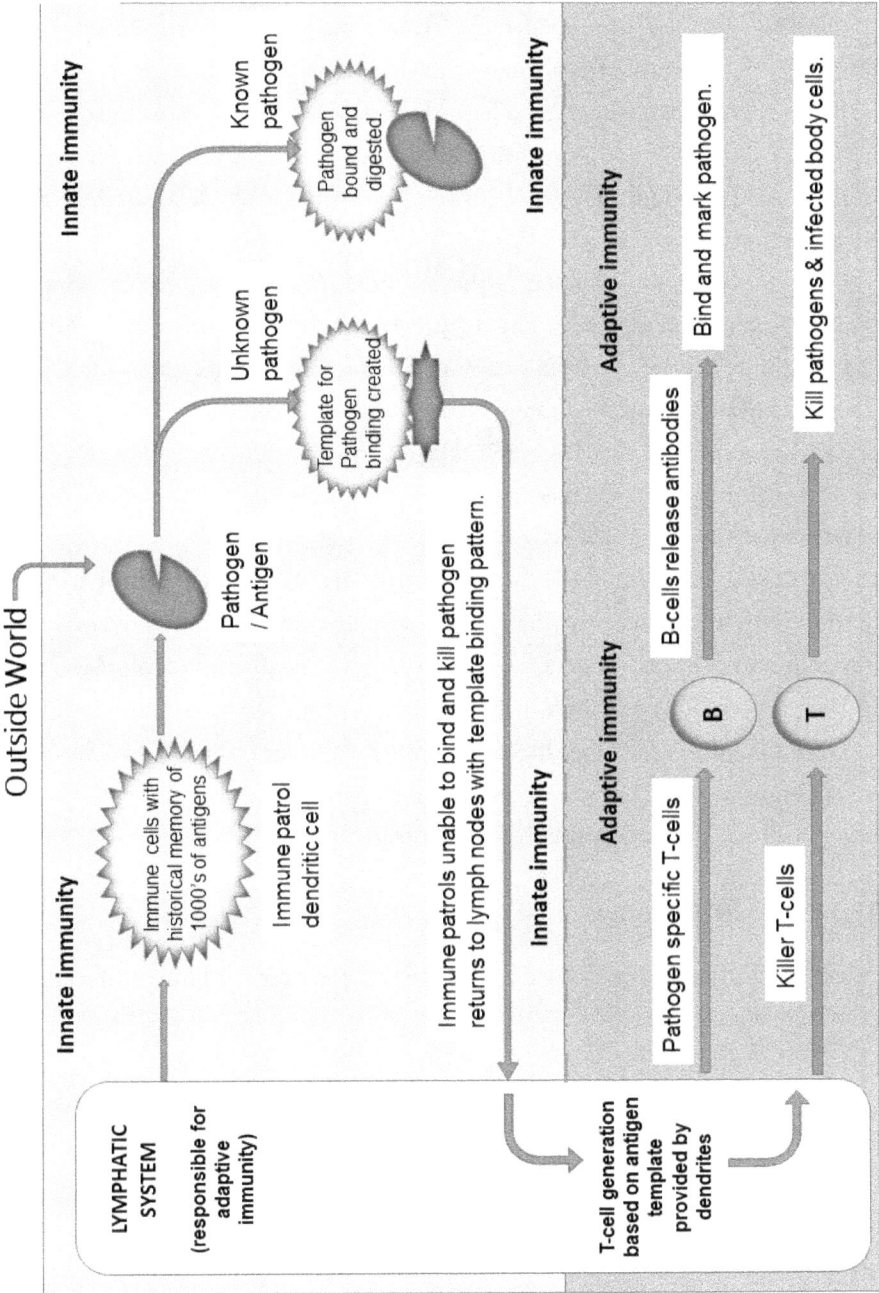

Fig.12.1: Simplified schematic of the immune system (Fig 3.2 repeated)

There's the first line of defense from invading microbes called innate immunity which comes from some of the basic barriers in the human body like skin, fluid in the eye, saliva, etc. These barriers, working alongside the dendritic immune cells at the tissue level with historical evolutionary knowledge capable of distinguishing body cells from invading microbes, provide a certain level of protection called innate immunity.

The second line of defense is the adaptive immune system involving the lymphatic system in the body. This adaptive part of the immune system provides the capability to fight new kinds of invasive microbes that the body has no previous knowledge of.

The concept that there is immunological memory in our bodies to disease-causing viruses and bacteria that can last anywhere from a few days to a few years to a lifetime is what is used to our advantage in designing vaccines. Vaccines are designed to create an immune response in the adaptive part of the immune system. This whole immune response works best when the adaptive immune system is activated by the innate immune system. Modern vaccines typically use small amounts of smaller parts of the virus or viral protein which may not elicit an immune response. Hence vaccines sometimes use other ingredients called adjuvants which help activate the innate immune system against the viral proteins introduced by vaccinations. This helps small doses of vaccine become more effective.

The Types of Vaccines

There are four main types of vaccines based on their composition and strategies used to make them:

- Live, attenuated vaccine
- Inactivated/killed vaccine
- Toxoid (inactivated toxin) vaccine
- Subunit, recombinant, polysaccharide, and conjugate vaccines

Table 12.1. lists the popular vaccines and the category they fall under.

Vaccine Type	List of Diseases
Live, attenuated vaccine:	Vaccinia (smallpox) Measles, mumps, rubella (MMR combined vaccine) Varicella (chickenpox) Influenza (nasal spray) Rotavirus Zoster (shingles) Yellow fever
Inactivated/killed vaccine:	Polio (IPV) Hepatitis A Rabies
Toxoid (inactivated toxin) vaccine:	Diphtheria, Tetanus (part of DTaP combined immunization)
Subunit/conjugate vaccine:	Hepatitis B Influenza (injection) Hemophilus influenzae type b (Hib) Pertussis (part of DTaP combined immunization) Pneumococcal Meningococcal Human papillomavirus (HPV)

Each type has strengths and limitations in its approach to inducing immune memory against specific types of viruses and bacteria.

Viruses cause disease by quickly multiplying to thousands of units per ml inside the body of a natural host. To create weakened viruses for human vaccines, one strategy is to create an active live human virus population and introduce it into a new host or medium like eggs, cultured tissue, or even other animals. Viruses are typically very selective to the host, and a human virus cannot thrive in one of these mediums. However, there tends to be some mutation in some of the original population that allow them to survive and multiply very slowly in this new medium. This creates a slightly modified strain of the original virus, one that is a slow multiplier. The new strain – when re-introduced in the original host – only retains this ability to multiply very slowly and does not have the ability to cause disease. This new strain of vaccines virus is what live vaccines are made up of. However, these so-called weakened vaccine viruses replicate well enough in humans to induce "memory B-cells" that protect against infection of the actual disease virus in the future. The advantage of live "weakened" vaccines is that one or two doses provide immunity that is usually lifelong.

The limitation of this approach is that these vaccines usually cannot be given to people with weakened immune systems.

Killed virus particle vaccines take an entirely different tack. Using this strategy, viruses are completely inactivated (or killed) with a chemical. By killing the virus, it cannot possibly reproduce itself or cause disease, but because the virus is still "seen" by the body, cells of the immune system that protect against disease are generated. Advantages include the fact that the vaccine cannot cause even a mild form of the disease that it prevents and that the vaccine can be given to people with weakened immune systems. However, the limitation of this approach is that it typically requires several doses to achieve immunity. There are also concerns about the quality control and safeguards on the kill process used in manufacturing, where if it's not a hundred percent thorough it could result in the live virus being administered as a vaccine.

A third approach uses bacteria. Some bacteria cause disease by making a harmful protein called a toxin. The toxin invades the bloodstream and is largely responsible for the symptoms of the disease. The protein-based toxin is rendered harmless (the toxin, once inactivated, is called a toxoid) and used as the antigen in the vaccine to elicit immunity. To increase the immune response, the toxoid is added to aluminum or calcium salts, which serve as adjuvants.

Subunit recombinant, polysaccharide, and conjugate vaccines – the fourth type of vaccines – is the classification type for many of the more recently developed vaccines, including DNA and RNA based vaccines. They use only a part of the virus in their design. The vaccine is composed of a protein that resides on the surface of the virus. This strategy can be used when an immune response to one part of the virus (or bacteria) is responsible for protection against disease. In bacterial vaccines it is also possible to use part of the sugar coating (or polysaccharide) of the bacteria. Protection against infection by certain bacteria is based on immunity to this sugar coating (and not the whole bacteria). However, because young children don't make a very good immune response to the sugar coating alone, the coating is linked to a harmless protein (thus a "conjugated polysaccharide" vaccine). In fact, many viral vaccines are also conjugate vaccines where a weak antigen is combined with a strong antigen so the immune response to the weak antigen in the vaccine is strong. One advantage of these subunit vaccines is that they can be given to people with weakened immunity as they don't contain the whole virus and therefore are not capable of causing the disease they vaccinate against. But the limitation of these vaccines is that they often need multiple doses to provide immunity and may require additional booster shots to get ongoing protection.

The reason I am offering this explanation about the making of vaccines is because the argument about the safety of vaccines is an emotionally charged topic. Numerous parents have noticed retrogression of previously mastered skills in their children after vaccinations, and feel strongly about them being the cause. Scientists and authorities keep brushing aside these concerns as coincidental or come up with other feeble excuses. If observation is the basis of all science, then this observation by parents needs to be acknowledged and explained, which has not happened so far. So, the question of vaccination safety for newborn kids remains a hard one for many parents.

Parents who know more about their child's health condition from birth may be in a better position to make informed decisions for their children if they have a better understanding of vaccines. Knowledge of the design and make up of these vaccines equips parents with important details needed for making just such an informed decision. It turns out that opposition to vaccines is typically directed against live virus vaccines and not against some of the others. Understanding why and how that manifests itself in the current controversy requires learning something of the history of vaccines.

Key Take Away: Covid-19's effect on Alzheimer patients reminds us of the devastating effects viruses can have on people with pre-existing brain conditions. The immune response to disease is comprised of innate immunity and adaptive immunity. Vaccines are designed to trigger immunological memory by activating the adaptive part of the immune system. We have seen how vaccines are classified into multiple types depending on how they are synthesized and the different strategies they use to create immune memory.

CHAPTER 13

The History of Vaccines

V accines have come a long way from the time when the first modern vaccines started making their appearance in the nineteenth century. Before then there were practices that amounted to vaccination against smallpox in China as early as 1000 AD and other such ancient practices were also known in Turkey and Africa.

The Enormous Success of Vaccines

The English physician and scientist Edward Jenner is credited with discovering the first modern vaccine in 1796 when he used cowpox (a disease similar to smallpox that infects cows) to create the first smallpox vaccine. Smallpox was known to kill up to 35% of people it infected and leave others scarred and blind. Over the next 200 years developments in vaccines and adoption around the world has resulted in smallpox being effectively declared eradicated from the world.

The practice of developing vaccinations for diseases accelerated after 1885 when French Chemist Luis Pasteur developed the first rabies vaccine. Soon vaccines were developed for numerous debilitating and deadly human diseases including vaccines for typhoid (1899), cholera (1911), diphtheria (1914), tuberculosis (1921), and tetanus (1924). In the mid-twentieth century vaccines for polio (1955), measles (1963), mumps (1967), and rubella (1969) were developed.

The polio vaccine was a classic example where the horrible disease led to its very swift adoption. In 1951 Dr. Jonas Salk discovered a way to create the polio vaccine; in US trials in April 1955, it was shown to be 80-90% effective. The vaccine was approved same day and in production by May 1955. Production methods were adjusted after a brief hiccup where some getting the vaccine were paralyzed, and the vaccine went on to reduce the number of paralytic polio cases to negligible levels within a decade. By 1994 polio was declared eradicated in the Americas.

With such a track record of success, vaccines became the most powerful disease fighting option in the hands of health officials. But typical immunity provided by many vaccines is not 100%. In many vaccines, effectiveness is more like 85-90%, so if an outbreak occurs it's still possible for some vaccinated individuals to be susceptible to disease, which is one reason health officials try to get as many people immunized as possible so as to keep any spread of disease under check. For obvious reasons it is also only possible to eradicate viruses that are exclusive to humans. In cases where the virus crosses over to other species or when the disease agent hides successfully in the environment (like in the case of food or water-borne diseases), it may not be possible to completely eradicate it. Some viruses can be particularly insidious and change frequently. This is the reason why we still need vaccines against some of these dangerous diseases even though many of the worst ones have been successfully eradicated. Vaccination is truly a glaring example of an instance where modern medicine has successfully triumphed over diseases that have plagued human beings for centuries.

While vaccine science has been advancing at a very rapid pace in recent times, our understanding of immunity and vaccines is still vague at best. Vaccines, particularly those involving live weakened viruses, are known to be risky when administered to immune-compromised individuals. On rare occasions they have been known to cause significant adverse reactions even in seemingly healthy individuals. Interestingly, the most significant side effects involve unwarranted immune reactions – immune attacks on specific tissues and cell types in the body. The most dangerous reactions are those that involve the nervous system and heart muscles, including anaphylactic shock. While any reactions might subside over time, certain effects can linger for a lifetime.

The Anti-Vaccine Movement

Opposition to vaccinations has existed for almost as long as vaccinations have existed. In fact, opposition predated vaccine injections during the times when the practice of variolation was the norm. But reasons for opposition have changed and evolved over time. Initially it was against the adverse effects of contaminated vaccines that ended up taking lives. Then there was opposition to the use of animal sources, mixed in with religious beliefs about interfering with God's agenda and fate. Add to this actual patient adverse experiences with vaccines, alternate scientific beliefs, lack of trust in health care professionals and there were plenty of reasons to go around as to why someone might be opposed to vaccines. But the net effect of these movements was that it made vaccines better and helped improve and streamline the vaccine manufacturing and administration process in general.

Fast forward to modern times and you'll find that most opposition to vaccines comes as a result of their implication in causing modern afflictions like allergies, auto immune disorders and autism. Since some of the killer diseases have been eradicated, it might be expected that the number of necessary vaccinations might drop. Instead, more and more diseases have been added to the list, including non-eradicable ones like the flu. These are perceived by some as attempts by the pharma industry to profit from a continuous revenue stream by introducing new and unnecessary vaccines. There are thousands, perhaps millions of viruses out there, and some of them can cause communicable diseases in humans while others keep mutating and crossing over from animals as well. How many diseases to vaccinate against and which ones to assume risk on, are hard to define and an ongoing source of debate.

The profile of the modern parent who has concerns about vaccinations is contrary to what pro-vaccine folks would like to portray them as. Parents who don't vaccinate kids tend to be affluent, better educated and typically people who want to do the right thing for their kids. These people understand the difference between live and other forms of vaccines. Given the absence of evidence or explanation for adverse outcomes these parents do not want their child to be a guinea pig when outcomes are pretty much luck of the draw. Their beliefs are reinforced by parents that notice retrogression of skills in their children after vaccines. As a result, clarifying the circumstances around vaccine injury and helping determine better criteria for vaccine contra-indication is a pressing issue.

Vaccines and Public Health Administrators

There's obviously been a lot of sweat and blood invested into the development of vaccines over the past 200 years and it hasn't come easy. Researchers and health officials who remain exceptionally aware of these struggles and hard-fought gains in the history of vaccine development continue to be the most ardent supporters of vaccines. Achieving a world free of deadly and debilitating diseases like smallpox and polio has been no mean feat, and pro-vaccine supporters fear these victories are being forgotten when the vaccination rates in the population start falling. But what's lost in the pro-vaccine lobby is the understanding that historically, the challenges put forward against vaccines have actually led to improvements in safety and other positive changes in their manufacture, distribution and use. Researchers are now being challenged with achieving what will truly be the next big chapter in the history of vaccines in developing better alternatives to live vaccines (and ridding vaccines of at least some of the allegations that have been lodged against them). In the age of artificial intelligence and genetic engineering this sort of development remains in the realm of possibility, given the right motivation to make it a reality.

At the same time, government public health officials often worry about contagious diseases reaching pandemic proportions – a situation they are tasked with avoiding. In this day and age, diseases can pretty much travel at the speed of airplanes. As Covid-19 has illustrated, controlling an outbreak of disease by isolating it at the source, particularly the very infectious and deadly viruses, can be a very difficult challenge for health officials anywhere in the world. Their options are pretty limited, with the main tools in their arsenal either to quickly figure out a cure or get a vaccine ready that can prevent the spread. There are limits to how much physical methods such as quarantine and controlling other modes of transmission can help.

Vaccines therefore have become a vital part of any government's repertoire of tools to prevent disease pandemics. They have been widely adopted around the world as the primary defense against what are now called 'preventable' diseases. Deadly and debilitating diseases like smallpox and polio have been eradicated thanks to the efficacy of vaccine programs around the world. The cost benefits and incidental benefits have been so real that it's hard to argue against the value they have brought on to modern society. The upside to vaccines are so many that the occasional issues with their use, particularly things like allergies and other side effects, have been relegated to the fringes. Governments simply cannot afford to have people unvaccinated just because of seemingly remote possibility of side effects. They tend to fight really hard against any notion that vaccines are to blame for any injury caused to an individual.

It is widely agreed that vaccine production needs strict quality controls and any lapse could lead to actually giving the disease to the vaccinated (at least in the case of live vaccines). Many such instances have happened throughout the history of vaccines, like when the polio vaccine caused paralysis in the early days of its adoption. In addition, dangerous concoctions have been produced and distributed as vaccines by unscrupulous charlatans in the past, which resulted in deaths and other tragic outcomes. As a result, vaccine production has been brought under the control of government health agencies over time. This has mostly alleviated any risks associated with vaccine production and quality control.

Vaccine Autism Lawsuits and the Omnibus Trial

But like any medicine, vaccines come with a lot of warnings noted on their labels and issues can crop up from time to time. In spite of their vastly improved safety, the warning label states that in certain rare occasions they do cause injury. But when impacted parents started taking on the vaccine manufacturers in court, manufacturers started leaving the business, in turn threatening the vaccine supply of the US. This prompted the US government to intervene with the National Childhood Vaccine Injury Act of 1986. Subsequently the Vaccine Injury Compensation Program (VICP) was created in the U.S. as a no fault alternative to the court system in an effort to bolster the vaccine supply while still providing out of court settlements for the most seriously impacted. The program investigates vaccine adverse effect complaints and approximately one in a million vaccinated cases have been receiving compensation.

In the late 1990s and early 2000s, more and more parents became aware of the program and worries increased about the perceived link between autism and vaccines. This resulted in more claims and increased success of cases regarding autism in vaccine court. Per the hrsa.gov website, in the 29 years from the time of creation in 1988, compensation to the tune of 3.7 billion has been paid.

As I will explain in the next chapter, visible retrogression happens after vaccines are administered in cases where there is prior brain injury. Although they are not the root cause, vaccines were blamed for autism in the early to mid-2000's and the rise in compensation demands threatened to destroy the VICP program. Over five thousand cases had been filed and were pending in US courts against vaccines prior to 2009.

To deal with the influx the government grouped these cases together into 6 representative class action suits and instituted a special court called the "Vaccine Omnibus hearings" to deal with them. The primary complaints were that mercury containing adjuvant (thimerosal) in vaccines and the MMR vaccine were causing autism. The 6 representative cases fell into 3 biological categories: MMR only, thimerosal only and combination of MMR-thimerosal as the cause in autism. The court denied a "preponderance of evidence" in all cases and absolved vaccines of any responsibility for autism. The loss of the plaintiffs in these Vaccine Omnibus hearings in 2010-2011 dealt a severe blow to the anti-vaxxers whose real-world observations did not pass the legal test. But the court did not stop there: they pointed at genetics as the cause for autism based on the defendants arguments rather than say they did not understand the true cause yet. In our world, it seems easiest to blame unknown causes as "genetics" rather than accept the truth as "unknown." This move by the special vaccine court ended up diverting valuable research dollars chasing genetic causes that do not exist.

Key Take Away: Vaccines have been enormously successful in reducing and eliminating the occurrence of a whole host of debilitating diseases in the 20th century. This great success has encouraged the pharma companies, medical community and health officials to push more and more vaccinations on the population, unmindful of the adverse effects they have on certain people. The anti-vaccine movement in modern times has been a response to the adverse effects people believe they suffer as a result of vaccinations, such as allergies and auto immune disorders. The failure of the autism omnibus proceedings in proving vaccines as the cause of autism has further strengthened the hands of the pro-vaccine crowd, while the anti-vaxxers continue to be wary of them due to their observations of retrogression in skills of their kids or occurrence of severe allergies and immune disorders after vaccines.

CHAPTER 14

The Vaccine Double Whammy – Cementing Prior Brain Damage

As much as vaccines have been an enormous success, parents have in many instances seen adverse reactions in their kids after vaccinations. Their views often get written off as nonsense by the pro-vaccine advocates in the media and are dealt with tougher mandates from health officials and the government, making it difficult to avoid vaccinations. After all, vaccine safety has been tested time and time again and adverse reactions are mild in the vast majority of cases while more severe reactions can be attributed to other pre-existing conditions and causes. But it's important to note that the anti-vaxxers are not all irrational idiots like the advocates and health officials and ill-informed media would like to paint them as, but rational everyday folks that were observant enough to notice cause and effect in their kids related to vaccinations. These are mostly people directly impacted by autism and developmental challenges in their kids or their immediate family and friends. The mental effects of autism emerge over a long time-frame as they relate to childhood development and sometimes vaccinations are the trigger for realizing what is really happening.

That was certainly the case with me. My kids were not very verbal when they were vaccinated prior to age 2, and by the time I realized that the 3rd year vaccinations had sent them back much further it had been a few months. The only adverse reactions I immediately noticed were skin rashes in my second son (which we were accustomed to since it had happened every time he received a vaccination). The pediatrician's office prescribed topical creams to take care of it and to our thinking that was the end of the story.

I was unaware of the adverse history of vaccinations in the US and the presence of the VICP and VAERS adverse effect reporting system prior to writing this book. In fact, most parents I have spoken to, do not know of the existence of the VICP or the VAERS programs. Even if I had known about them chances are, I wouldn't have reported anything – it was just a skin rash after all. Parents have to know about autism, anticipate and watch for it carefully at such an early age to be able to notice the effects. Health officials and vaccine advocates often point to the lack of reporting in the VAERS as a factor in their justification of the lack of adverse reactions. But even for the most observant parents the lack of awareness of the existence of these systems and the difficulty in anticipating the invisible mental and psychological effects on kids 3 years old or less is daunting. The cause and effects are hard to identify and correlate; unless you believe autism is caused by vaccines and watch for it, it's hard to catch. If and when retrogression happens by the time you do realize what's happening it's often much later.

The MMR Vaccine

Most vaccines do come with warnings around the potential for injury, but medical practitioners are mostly trained to push vaccines on everyone with their 'vaccines are safe for everyone' mentality and tend to not take any of these warnings into consideration. These vaccines are typically administered by nurses and not doctors, and even if nurses did want to warn patients, they are not allowed to offer medical advice.

Yet the proof of the danger live vaccines like the MMR represent for brain damaged individuals is pretty much hidden in plain sight. The first line of the MMR warnings section clearly states prior brain injury being a risk:

WARNINGS

Due caution should be employed in administration of M-M-R II to persons with a history of cerebral injury, individual or family histories of convulsions, or any other condition in which stress due to fever should be avoided. The physician should be alert to the temperature elevation which may occur following vaccination (see ADVERSE REACTIONS).

Hypersensitivity to Eggs

Live measles vaccine and live mumps vaccine are produced in chick embryo cell culture. Persons with a history of anaphylactic, anaphylactoid, or other immediate reactions (e.g., hives, swelling of the mouth and throat, difficulty breathing, hypotension, or shock) subsequent to egg ingestion may be at an enhanced risk of immediate-type hypersensitivity reactions after receiving vaccines containing traces of chick embryo antigen. The potential risk to benefit ratio should be carefully evaluated before considering vaccination in such cases. Such individuals may be vaccinated with extreme caution, having adequate treatment on hand should a reaction occur (see PRECAUTIONS).{46}

However, the AAP has stated, "Most children with a history of anaphylactic reactions to eggs have no untoward reactions to measles or MMR vaccine. Persons are not at increased risk if they have egg allergies that are not anaphylactic, and they should be vaccinated in the usual manner. In addition, skin testing of egg-allergic children with vaccine has not been predictive of which children will have an immediate hypersensitivity reaction...Persons with allergies to chickens or chicken feathers are not at increased risk of reaction to the vaccine."{47}

Hypersensitivity to Neomycin

The AAP states, "Persons who have experienced anaphylactic reactions to topically or systemically administered neomycin should not receive measles vaccine. Most often, however, neomycin allergy manifests as a contact dermatitis, which is a delayed-type (cell-mediated) immune response rather than anaphylaxis. In such persons, an adverse reaction to neomycin in the vaccine would be an erythematous, pruritic nodule or papule, 48 to 96 hours after vaccination. A history of contact dermatitis to neomycin is not a contraindication to receiving measles vaccine."{47}

Thrombocytopenia

Individuals with current thrombocytopenia may develop more severe thrombocytopenia following vaccination. In addition, individuals who experienced thrombocytopenia with the first dose of M-M-R II (or its component vaccines) may develop thrombocytopenia with repeat doses. Serologic status may be evaluated to determine whether or not additional doses of vaccine are needed. The potential risk to benefit ratio should be carefully evaluated before considering vaccination in such cases (see ADVERSE REACTIONS).

"Due caution" out here is a very vague term. This should mean avoid MMRII for individuals with with brain injury altogether

Fig. 14.1: MMR combined vaccine label

Admittedly the phrase "due caution" in this statement is still pretty vague and only points to stress due to fever and not to direct impacts of live vaccine viruses on an injured brain. Phrases like that lend themselves to faulty interpretation by pediatricians brainwashed into believing vaccines are fine for everybody and people who avoid it are only being irrational. The label should clearly state that the vaccine needs to be avoided for pre-existing brain injury.

Of all the vaccines children are given these days, the measles vaccine holds a special place in the minds of anti-vaxxers. This is due to the observations of immediate retrogressive effects on their children by autism and ADHD impacted parents. My research into the literature helps me come up with the reasons why this is the case.

Viruses that Cross the BBB and Those that Don't

Viral diseases present the scariest of challenges to modern medicine as witnessed in the Covid-19 pandemic. Some viruses are quite harmless and seem to pass through the body without creating a disease or triggering an immune response. Some others cause minor illness until they are fought off by the immune system. Then there are others that can cause severe illness and kill or leave us with long term debilitations. The difference seems to come mostly from whether these viruses have evolved mechanisms to cross the blood brain barrier (BBB) or not. Of course, most viruses would invade the central nervous system (CNS) across the BBB if given the chance as a result of conditions like immunosuppression, severe systemic infection or prolonged presence inside the body. Many viruses are tissue specific and lock on to specific receptors on certain cell types in our body. This is the reason we have different types of diseases each with its own set of symptoms. The following viruses in table 14.1 typically affect certain specific organ systems in the body and come with corresponding symptoms.

Table 14.1 Viruses that affect different parts of the body.

Viruses	Primary Affected Systems	Rare CNS Involvement?
Respiratory Viruses		
Rhinoviruses (Common Cold)	Respiratory (Nasal, Upper Airway)	No
Seasonal Coronaviruses (229E, OC43, HKU1, NL63)	Respiratory (Upper & Lower)	Rare (COVID-19 can cause neuroinflammation)
Influenza A & B	Respiratory (Flu)	Rare (Severe cases may cause encephalopathy)
Parainfluenza Viruses (PIV 1-4)	Respiratory (Croup, Bronchiolitis)	No
Respiratory Syncytial Virus (RSV), Metapneumovirus	Respiratory (Bronchiolitis, Pneumonia)	No
Adenoviruses (Types 1-7)	Respiratory, GI, Conjunctiva	Rare (Certain strains can cause meningitis)

Gastro Intestinal Viruses		
Norovirus, Sapovirus	Gastrointestinal (Viral Gastroenteritis)	No
Rotavirus	Gastrointestinal (Severe Diarrhea)	No
Hepatic Viruses		
Hepatitis C Virus (HCV)	Hepatic (Liver)	Rare (indirect neuro effects in liver failure)
Hepatitis B Virus (HBV)	Hepatic (Liver)	Rare (associated with hepatic encephalopathy)
Hepatitis E Virus (HEV)	Hepatic (Liver)	Rare
Miscellaneous Viruses		
Human Papillomavirus (HPV)	Skin, Mucosa (Warts, Cervical Cancer)	No
Parvovirus B19	Hematologic (Fifth Disease, Aplastic Crisis)	Rare (can cause fetal hydrops)
Human Herpesvirus 7 (HHV-7)	Skin (Roseola-like illness)	Rare
Human T-lymphotropic Virus (HTLV-1, HTLV-2)	Hematologic, Neuromuscular	Rare (HTLV-1 can cause myelopathy)

Most of these viruses lack the specific abilities necessary to directly cross the BBB but may indirectly affect the brain. Any neurological symptoms from these viruses are usually due to immune responses, inflammation, or metabolic dysfunction rather than direct invasion of the brain.

Certain other viruses however have evolved mechanisms where they directly attack the endothelial cells of the BBB. Some use a trojan horse mechanism like infecting immune cells like macrophages that can traverse the CNS, or travel along the peripheral nerves. Viruses like measles and certain arboviruses trigger inflammation causing BBB disruption and thereby gain entry into the brain.

Table 14.2: Key CNS-Infecting Viruses

Virus Family	Examples	Primary CNS Diseases
Herpesviruses	Herpes Simplex (HSV-1, HSV-2) Varicella Zooster (VZV, HHV-3) Epstein-Barr (EBV, HHV-4) Cytomegalovirus (CMV, HHV-5) Human Herpesvirus 6(HHV-6)	Encephalitis, meningitis
Enteroviruses	Poliovirus, Coxsackieviruses (A and B), Echoviruses	Meningitis, poliomyelitis
Arboviruses	West Nile Virus (WNV) Japanese Encephalitis Virus (JEV) Zika Virus Dengue Virus Chikungunya Virus St. Louis Encephalitis Virus (SLEV) Eastern and Western Equine Encephalitis Viruses (EEEV, WEEV) La Crosse Virus	Encephalitis, congenital defects
Rhabdoviruses	Rabies Virus	Fatal encephalitis
Orthomyxoviruses	Influenza	Rare encephalopathy
Paramyxoviruses	Measles, Mumps, Nipah	SSPE, encephalitis, meningitis
Retroviruses	Human Immunodeficiency Virus (HIV)	HAND, opportunistic CNS infections
Arenaviruses	Lymphocytic Choriomeningitis Virus (LCMV)	Meningitis, encephalitis
Bunyaviruses	Rift Valley Fever Virus (RVFV)	Encephalitis
Filoviruses	Ebola, Marburg	Hemorrhagic encephalopathy
Coronaviruses	SARS-CoV-2	Neuro inflammation, Altered BBB

As we can see, the more dangerous and deadly diseases are caused by viruses that can cross the BBB, into the immune privileged areas of the brain. These are also the main diseases that we vaccinate against. These vaccines, particularly the live vaccines of these BBB crossing viruses remain the subject of controversy in autism causation, which is a brain development disorder.

Vaccines & Viral Latency – Viruses that Come and Never Leave

The measles virus, like the polio virus and certain others, is capable of attacking the endothelial cells that form the blood brain barrier directly and get past the tight junctions of the endothelial cells of the barrier. As a result, the measles virus establishes a lifelong latency in the neuron cells of the body. Viral latency is known to inhibit/consume the nerve growth factor (NGF) at least in the case of Herpes Simplex[14.1] (HSV1) and could be similar with measles, which at the early ages potentially stops brain development in its tracks and turns the clock back on development. Such a lifelong latency could result in enduring effects for the life of the impacted individual.

Viral latency can even occur in the neuron cells of the brain, when the live virus in the live vaccine interacts with the neuron cells of the brain, by getting past a damaged blood brain barrier. Such latency is probably causing what is sometimes referred to as mitochondrial dysfunction. Mitochondria are organelles in the cells that are responsible for generating cellular energy molecules called ATP. There are other very important functions including cellular signaling functions that mitochondria are involved in. When viral latencies resulting from the compromised blood brain barriers of a damaged brain interact with these various functions in neuron cells, they cause whole body dysfunctions at various levels, including brain fog, lethargy/hyperactivity, and general neuro muscular weakness in individuals suffering from autism from traumatic brain injury at birth.

Some of the viruses that infect the human body (particularly the herpes virus family but also many other virus types) establish a lifelong latency and never get eradicated from the body. This leaves open the possibility that they become active later in life or just sit around in certain body cells causing other diseases where the causative factors haven't been established. They do this by putting out material in cell cytoplasm (episomal latency) or by injecting material in the DNA in the cell nucleus (proviral latency). Certain viruses of the herpes virus family (Herpesviridae) including chicken pox, Herpes simplex viruses (HSV-1, HSV-2), Human herpes virus 6 (HHV-6A, HHV-6B) all establish episomal latencies in neuron cells and are suspected in a lot of diseases where the disease associations haven't been proven. Proviral latency is the reason the HIV-AIDS virus has remained almost impossible to completely cure.

Interestingly, it's not only the live vaccines that come with this warning, but even other vaccines like DTP come with a warning of neurological side effects. In these cases, it's potentially the immune response, fever and predisposition to seizures that seem to be a factor. This is where the risk of high fevers that can literally 'fry the brain' causing damage, becoming the cause of neurological issues. However, in these cases, the effects may not bring on lifelong debilitations. Only live viruses capable of surviving in immune privileged areas affecting neurons and establishing a neuronal latency are suspects in stopping of the brain healing processes following exposure to them.

Needless to say, live vaccines as an immunization strategy definitely need to be re-considered. These live vaccines and their production methods have remained the same for decades and in the wake of newer developments in the areas of protein and genetic engineering it's time to re-engineer them to be non-live virus vaccines. But until a way around live vaccines is found; they are probably still something that will stay with us as the preferred method of health officials. It's true that alternate methods do not afford the lifelong immunity that live vaccines provide, but lifelong immunity also means introduction of viruses that establish a latency in the body of the immunized.

Autism Cemented by Live Vaccine Virus & TBI interaction

Dealing with 2 kids on the spectrum and by virtue of my first-hand observation of their development right from pregnancy and birth – combined with my research into anything and everything out there that could help identify the roots of my kids' problems – have led me to arrive at some conclusions on the exact etiology of their condition. My kids sustained traumatic brain injury by way of Pitocin abuse. Even though they were already delayed as a result of their birth injuries, their damaged brains tried to recover and they were beginning to show some progress with language and interaction. The vaccinations they were subjected actually kept sending them backwards at every stage with the eventual loss of those minimal verbal interactions after the third-year vaccinations. Looking back, they were improving and showing signs of progress but then retrogressed with every bout of vaccinations until we stopped vaccinations when my second boy was age 3. To this day we still notice some retrogression of skills and increase in behaviors after bouts of simple viral illnesses like the common cold. Now of course it is obvious to me that the interaction of viruses with their brains is having an impact.

We had some viral antibody testing done on our boys where we found my first son had a high level of measles antibodies while my second boy had a high level of HHV6 (Human Herpes Virus 6) antibodies. While measles antibodies might be from the vaccine viruses, the HHV6 is a virus that pervades about 98-100% of all human populations without causing adverse reactions. We now keep them on long term antiviral medication which helps them with their stimming behaviors and helps them focus better. Such antiviral medications are not a cure and do not result in the reversal of the damage caused by vaccines and autism; indeed, they offer only a slight improvement compared to the significant retro-gressions suffered after vaccinations.

Having talked to numerous parents about their experiences leads me to the conclusion that vaccines are the second part of a double whammy on a child's brain in the early years of life reinforcing the brain injuries at birth that are the cause of autism. Kids suffering brain damage during the birth process begin to recover (with girls recovering better than boys due to the brain protective nature of estrogen and potential redundancy in brain functionality in girls). But vac-cinations stop that recovery in its tracks (particularly the live vaccines which alter the brain protein chemistry in unfavorable ways).

A damaged brain with large areas of injury sustained at birth is a maze of dead and damaged neurons, scar tissue, reduced blood flows, and a compromised blood brain barrier, lodged inside a body working hard to grow new pathways to heal the damage. The glial cells of the brain are responsible for both brain im-munity and the local wound healing process. Glial scars are required to seal the site of injury, protect the damaged neural tissue, prevent an overwhelming inflammatory response, and to re-establish the blood brain barrier. But these same scars are known to inhibit the regrowth of neurons through the damaged areas.

The compromised blood brain barrier and scar tissue might represent entry points where viruses might penetrate the CNS including immune privileged areas like the white matter. Live vaccines and other ubiquitous worldly viruses potentially become firmly entrenched in immune privileged areas, scar tissue and other low blood supply areas of the damaged brain and successfully hide away from the reach of the body's antibody defense mechanisms. In this safe environment of the damaged brain, these viruses might also keep multiplying at a slow rate and keep spilling virus particles into the active parts of the brain and body, triggering constant antibody responses. It is possible that neurons surrounded by the constant presence of either virus or virus antibodies are deprived of nutrients and inputs required for their proper functioning. It is also possible the virus or antibody particles interfere with the synapses connecting neurons by accumulating at these electrically rich junctions, thus impeding electrical impulse signals from traveling through critical connection routes in the already damaged brain, resulting in the worsening of brain functionality with viral exposure. Add to this the ACAID phenomenon described earlier about how viruses can obtain whole body immune privilege by entering certain vital areas of the body and you can see why viruses in any form are potentially catastrophic for children with autism from traumatic brain injury.

There could be further complexities in how these mechanisms actually work. For example, it's known that viruses like measles already have a brain impact listed as one of their effects on the body. The statistics say 33 out of every 100,000 individuals who actually got measles end up with CNS damage and mental retardation. Diseases like measles, chicken pox etc., are known to permanently change your body by establishing a latency, causing long term effects like allergies in a person that previously did not have such allergies. The measles vaccine actually contains 13 different known variants of the measles causing virus, which might cause this allergy effect to be magnified even further. These allergies (particularly the food allergies) in turn obstruct the absorption cycles of vital nutrients by the body, resulting in an imbalance of chemicals in the body and brain. Such interference in absorption functions by these gut allergies at a critical time in brain development could then be another mechanism that can further negatively impact the body's attempts at recovery from brain injury. The relationships between TBI and gut dysbiosis have now been borne out by numerous recent studies, even in adults[14.4, 14.5]. Fig 14.2. summarizes this interaction between viruses possibly including the weakened live viruses found in live vaccines and the damaged brain and a pathway for vaccines and viruses in general to compound autism.

Autism from TBI at Birth Compounded by Viral Interactions

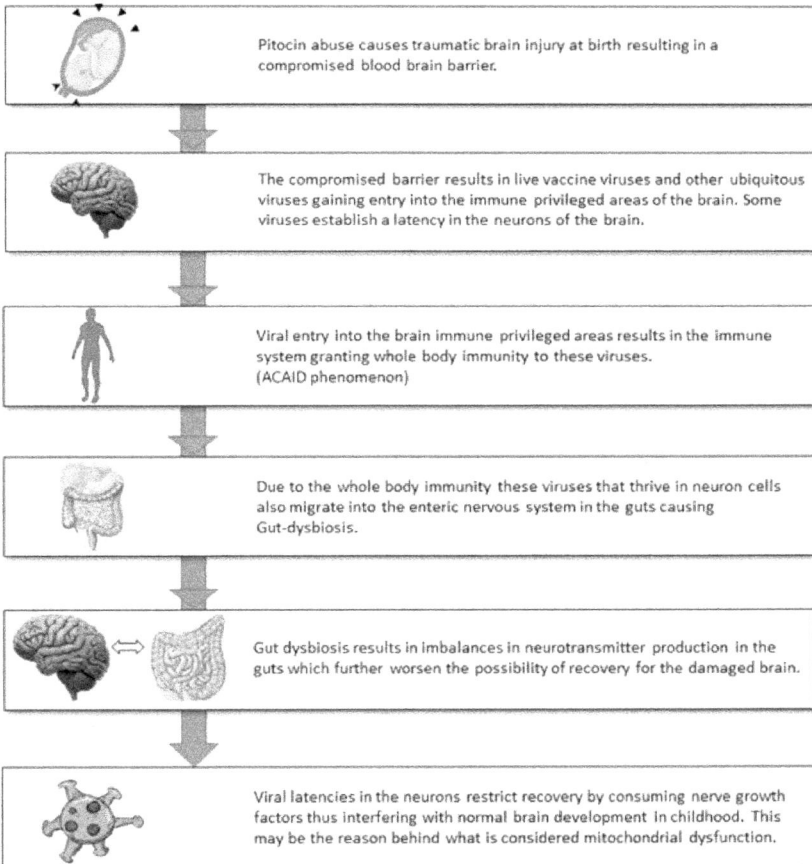

Pitocin abuse causes traumatic brain injury at birth resulting in a compromised blood brain barrier.

The compromised barrier results in live vaccine viruses and other ubiquitous viruses gaining entry into the immune privileged areas of the brain. Some viruses establish a latency in the neurons of the brain.

Viral entry into the brain immune privileged areas results in the immune system granting whole body immunity to these viruses. (ACAID phenomenon)

Due to the whole body immunity these viruses that thrive in neuron cells also migrate into the enteric nervous system in the guts causing Gut-dysbiosis.

Gut dysbiosis results in imbalances in neurotransmitter production in the guts which further worsen the possibility of recovery for the damaged brain.

Viral latencies in the neurons restrict recovery by consuming nerve growth factors thus interfering with normal brain development in childhood. This may be the reason behind what is considered mitochondrial dysfunction.

Fig 14.2: Viral interaction with pre-existing brain injury, causing gut-dysbiosis.

Thus, live vaccine viruses, inflammatory responses and antibody interference might actually have an impact on early brain development, particularly where a previously damaged brain is involved. This explains why only a small fraction of parents observe retrogression of skills in their kids after vaccination and why only certain people are impacted (and not everybody reacts the same way to vaccination). These impacted kids might have recuperated from their brain damage had they not been subjected to a constant barrage of viral vaccines in early childhood, coinciding with the time of maximum brain development. This period is also the window during which the maximum possibility for recovery from brain injury exists. Thus, in cases of pre-existing brain injury vaccines actually represent the second blow to a developing brain causing the autism epidemic.

Diseases, Vaccines and Allergies

Most vaccines come with warnings of allergies including rare occurrence of anaphylactic shock. The science behind immunity, vaccines and their interactions with our bodies is very complex, but the logical explanation to vaccine related allergy effects is actually straightforward. Some viruses pass through our bodies without causing disease. They lack the right protein structure to invade our body cells and trigger an immune response. Some others evade the immune system by staying benign. Then some others have proteins that help them invade certain body cells and replicate out of control triggering disease and an immune response.

Some viruses are eliminated from the body by the immune system, and some others continue to hide in our bodies establishing episomal and proviral latencies in certain cells of our bodies as described previously. In cases where the viruses are completely eliminated from the body, the immune memory doesn't typically last too long. That's simply the way the human body is designed and the way the immune system works. A long term continuous inflammatory immune response is detrimental to the body and the immune system itself. Once the invading antigen is subdued, the immune response is scaled back and the activated immune system becomes inactive with innate immunity taking over.

Some diseases like measles and chicken pox provide lifelong immunity, simply because the virus becomes latent and continues to hide in certain parts of the body and have to be continuously kept under check by the immune system. The immune system achieves this by maintaining a high level of antibodies to the disease at all times. This maintenance of higher levels of antibodies is the reason for long term allergies. Shingles for example is a disease caused by the re-activation of the chicken pox (varicella) virus later in life when the immune system loses its grip on the virus.

My observation has been that diseases which produce long term immunity also cause allergies that stay for the life of the individual. Due to their establishing latency in the body and the need for long term suppression, the affected persons immune system itself gets changed in ways that result in a lifetime of allergies. Thus, long term immunity equates to a lifetime of allergies. If such allergies happen due to viral latencies in the neurons of the brain and the enteric neurons of the gut, due to pre-existing brain damage, the result can be an exacerbation of autism symptoms and prevention of damage healing.

The deal with vaccines is that vaccine manufacturers, health officials and everybody else for that matter, want vaccines to provide lifelong immunity. Nobody wants to be getting frequent vaccines (getting frequent vaccines itself has been shown to be counterproductive). Long term efficacy is actually difficult to create, so manufacturers add numerous other ingredients to the vaccines to achieve a high level of immune response and that long term immunity. Unfortunately, such immunity is achieved from a constant high level of antibodies and the result is the accompanying allergies and inflammatory diseases.

What Should Parents Do?

The compulsions of modern society where mothers are part of the workforce also means newborn infants and babies are forced into daycare where they can unwittingly spread diseases to epidemic proportions. The modern answer to this problem has been to vaccinate kids. The sheer number of diseases and vaccines a current-day human infant will be vaccinated against has grown 10-fold since the 80's. While any disease left undiagnosed, unsupported or untreated can turn deadly, it has become a matter of schedule and convenience to vaccinate. But with the vaccine autism relationship making headlines parents with awareness of adverse effects have begun making a choice not to vaccinate. The truth remains that nobody wants to become a part of the minority statistic, where a disease turned deadly or end up with a lifelong debilitation for their child. Most parents are caught up in the conflicting information about the vaccine autism relationship and the need to protect their babies from debilitating and life-threatening diseases.

Modern hygiene standards and family circumstances can allow some of these vaccines to be delayed. In cases where a mom, dad or other caretaker are looking after a new born at home, it may be possible to work with a pediatrician to delay some of the live virus vaccines. However, if a child is going to be in a day care situation, parents' options may be limited, which is where their knowledge and commonsense becomes paramount. The vaccine schedule is made with the earliest possible vaccine administration ages in mind. The Center for Disease Control (CDC) publishes a vaccination schedule and also possible contra-indications to vaccines. It is advisable for parents to go through the schedule, study the contra-indications, identify the live vaccines in there and figure out the best course of action for them with their pediatrician with due consideration of the birth circumstances. The caveat is most pediatricians are trained about the positives of vaccination and not the other side of the story. You may have to interview them for their point of view.

The real risk and most important factor with the vaccine decision for your child is the potential for reinjuring their brains due to the live virus found in many vaccines. Some criteria for new parents looking to vaccinate your babies is to look back at your birth experience for possibilities of brain damage:

- Were you induced for more than 4-5 hours?
- Did you have severe blood pressure/ gestational diabetes issues?
- Was the baby premature for any reason where doctors suspected neuro issues?
- Did the mother have infections/fevers during pregnancy?
- Were you C-sectioned due to fetal distress of any kind?

While not be an exhaustive list, if you answered yes to any of these questions, then it is possible your child has brain damage. As a parent you know if you had a traumatic birth for any reason, in which case it might make sense to wait on the live vaccines and any other vaccines like DTP with listed neurologic side effects until after age 6, by which time brain development is past the phase of maximum development. By then you would know for sure if the child has recovered from any possible brain injury sustained at birth. If a child has development issues past age 6 in spite of not being subjected to live vaccines, you might consider keeping him or her away from vaccines for the rest of their lives and hope they get 'herd protection' from these viruses by way of healthy individuals around them being all vaccinated.

Parents and pediatricians need to be aware of the arguments for and against vaccinations and make an informed decision on a case-by-case basis. There is absolutely no reason for parents that had a natural, trouble-free pregnancy and birth to keep their kids away from vaccines. In their case the effects of getting the disease are far worse than the effects of the vaccines. Indeed, it's the responsibility of those fortunate parents who had a problem-free delivery or had expert OB/GYNs that helped navigate their pregnancy and delivery without brain damage to vaccinate their kids so as to offer herd protection to the unfortunate ones that suffered brain damage at birth.

Key Take Away: While vaccines may not be directly responsible for autism, when pre-existing brain damage exists, vaccines and their interactions with a previously damaged brain results in further reduction in brain capacity that is noticed by parents as retrogression in development. This is particularly true of live vaccines like measles where the viruses create a neuronal viral latency. Pediatricians, medical providers and health officials need to stop being obstinate about vaccinating all kids and instead take into consideration birth trauma circumstances and (at the least) avoid live vaccines for such high-risk kids.

PART IV

The Learning

In this section we learn about the four different "tracks" of complications which are the true causes leading to autism and related disorders. We also investigate the possible treatment options based on our understanding of the causes. While a complete recovery may not be possible, with the current state of medical technology, it is important to foster and advocate for new technologies that pursue the possibility of a full recovery.

CHAPTER 15

The Multiple Pathways to Perinatal Brain Injury and Autism

In talking to other impacted parents over the years and based on my own knowledge of what happened to my boys, I have been able to draw conclusions on the different causative pathways to autism and other neurological disorders. I have put together my conclusions based on some probing questions I had asked other parents and their descriptions of their circumstances and experience from pregnancy through birth and beyond. The actual percentage of cases in each pathway is based on my small sampling of data, so that could vary if studied at a more regional or national level, although it is probably still ballpark. The more I have investigated these questions, the more I realize the answers can only come from impacted parents. Research studies are typically focused on specific causative factors while (as you will see here) the causes are just as much a broad spectrum of reasons as the consequences are. These causes and diagnosis can come over prolonged periods of time, which can only be pinned down by parents and caregivers associated with the impacted individual over the entire period. Obstetric malpractice also plays a significant role, something academic research never wants to touch with a 10-foot pole.

I have identified the following four broad causative pathways into which I can categorize most of the causes of neurodevelopmental challenges in children. Three of these lead to the condition of autism with the fourth. But once the cause is known then it becomes a disease not a disorder. So lets address that in the next few pages. These tracks in order of frequency of occurrence would be as follows.

1. **Traumatic Brain Injury at Birth, from abusive interventions.**

   a. Induced contractions beyond the 72 contraction count limits prescribed by the ACOG, continued all the way to vaginal delivery or late C-section after too many contractions.

   b. Unaddressed hypertonic contractions during induction.

   c. Forceps or vacuum extraction: These instruments can cause head injuries if used improperly.

2. **Perinatal Hypoxic brain injury from numerous birth conditions.**

   d. Nuchal umbilical cord around the baby's neck causing hypoxic ischemia in utero.

   e. Fetal distress during natural labor, or labor induction.

   f. Sent to emergency C-section upon detection of fetal distress during check-up.

   g. Placental abruption during labor or labor induction.

   h. Meconium aspiration creating undetected respiratory distress in the first few weeks of life.

   i. Very premature birth with undeveloped lungs

3. **Abnormal chemical or biological uterine environment during pregnancy.**

   j. Maternal medications during pregnancy, including hormonal, psychiatric and others including those deemed safe for pregnancy.

   k. Maternal uterine infections and sickness during pregnancy

   l. Extreme mental stress of the mother during pregnancy

   m. Severe gestational diabetes in mother.

   n. Extremely high blood pressure in mother.

   ▸ TBI at birth caused by obstetric negligence (50%)
   ▸ Non-Autistic Genetic Disorders (10%)
   ▸ Maternal complications during pregnancy (10%)
   ▸ Natural delivery trauma at birth (30%)

While there is no preventing genetic disorders, the others are causes that expert OB/GYNs can help their patients successfully navigate through with proper pregnancy and obstetrics care; indeed, minimizing these risks is one of the reasons people go to hospitals for birth in the first place. Figure 15.1 summarizes the four major neuro disorder tracks.

The DSM definitions of the autism spectrum have changed over time and they are now in their 5th iteration. I believe this is due to trying to define it from the symptomatic side instead of trying to name it from the root cause side of the issue. This kind of root cause diagnosis-based naming may help doctors identify and treat the causes of the symptoms better, resulting in earlier intervention and better outcomes for the impacted individuals. For example, symptoms are slightly different based on the circumstances causing the autism. Boys with traumatic brain injury from Pitocin abuse tend to have more behavior issues (e.g. flapping and visual and vocal stimming) compared to boys with hypoxic damage from cord complications. Boys with hypoxic damage tend to have more memory, learning, anxiety, anger control issues, while the problem with boys with traumatic brain injury tends to be one of hyperactivity and lack of focus more than memory or ability to learn. Traumatic brain injury tends to impact language ability a lot more than hypoxic damage.

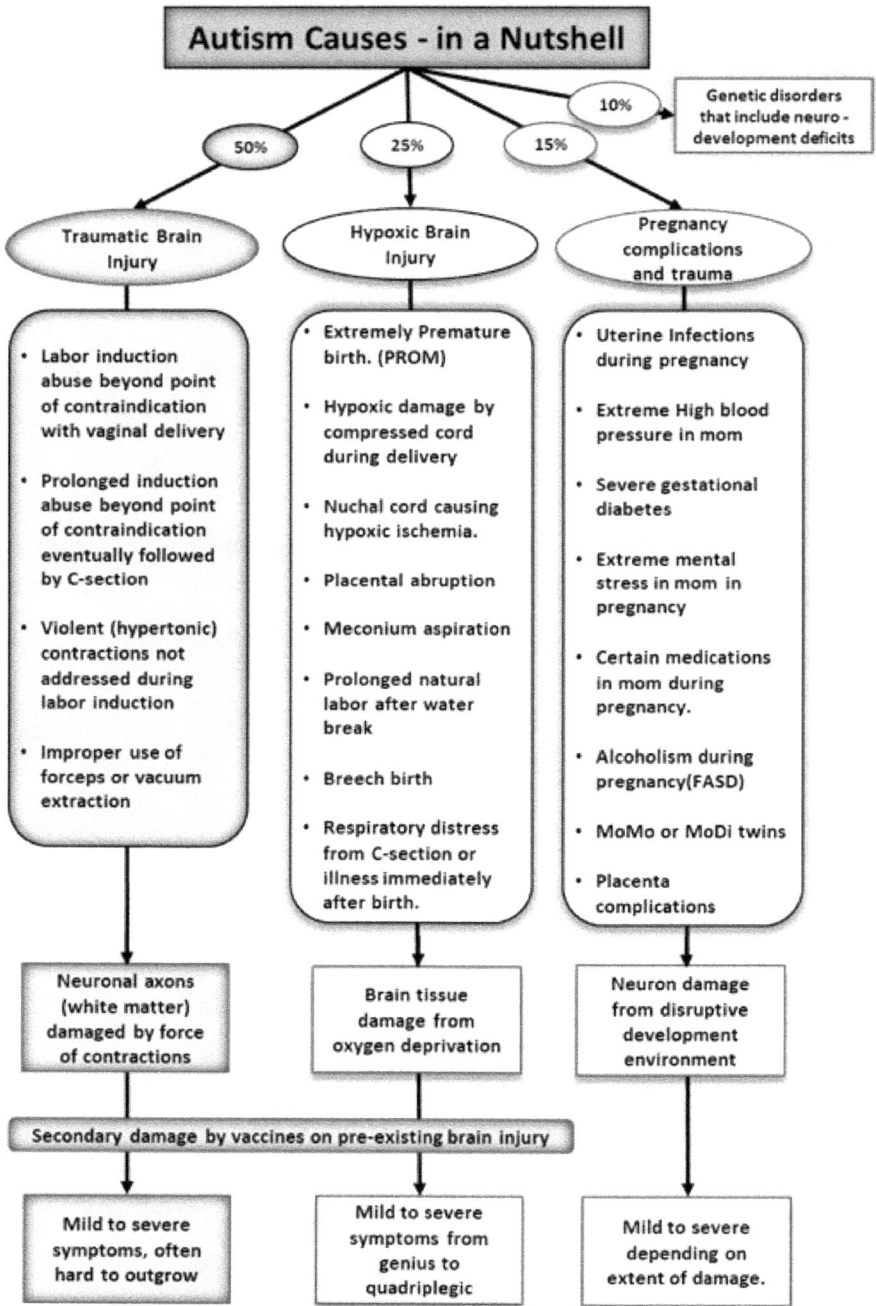

Fig. 15.1: Illustration of the various tracks.

In order to better explain the causes of autism and remove confusions related to attributing autism to genetic causes, I propose the following four new categorizations of autism for the four paths identified above, making these more of diseases with known etiology vs disorder of unknown origins. Such categorization might help better diagnostics and more effective treatment of these separate causes of brain damage

Genic-Autism: Genetic mutations causing neurodevelopmental disorders in a child. A more formal definition would be "neurodevelopmental disorder traceable to genetic deficiencies."

Gestic-Autism: Gestational or pregnancy complications creating developmental disorders in a child. A more formal definition would be "a neurodevelopmental disorder on the Autism spectrum traceable to complications during pregnancy."

Hypoxic-Autism: Birth complications creating developmental disorders in a child. A formal definition would be "a neurodevelopmental disorder on the Autism spectrum traceable to complications during birth."

Tebic(T.B.I)-Autism: Perinatal (at or near birth) traumatic brain injury or iatrogenic brain injury resulting in developmental disorders in a child. A formal definition would be "a neurodevelopmental disorder in the Autism spectrum traceable to faulty interventions, leading to traumatic brain injury to the child during delivery"

Path 1: Genic Autism

Genetic causes are usually beyond the control of people and science and a matter of destiny. They are known to happen as a result of in-breeding within a genetic pool. Correlations have been established, which point to genetic damage from environmental chemicals, viruses or age of parents. Sometimes there are genetic traits that run in families. But modern science can tailor specialized cures in some cases using gene therapies where the cause is identified by gene mapping, within the genome of the impacted individual. The percentage of these cases among the total population have remained fairly small and very constant over time. Only a small subset of genetic disorders cause neurodevelopmental deficits. Their symptoms tend to be very different from autism, but they are often confused with Autism due to symptomatic definition of autism and similarities in how they impact neurodevelopment.

Down's Syndrome: This is the most common genetic abnormality with mental health implications and occurs in about 1 in 1000 individuals. Normally people have 23 pairs of chromosomes in the nucleus of their body cells. Down's syndrome happens when an extra full or partial copy of chromosome 21 appears in the cells of the person due to the genetic copy process going wrong at conception. It causes distinctive features in the eyes and nose, smaller ears, hands, legs and other conditions affecting mostly hearing, the heart, and sleep. Their health challenges can sometimes keep them from living a long life and they sometimes have learning difficulties, but children with the condition are capable of speech and even achieve limited independence in adulthood. Its occurrence has been correlated to the age of the mother. However, the same mother can have subsequent babies that don't have the syndrome, which makes it despite such correlation a pure game of chance. Down's syndrome is not autism but approximately 20% of kids with it are also said to have an autism diagnosis.

Screening for presence of Downs syndrome during pregnancy is now available and utilized almost routinely along with screening for other birth defects in many parts of the world. At about 10-14 weeks of pregnancy an ultrasound to detect fluid collection at the back of the baby's neck, combined with maternal blood testing is used as an indicator. Genetic testing of amniotic fluid in the 15-20 weeks of pregnancy using a procedure called amniocentesis can confirm the presence of this syndrome and others. Parents mostly opt to abort the pregnancy if such a defect is detected and this has resulted in a ethical dilemma and debate in many countries. Some other countries have claimed total elimination of Downs syndrome births as a result of such testing.

Craniosynostosis: The human skull (cranium) is composed of 22 different bones encasing the brain and forming the facial features. Of these, 8 bones are cranial bone plates that encase the brain. These are held together by unique joints called sutures, which are made of thick connective tissue. They're irregularly shaped, allowing them to tightly join all the uniquely shaped cranial bones. The sutures don't fuse until adulthood, which allows your brain to continue growing during childhood and adolescence. Craniosynostosis is a malformation that involves the early closure of one or more sutures of the skull, usually prior to birth. Craniosynostosis may occur in isolation or this condition may be associated with other abnormalities as part of a syndrome.

There are close to 200 known genetic disorders which include craniosynostosis as one of the effects. These syndromes are primarily differentiated by the type of suture and gene mutation involved. One in 2500 births are known to involve craniosynostosis. Natural birth requires that these bones be separable so that they can take the right shape to help the baby make it safely through the birth canal without injury to the brain. Fused cranial plates at birth can result in brain injury through crushing and deformation of the head. Some of the underlying conditions that cause craniosynostosis can also cause neurodevelopmental disorders.

Dyslexia: Dyslexia is a learning disorder that involves difficulty reading due to problems identifying speech sounds and learning how they relate to letters and words (decoding). Also called reading disability, dyslexia affects areas of the brain that process language. It tends to run in families which is why it is categorized as a genetic disorder. Studies supported by the UK MRC, the Wellcome Trust, Yale and the NIH have identified a few genes responsible for the learning disability. Just as in autism it can involve speech deficiencies in addition to reading. However, speech difficulty in autism tends to be due to lack of focus and slow processing speed rather than underlying language reading abilities. It is said that about 1 in 4500 newborns is diagnosed with dyslexia.

There are over 250 other genetic defects like fragile X syndrome that are very rare, each with its own specific set of symptoms, some including impacts to brain development. Underlying genetic conditions can also cause several neurodegenerative and metabolic conditions that slowly progress over time. One final class genetic disorder that merit mention here are the brain cephalies, many of which are listed in Figure 11.1 in the chapter on MRI as they are easily identified by MRI scans. One interesting example of a microcephaly is the *Microcephaly-capillary malformation (MIC-CAP) syndrome.* The MIC-CAP syndrome is caused by a mutation in the STAMBP gene causing microcephaly, an abnormally small head resulting from problems with brain development during pregnancy. Mutations to this gene can result in cells dying during development, affecting the entire development process.

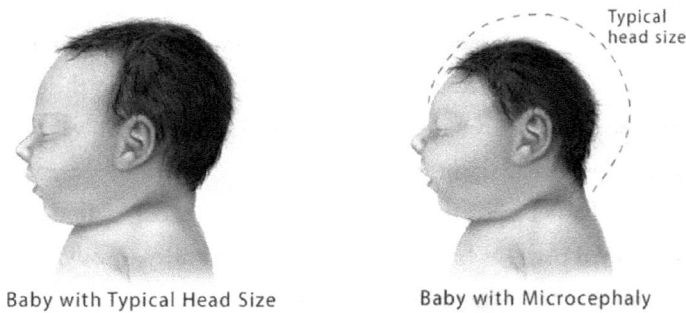

Baby with Typical Head Size   Baby with Microcephaly

Fig. 15.2: Difference in head sizes normal vs microcephaly.

Microcephaly is also caused by various other factors and it is distinct from autism or any of the other typical developmental disorders. Kids with autism have normal head sizes and exhibit no other bodily disorders except those stemming from brain damage and related malfunctioning.

***Maternal genetics vis-à-vis pregnancy*:** This is the only real genetic issue that is fairly widespread and is a cause of autism symptoms in some children. This has to do with the ability of the mother to support the baby in the third trimester of pregnancy. Some mothers have traits running in the family where they have a tendency to lose the fetus late in the pregnancy. The exact causes are unclear, but it could be due to various circumstances mostly related to placental issues (and brain damage is typically caused by insufficient oxygen that is supplied through the placenta and the umbilical cord). This typically results in the death of the baby, but in the rare occasion that this is caught ahead of time during an office visit where the baby is already in distress, the result could be a baby with hypoxic/ischemic brain damage with an eventual autism diagnosis.

Path 2: Gestic Autism

Maternal Complications: It is traditional wisdom and common knowledge that pregnant women need to be well cared for, with good food and emotional support during her pregnancy to ensure the best outcomes for the baby. Recent studies in the field of epigenetics suggest that a mother's experiences and habits during pregnancy can play a role in activating or de-activating genes in the fetus, which can play a significant role in the future life of the baby. A lot of these changes show up in the long term and do not impact the immediate birth outcome significantly. This is also the reason modern medicine recommends prenatal vitamins to ensure there are no chances of vitamin deficiencies in mothers as these can impact fetal development.

A pregnant woman's body undergoes a lot of changes as it prepares for the nourishment, growth and delivery of a baby. Some pregnancy related changes in the mother's body, like developing high blood pressure or gestational diabetes or both can happen and they can have impacts on the fetus and birth. In most cases, the impacts of maternal complications are small, and a lot of times impacted kids are able to speak, but have other characteristics like social anxiety, emotional extremes and such. These are diagnosed as higher functioning autism, but in worst case scenarios when the mother contracts diseases such as cytomegalovirus infection, herpes simplex virus infection, rubella, hepatitis B, syphilis or some food borne illnesses such as listeriosis or toxoplasmosis, it can result in serious negative outcomes for the baby including mental retardation, microcephaly, cerebral palsy, or even stillbirths. Zika is one such new virus that made headlines for the impact it had on brain growth in babies of pregnant mothers who contracted the illness. When there is no occurrence of any of these effects, maternal complications mostly result in milder forms of development delays which can be treated very well with early intervention programs.

High blood pressure: High blood pressure during pregnancy if not stress-related is mostly an attempt by the mother's body to ensure the fetus is adequately supplied with oxygenated blood and nutrients. It can be a reflection of how strongly the placenta is attached to the blood supply and how well supplied it really is. As the baby grows bigger, the demands on the mother's body to keep it supplied with nutrients increases as well. If the placenta for some reason is not tapped well enough into the mother's blood supply through the uterus then it can result in the body trying hard to compensate by a higher blood pressure. Thus, high blood pressure can be an indication the fetus may not be getting enough oxygen and nutrients flowing through. It is particularly common toward the 3rd trimester, and although most babies do not have any complications from this, in the most seriously impacted (where the blood reaching the fetal brain is not sufficient) the results can be autism symptoms.

Gestational diabetes in mother: Higher blood sugar levels in mothers means the baby's pancreas has to work harder to control its sugar levels. The higher sugar levels also mean higher fat storage in the baby, making for bigger babies. Such babies are at risk of hypoglycemia when that sugar level drops drastically after birth as the pancreas adjusts to the more normal levels. A bigger baby can also lead to birth complications in vaginal delivery. When the mother takes medications to keep her blood sugar under control, the impacts of the medication on the baby are not clearly understood. There can be additional effects caused by using sugar substitutes: for example, aspartame is a neurotransmitter. When used by the mother as a sweetener to replace sugar to control her gestational diabetes, it could impact the fetus by neurotransmitter overdose (excitotoxicity) causing neuron apoptosis (suicide) or possibly inhibit neurogenesis in the fetal brain.

Although I do not have a lot of data to prove it, another interesting outcome that I have sometimes observed is differences in birth when the mother has gestational diabetes: C-section babies turn out fine while babies delivered vaginally develop autism. Perhaps the diabetes and high sugar levels in the mother make the neurons in the baby's brain brittle or in some other way more susceptible to damage when subject to the pressures of vaginal delivery.

A skilled obstetrician can help mothers navigate this risk through managing the diabetes with restrictive diets and food regimens, controlling the natural weight gain in pregnancy and lifestyle changes which can help control diabetes without medications and result in a healthy baby.

Obesity in mother: This is a tough one to single out, simply because mothers that are very obese prior to pregnancy tend to have a lot of the other complications described here during pregnancy and it is actually very difficult to ascertain the true cause of the child's complications. But regardless of whatever complications in the mother's health that might be causing the mother's obesity, like hormonal imbalances, metabolic disorders, mental challenges, etc., these can also cause elevated blood pressure, gestational diabetes, etc. However, at the hands of an exceptionally capable obstetrician many such mothers can navigate their pregnancy very successfully and deliver healthy normal babies in many cases.

Path 3: Hypoxic Autism

Birth (parturition) trauma, particularly oxygen deprivation (asphyxia) due to factors ranging from cord prolapse to complications of twin birth ranks as the second-highest cause of autism. The lifelong neurological consequences of in-utero asphyxia are very well known to the medical community and very well documented. These complications that happen naturally are the primary reason why a hospital birth with careful monitoring of the fetus is warranted in the first place. Typically, outside of accidental complications like nuchal cords described below, most mothers that have maintained a healthy lifestyle prior to and during pregnancy tend not to run into most of these complications in their babies.

Extremely premature birth: Babies born very premature (before 37 weeks of pregnancy) do not have a fully functional body ready to take on the challenges of the world. When they leave the protection of the mother's womb ahead of time, their lungs are not fully developed. This can lead to deficiencies in their vital oxygen supply necessary to sustain the rest of the body and can have permanent adverse effects on the future of the child. The more premature a baby the more the possibility of permanent brain damage. As the organ consuming the most oxygen, the brain is the most vulnerable to hypoxic damage.

Umbilical Cord Issues: Umbilical cord issues tend to be more common than they're given credit for, and when they do not cause the stillbirth of the baby, they contribute to a significant fraction of autism impacted kids.

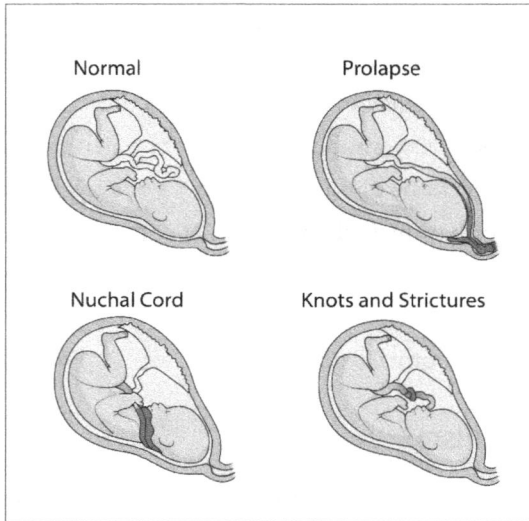

Fig. 15.3: Umbilical Cord Issues

The fetus derives its oxygen and nutrients from its mother while in the womb. A compressed cord most often happens when the cord is prolapsed or stuck in the birth canal ahead of the baby. When this happens, it can cause compression in the cord, cutting the flow of vital oxygen to the baby, which if left untreated can result in hypoxic brain damage and even death of the baby in what is called a cord accident

Nuchal cords happen when the baby gets tangled in the umbilical cord while swimming in the womb. The umbilical cord is 20-24 inches long typically, but long cords of 32 inches or more are known to occur. The longer cords can tangle around the baby and end up looping around the neck. They typically untangle by themselves in the buoyant fluid-filled environment of the womb. When the umbilical cord knots around itself or gets kinked in some very rare instances, it can again restrict blood flow and gas exchange between the mother and fetus, resulting in hypoxic brain injury.

Since the baby is not breathing through the lungs yet, a cord around the neck is not usually a problem. But the problem occurs when the cord tightens and compresses to a point where the oxygen flow through the cord is impacted, particularly when the cord is still around the neck while the baby makes its way through the birth canal. The blood flow through the neck to the fetal brain can also be constricted and such constriction of blood flow to any part of the body is called ischemia. Thus, an injury involving both lack of oxygen in the blood itself (hypoxia) and lack of blood flow (ischemia) leads to what is called hypoxic-ischemic injury. This happens in less than 2% of births, but when it happens, it can result in stillbirths and babies that are born with an extreme blue or dark skin tone due to lack of oxygen. Boys in particular tend to be later diagnosed with autism. Cord accidents are known to be responsible for about 10% of all stillbirths.

Fetal distress in late-stage pregnancy and labor: As the baby grows bigger, more nutrition and oxygen are needed to keep the baby healthy. While it is not a problem in most cases, sometimes other maternal complications like high blood pressure, placenta complications, external trauma or maternal habits might result in the fetus not getting sufficient oxygen leading to distress which might result in a doctor recommending an emergency C-section during one of the prenatal checkups. Such kids born from distress might suffer neurodevelopmental delays.

Placental abruption: This is the placenta detaching from uterus before baby is born. While this is extremely rare, it is known to happen where the placenta partially detaches causing internal or external bleeding. It can happen anytime during pregnancy, but the propensity is more in the perinatal stages.

While it is known to occur only less than 1% of cases, it can cause death of the baby from insufficient oxygen and nutrient supply. In milder cases it can lead to growth restriction, fetal distress, acidosis and lead to brain damage in the baby.

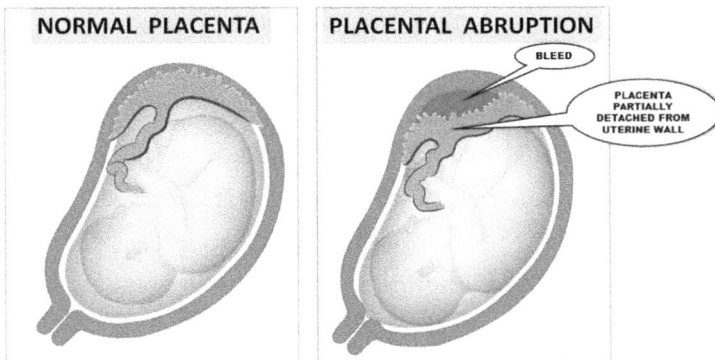

Fig. 15.4: Normal placenta vs abruption.

Ductus arteriosus premature closure: A special blood vessel in fetuses helps bypass the nonfunctioning lungs before birth. This is supposed to close after birth and become a remnant ligament. But premature closure is known to occur mainly as a side effect of maternal medications. A premature partial closure affects the heart, circulation and oxygenation with adverse effects.

Cholestasis or jaundice as a result of pregnancy: Blocking of the bile duct in the mother due to side effects of medication or other causes results in jaundice in mother and baby during pregnancy. This condition is associated with an increased risk of premature delivery and even stillbirth. Some infants born to mothers with intrahepatic cholestasis have a slow heart rate and suffer from a lack of oxygen during delivery, leading to fetal distress and all the other complications that arise from it including neurodevelopmental disorders.

Cephalopelvic disproportion (CPD): This occurs when the head of the baby is considered too large to fit in through the mother's pelvis. Both the pelvic bone structure and the head of the baby are designed to give. Even with a 10cm dilation for the head to emerge from the cervix and allowing for some skull coning, there is still obviously a minimum pelvic diameter necessary for a baby to pass through, and at times there are still complications. CPD is a problem that's been neglected by modern obstetrics and remains one of the most frequent reasons for C-sections, but it also presents one of the most common risks of brain damage to a baby when doctors try for vaginal delivery in these cases.

Prolonged natural labor after water break: Doctors disagree on how long after a woman's water breaks that a baby needs to be delivered for achieving best health outcomes for the baby. Recommendations vary from about 12 to about 72 hours after the amnion ruptures for the baby to be delivered. The lack of amniotic fluid heightens certain other risks if the baby doesn't come soon and labor gets stuck. Some of the risks to the baby include infection and a higher possibility of cord compression from the lack of protection of the amniotic fluid. Prolonged labor may cause one of these other situations leading to hypoxic brain damage or could result in traumatic damage from the force of uterine contractions.

***Meconium Aspiration Syndrome (MAS)*:** Meconium is a dark green sticky substance that accumulates in the intestines of a fetus, comprised of gastrointestinal secretions and other waste accumulated mostly during the third trimester from its limited metabolic functions. Meconium is passed typically within 24 to 48 hours of birth under normal circumstances. However, some fetuses tend to pass the meconium while still in the fluid-filled amniotic sac, which is suspected to potentially cause fetal distress due to hypoxia. In about 5% of fetuses exposed to meconium, when the fluid-filled lungs of the fetus transition to the air breathing organs of the child difficulties emerge due to factors like blocked air passages, inflammation, infection, and lung surfactant inactivation. Development of MAS as a neonate has been shown to be related to longer-term neurodevelopmental disorders such as autism.

***Multiple births (twins or more)*:** Twin births can add an additional layer of complexity to the already intricate and complex pregnancy process. Dizygotic or fraternal twins are formed from 2 eggs and embryos and always have separate placentas and amniotic sacs. In the case of monozygotic twins or multiples where a single egg splits after a few days after conception, they might come with shared or separate placentas and share the chorion or the outer layer of the amniotic sac while have their own amnion or internal layer of the fluid-filled amniotic sac. Most twins or multiples come with their own placentas, their own amniotic sacs and umbilical cords. Monoamniotic-monochorionic (MoMo) twins with shared placentas chorion and amniotic sacs occur in less than 1 percent of twin births. MoMo twins are at extremely high risk for cord entanglement, cord compression, and other complications that can lead to autism.

Navigating these complexities skillfully are what OB/GYN's are trained to do, with full awareness of the consequences of not making timely decisions. These are the reasons why we go to the hospital for birthing in the first place. Most OB/GYNs tend to make the right decisions and are trained to save the life of the baby, but sometimes their inaction can result in loss of valuable time and the health of the baby suffers as a result, even when the baby is delivered live. The mental health of babies is something many OB/GYNs seem to take lightly, using neuroplasticity as the excuse for allowing the brains of babies to take a beating during birth. Consequently, perinatal malpractice has become fairly rampant.

Path 4: Tebic Autism / Autism Iatrogenic

Contraction Abuse: As a play on the acronym TBI and its pronunciation as Tee-Bee-Eye, and given its predominance as a cause of autism, I would call it Tebic Autism to describe autism caused by TBI or Traumatic Brain Injury, mostly from contraction abuse, but also from other traumatic injury from the likes of damage from forceps or other mechanical means during delivery. Brain damage from conditions like craniosynostosis might also fit the bill of traumatic brain injury, where the skull plates are fused and the baby cannot be pushed out through the birth canal and attempting to do so causes skull plates to break and cause injury to the brain.

This path to autism represents the highest number of autism cases out there. I estimate at least about 50% of the cases of autism in the US are due to birth injury of this variety. Indeed, all the prior reasons, risks and pathways have existed for centuries and cannot explain the recent meteoric rise of the number of cases of autism. This is the single reason why autism is so much more prevalent in western countries and also the reason why autism is on the rise.

The dangers of Pitocin are described right on the label of this drug. It has become the most abused medication in maternity wards across the country. Unfortunately, there's a lot of people including health care professionals who do not understand the induced labor process as much as they should. When a drug becomes so common, it is easy to let one's guard down and start treating it as the 'safest' thing out there, forgetting the warnings on the label. Unfortunately for parents and their kids impacted from Pitocin, the other routes to autism obscure the reality of the prevalence of this pathway.

The single most important line on the label about the circumstances for contra-indications of Pitocin use that OB/GYNs don't pay attention to is this:

> **5. Where adequate uterine activity fails to achieve satisfactory progress.**

"Satisfactory progress" is subject to interpretation. As mentioned previously the ACOG have clarified this as 72 continuous contractions. Most maternity wards interpret it as about 4-6 hours of labor induction at a low dosage with a contraction rate of 2 or 3 contractions per 10 minutes without progress to complete cervical dilation. What it doesn't explicitly say is what happens if you cross that limit. In many cases, in the absence of any other adverse reactions like fetal distress, some OB/GYNs have resorted to increasing the Pitocin dosage instead of resorting to a C-section or at least stopping the induction.

Continuing induction at this point is a sure shot way to damage the fetal brain through physical trauma that leads to scarring in the white matter of the brain – the fundamental networks of neurons that become the foundation that the future neuronal network will be built on. And unlike an adverse chemical reaction, physical trauma is guaranteed to happen to any fetus subject to Pitocin abuse. Any variations depend on the how much further beyond contra-indication the induction lasted, the size of the baby and the pushing involved.

Indeed, this is almost the only situation where I have seen girls develop autism (although their numbers are fewer due to their ability to recover from the injury faster due to the brain protective nature of estrogen). It is fairly common to find the same mother induced the same way have one boy on the autism spectrum and a girl that might be fairly normal although these might also turn out to be the hidden girls of the autism spectrum.

What's most unfortunate about this condition is that these OB/GYNs proceed with induction in the absence of other risk factors like fetal distress. The impacted individuals are the healthiest mothers and healthiest babies who are targeted for induction due to their low-risk pregnancy and end up paying a penalty for their good health at the hands of these OB/GYNs and their labor induction drug abuse.

Almost every article you find on the internet from doctors and researchers out there about the Pitocin – autism linkage talks about the chemical effects of the oxytocin hormone on the fetal brain as somehow being the explanation for autism. That is the result of the ACOG gaming the headlines to say Pitocin does not cause autism and citing flawed research papers providing this alternate mechanism, that does not cause autism and hence true, but hijacks the headlines about Pitocin causing autism What they don't talk about is the sheer trauma that artificially induced contractions can produce on the fetal brain causing traumatic brain injury. It's not a chemical adverse reaction but the effect of the physics of the sheer force of artificial contractions hammering an infant head first on a non-effacing cervix.

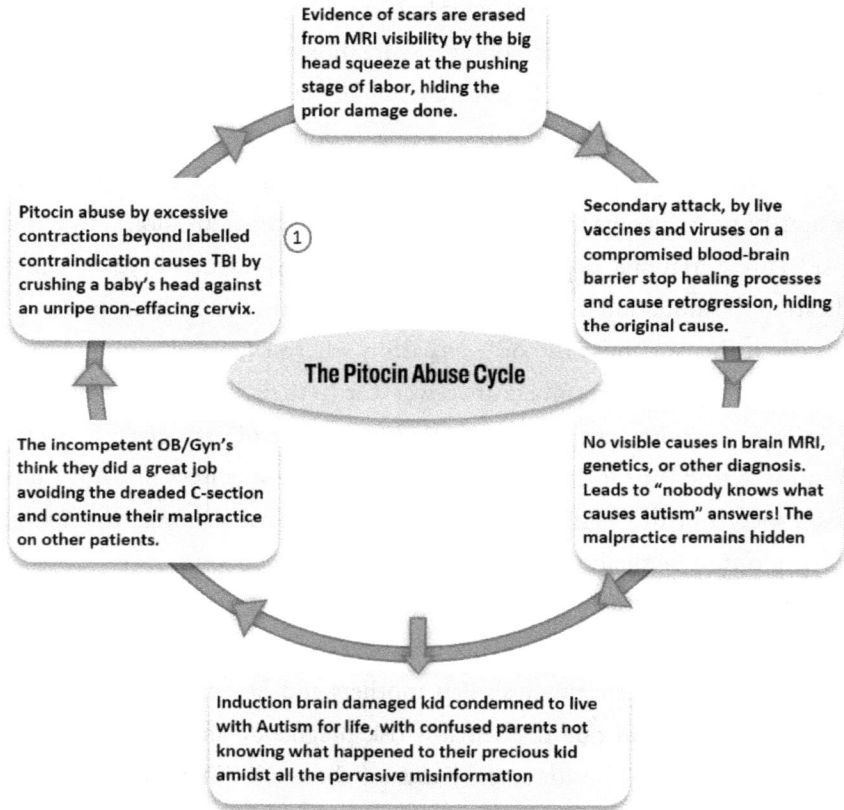

Evidence of scars are erased from MRI visibility by the big head squeeze at the pushing stage of labor, hiding the prior damage done.

Pitocin abuse by excessive contractions beyond labelled contraindication causes TBI by crushing a baby's head against an unripe non-effacing cervix.

Secondary attack, by live vaccines and viruses on a compromised blood-brain barrier stop healing processes and cause retrogression, hiding the original cause.

The Pitocin Abuse Cycle

The incompetent OB/Gyn's think they did a great job avoiding the dreaded C-section and continue their malpractice on other patients.

No visible causes in brain MRI, genetics, or other diagnosis. Leads to "nobody knows what causes autism" answers! The malpractice remains hidden

Induction brain damaged kid condemned to live with Autism for life, with confused parents not knowing what happened to their precious kid amidst all the pervasive misinformation

Fig. 15.5: Pitocin Abuse Cycle

Some conscientious researchers and OB/GYNs have tried to critique the practice in their hospitals. One such paper written by British researchers Karl Oláh and Phillip Steer is titled "The use and abuse of oxytocin" in the Journal of the Royal College of OB/GYNs[8.4] and goes into detail of how nurses do not understand the terminology involved in induced labor and the mistakes and misinterpretation in cardiotocography. They elaborate on the methods, intricacies and outcomes of asphyxia in many of the deliveries when strict guidelines and careful monitoring is not practiced. But for the most part the issue has been ignored as it falls under 'medical malpractice' and would break the taboo of doctors blaming other doctors and exposing their malpractice. And like everything else in the obstetrics world , the full version of this paper by Olah and Steer is locked up behind institutional access and pay walls to keep it from the prying eyes of parents. More testimony to the fact that even a research paper pointing fingers at obstetric practices gets hidden from the public. This kind of behavior has caused the burden of proof for birth malpractice to shift squarely onto the shoulders of impacted parents.

Tebic Autism or Iatrogenic autism can be eliminated once the recognition of contraction abuse gains common acceptance and interventions that can cause traumatic brain injury are avoided. This birth injury cause of autism is the true reason why autism is taking on epidemic proportions, as OB/GYN's continue to unleash labor induction abuse targeting healthy mothers with healthy pregnancies perpetuating this birth injury in ever increasing numbers.

Key Take Away: Four different causative pathways to autism are cataloged and a clearer labeling of autism subcategories is proposed, distinguishing autism from genetic disorders and establishing its roots in pregnancy and birth. Adopting such categorization could lead to better understanding of an individual's condition, better categorization of symptoms and lead to more directed treatments overall. The complications of birth are discussed and the role of perinatal birth injury in contributing to the autism epidemic is clearly identified.

CHAPTER 16

Treatment Possibilities

mpacted parents are desperate enough and pushed to a limit where they can fall prey to buying into anything that is touted as a possible cure. There are numerous websites with testimonials from people touting false promises. The internet can be a dangerous place where parents who are not discerning enough stand to lose thousands in hard-earned money and valuable time pursuing a path that bears no results and sometimes might actually cause more harm or damage their kid even further.

While some cases of these testimonials may be true, they are potentially one-off cases where the cause for the autism symptoms may not have been traumatic brain injury or hypoxia but one of the causes curable by other means such as Pandas, pans, Lyme disease or just an allergy that needed to be controlled. Unfortunately, medical science falls short when it comes to a cure to autism caused by TBI and hypoxia. In a cruel world where medical sciences bluntly tell parents "There's no cure for autism," hope turns to desperation. It's the last thing any impacted parent wants to hear. They would rather hold onto hope that their kids will be better one day and work toward it. As the character of Tim Robbins in the movie *The Shawshank Redemption* says, "Hope is a good thing, maybe the best of things, and no good thing ever dies."

Challenges to Brain Damage Recovery

We know that brain damage at birth is the cause of neurodevelopmental delays including autism, ADD, ADHD, etc. Consider Fig 16.1a and 16.1b showing fetal brain development and a picture of a child's brain in cross-section vs a young adult brain. The biggest physical change is the increase in folds of the brain. At 9 months from conception close to birth, the brain has already developed the basic folded cerebral structure. With age cerebral ridges become more pronounced as the development of new skills requires growth of more grey matter within the limited cranial space. More folds help accommodate the increased volume of grey matter on the cerebral surface to house all those additional neuron bodies that make up the grey matter in a process called gyrification. As the brain undergoes more experiential learning with age, more grey matter develops to store all those additional skills and information.

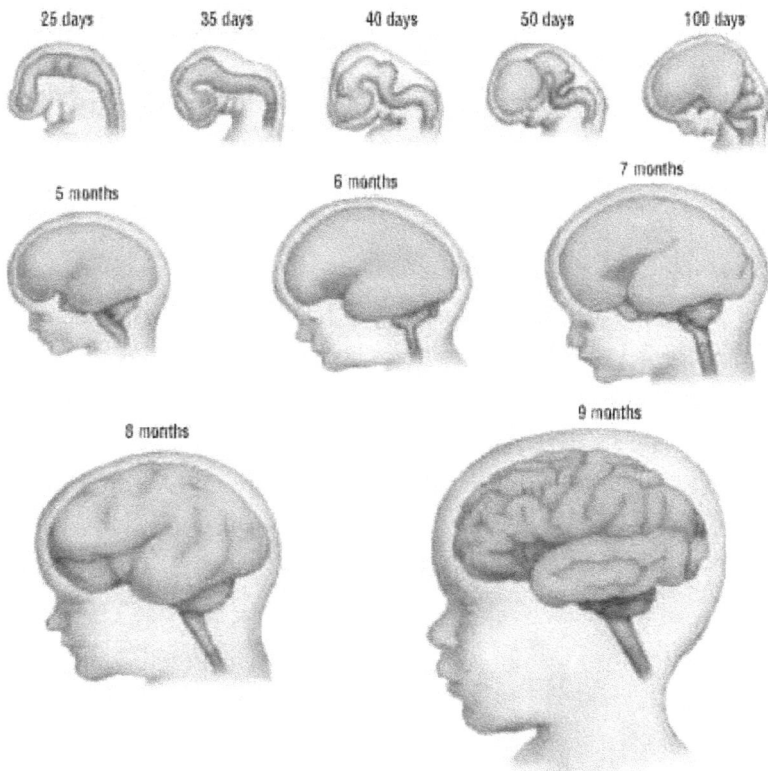

Fig. 16.1a: Fetal brain growth.

BRAIN GYRIFICATION WITH AGE

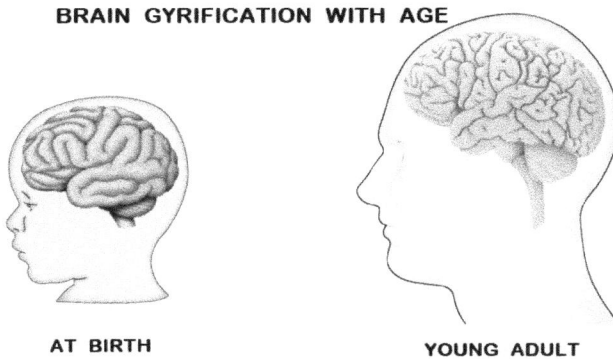

AT BIRTH   YOUNG ADULT

Fig 16.1b: Increased brain folds with age.

As seen in the pictures during fetal development and from birth through adulthood this increase in ridges on the brain surface is what happens in normal brain development, in a process called gyrification as the brain makes more surface area to accommodate more learnt skills.

Coordination of multiple grey matter areas involves the neural connections in the white matter, which connect the different areas of grey matter. For example, speech involves auditory processing, visual processing, cognition and memory – each of which by itself involves multiple areas of grey matter, each working with other areas it is connected to by white matter.

In a damaged brain such experiential learning is pretty restricted. This is because the foundational networks that connect the visual, auditory, memory and sensory processing are damaged, resulting in the grey matter areas needed to participate in an activity not communicating correctly. Worldly viruses crossing the compromised blood brain barrier create further imbalances in brain signaling and neuron function.

Autism resulting from brain damage to either the grey matter or white matter areas (or both) followed by a double whammy from live viruses gaining control of immune privileged areas, means that any cure needs to address the remediation of such damage:

▸ Help repair and recover from brain trauma;

▸ Help regrowth of neurons;

▶ Help with the removal of scar tissue;

▶ Help re-establish damaged connections between neurons and create new pathways;

▶ Reduce inflammation and protect from continuing damage due to viral antigens and toxins.

▶ Help re-establish brain chemical balance.

This knowledge can help parents evaluate any cures and therapies for their effects on some of these possible recovery pathways.

For example, the damaged blood brain barrier also explains the sensitivity of kids on the autism spectrum to environmental contaminants and the many arguments about external environmental factors being the cause of autism. Kids with TBI show incremental improvements when treated with natural or medical chelating agents designed to remove certain environmental toxins, although there are no major improvements in cases where there is no significant exposure. Thus, treatments directed purely towards removal of such toxins have not been widely successful. But it does make sense to keep individuals with TBI away from environmental toxins given their sensitivity to such toxins.

While there are no treatments that can address regrowth of neurons that could help with full recovery at the time of this writing, there are still things parents can do to help the natural recovery processes of the body and brain in cases of traumatic and hypoxic damage to the brain. To evaluate the best treatments and help currently available out there, it is useful to categorize these treatments based on their purported overall effect on the damaged brain.

Importance of Early Intervention

But before categorizing treatments it's important to note that early intervention is known to be an absolute necessity when it comes to seeing improvements in developmentally delayed children. Significant brain changes happen very early in childhood with development plateauing by about age 25. This is true even in normal neurological development, so for parents of challenged children it's a race against the clock if they want their children to recover from their developmental issues. The following graph by the Harvard University Center on the Developing Child illustrates this point.

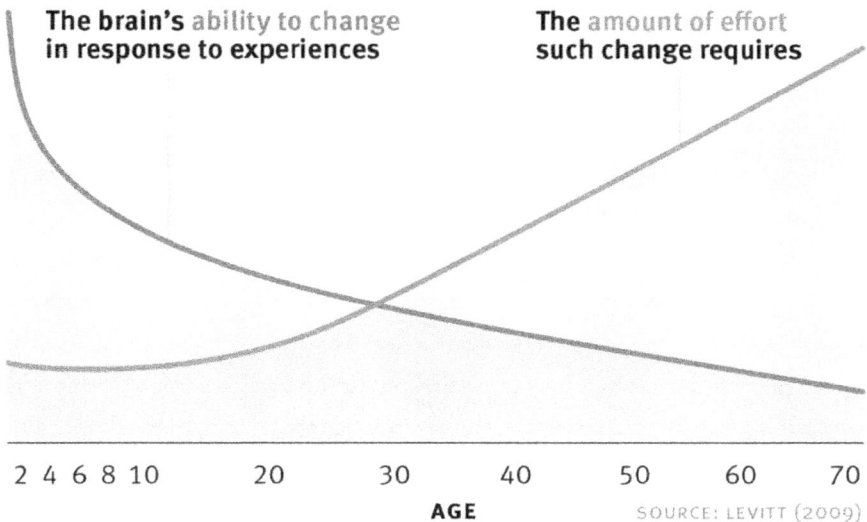

The brain's ability to change in response to experiences

The amount of effort such change requires

2 4 6 8 10   20   30   40   50   60   70

AGE

SOURCE: LEVITT (2009)

Center on the Developing Child 🛡 HARVARD UNIVERSITY   www.developingchild.harvard.edu

Fig. 16.2: The brain's ability to change/learn with age.

As you can see in Figure 11.2, the ability of the brain to change in response to external stimuli diminishes drastically with age and beyond the mid to late 20's, effecting any change would require an enormous amount of effort and even then, very little potential for change actually exists beyond that point in time. Unfortunately, most parents catch autism in their children very late (typically past age 3). Any progress would also depend on where a child starts and how much brain damage, he or she has sustained and which specific pathways might be affected.

Another really early intervention could come right after birth. Currently an MRI scan is not ordered other than in cases of obvious brain damage as in cerebral palsy. But a recent study by the US and UK (MARBLE study by Imperial college and NIH) have shown that a 15-minute MRI scan immediately after birth can predict future development delays to a 98% accuracy. So, modifying the standard of care to include an MRI scan at least in cases where the Apgar score is less than 10 would go a long way in identifying brain damage early. In recent times use of cooling blanket therapy to induce controlled hypothermia in babies with suspected brain damage has been shown to help with brain damage recovery] The infant is subjected to a reduced temperature of a few degrees by placing him or her on a mat that reduces their body temperature by a few degrees. The resulting hypothermia makes the body focus on core functions only, thus helping recovery from brain damage.

In our case for example our pediatrician Dr Joe had identified our first boy had sustained brain damage within 2 hours of birth. I saw all he did was holding the baby very adeptly in one hand while touching him with his ball point pen at various points and watched for the baby's response. His observation was his reflexes were poor, because he was induced for so long. And his statements at that point "I don't understand, why they still keep doing this (prolonged induction)" went a long way in understanding the malpractice that had happened once I recollected these events years later upon seeing brain damage in the MRI scan. Would my boy have fared better if he had immediately been given this cooling therapy once Dr Joe found this damage had occurred? This cooling therapy might only work for hypoxic damage and perhaps not trauma and it was not available back in 2007, but it is available now and it is important that it should become part of the very early intervention for cases of suspected brain damage. My expectation is such intervention could work from birth all the way up to when the first vaccines are administered that might muddy the waters when it comes to brain damage.

While babies' bodies work different from adults and the presence of any neuronal viral latencies in adults could have an impact on the outcome, the possibility of medically induced hypothermia, working for brain damage recovery in older kids and adults is something that deserves the attention of the research community.

Based on the fact that we are dealing with brain damage it is obvious that treatment options need to be addressing the root causes for them to actually work. That narrows down the field considerably in terms of treatments that help and ones that don't. The ones that might work can be categorized into the following three categories as summarized in table 16.1.

Table 16.1

Neuroplasticity based treatments	Biomedical treatments	Future treatments - neuron re-generation
These treatments are based on the fact that the undamaged parts of the brain are capable of learning new skills with training and the brain can repair itself.	Treatments based on reducing inflammation in the brain from allergies, viruses, antibodies or altering the brain chemical environment using supplements, hormones. neurotransmitters etc.	These are currently under study and no treatments are currently available capable of this yet, underscoring the importance of fast tracking of such research.
* Applied Behavior Analysis * Occupational Therapy * Speech Therapy * Computerized brain games. * Neurofeedback * Auditory Integration Training	* Antiviral medications * Neuro medications * Gluten Casein free diets * DAN allergy treatments * Stem cell treatments * HBOT (sometimes)	* Tissue Nano transfection * In vivo re-programming * Neuronal stem cells * Cure neuronal viral latencies * Tissue regeneration by QMRT

We will discuss some of these treatments in the upcoming chapters.

Key Take Away: Only treatments capable of producing brain damage recovery effects can actually be useful in helping autism symptoms. Parents need to stay away from any treatments that profess to cure the condition without credible pathways to helping the damaged brain perform better. A framework for credible pathways to brain damage recovery is established in this chapter.

CHAPTER 17

Neuroplasticity Based Treatments

This ability of the brain to change in response to external experiences is called neuroplasticity. Early interventions are mostly of the neuroplasticity type, but if they go hand in hand with biomedical and food interventions (discussed in the next chapter), the results are typically better. There is a need to approach the problem from various angles as there is no single easy solution to the problem. Instead, every therapy helps with a certain aspect of deficit and parents can only hope that there is some synergy between the various treatments resulting in reasonable overall improvement.

Neuroplasticity therapies are aimed at helping the brain establish new pathways to replace damaged ones. They involve using neuroplasticity to learn skills that have been lost or never developed due to damage to grey matter or broken white matter pathways resulting in lack of communication among grey matter areas.

The following are treatments and outcomes that I have personally worked on, or know first-hand of parents that have tried these. Efficacy of these treatments usually depends on whether an individual is in a position to benefit from these or not, and is often a matter of where someone starts. Even in my own case, with two similarly damaged boys, treatments helping one of them don't seem to be helping the other and vice versa due to the difference in the extent of the damage.

Parents are advised to use their best judgment before spending money on any of these. It's hard to restrain yourself from going above and beyond to try and do the best for your child, but it's important to not go overboard since it might only bring disappointment if you do, as individual results vary and none of these is a complete aid to recovery from the condition. Prior knowledge of these treatments will help parents anticipate possible outcomes and goals for their particular child and situation.

Applied Behavior Analysis (ABA) Therapy

If you are an autism parent, you likely deal with ABA therapists more than any other personnel. Applied behavior analysis is defined as "the process of systematically applying interventions based upon the principles of learning theory to improve socially significant behaviors to a meaningful degree, and to demonstrate that the interventions employed are responsible for the improvement in behavior" (Baer, Wolf & Risley, 1968; Sulzer-Azaroff & Mayer, 1991). This systematic approach does help in bringing some behavioral improvements (mostly in the form of compliance), which is an important characteristic missing from kids on the spectrum. This is definitely the first step to helping autism spectrum kids and so I list this first.

The success of ABA therapy to a large extent depends on the capabilities of the therapist to identify the exact deficits in the child and apply the principles of ABA to address them. It takes exceptional commitment on the part of the therapist and a reasonable functioning level of the child, for ABA to work. But ABA therapy can only go so far. Like everything here, it is not really a cure but just one cog in the complex array of tools parents should consider to help their child's damaged brain learn and establish new neuronal pathways of learning.

Many ABA centers are good at bringing about considerable improvements in children on the autism spectrum, and strive to continually build on newly achieved skills. However, a recent phenomenon has been that ABA therapy centers have now become a popular business growing alongside the increase of autism particularly in the US. While it can be a good thing and add to the choices for impacted parents, some of these are turning out to be rip-off programs that add no additional value than traditional daycare but come with a hefty price tag. Insurance coverage of ABA due to hard fought victories by parents that have gone before has meant growth of these ABA centers whose main specialization seems to be their ability to efficiently bill insurance to the fullest rather than their ability to help their clients. Parents need to be watchful of these types of centers and choose these settings carefully based on their track record and monitor their kids progress very carefully.

Occupational Therapy

Occupational therapy aimed at developing the motor skills of a child can bring on great improvements in the brain of a child on the autism spectrum. Motor coordination and movement tends to be a feedback loop to the brain, which when given such movement inputs tends to learn from them. While it happens automatically in children, a child on the spectrum needs this kind of therapy to help them get out of the shortcuts and other workarounds their brains tend to create to bypass having to use the damaged parts of their brains. Engaging in any kind of physical sports activity can have the most therapeutic value for kids with ASD. With occupational therapy the therapist evaluates various ranges of motion, from gross to fine motor skills, and engages in therapy directed at improving the motor skill deficits found.

A child's normal motor development needs to go from head to toe, from shoulder out to the fingers. They are first able to hold their head up on their shoulders, flip around on their belly, start using their shoulders to move their body as the first step to crawling, then use their legs to start crawling. With kids suffering from brain damage, the first signs (outside of low Apgar scores after birth) is the failure to develop motor skills out of developmental order. These little nuances of motor development (if caught) can be indicative of other problems down the road.

It should be noted that a damaged brain also makes these kids susceptible to brain hemorrhage risks later in life as adults, particularly if they develop other conditions like high blood pressure and depression. This can be the cause of sudden death, causing even more pain to loved ones. Although children on the spectrum will not typically suggest it themselves, it is a good idea for parents to cultivate interest in their kid in a pastime that involves physical activity early on so they can maintain good physical health, which in turn keeps their mental health from worsening as the years go by. It might just be a simple habit they can do even by themselves like walking or running on a treadmill while watching something on TV or playing a simple solo game like shooting basketball.

Learning therapy – Visualizing and verbalizing

The Lindamood-Bell system originated by Charles and Pat Lindamood and Nanci Bell has been helping kids with learning difficulties in reading and comprehending for over 3 decades. While it is not specifically oriented toward kids on the autism spectrum, sensory-cognitive instruction has proven successful for individuals with learning challenges, including ADHD and autism, and high functioning kids on the spectrum can benefit from this type of learning. Their instruction is based on a theory of cognition. There is a conscious effort to think in pictures, which is apparently lacking in kids with autism, thanks to damaged or detached areas of the brain needed for imagination. It should be noted that this kind of therapy can also be expensive for families since learning is typically not covered by insurance and quality one on one therapy such as this tends to be pricey, putting it out of reach for many families.

Computerized Brain Training Games

An individual's ability to learn comes from their ability to observe, focus and discern visual and auditory inputs to the highest level of detail, use that for pattern recognition and incorporate that understanding into existing knowledge. When it comes to individuals with autism one or more of these functions is lacking (or is working sub-optimally) due to brain damage. It is quite possible that brain training games can be designed to address some of these deficits.

The companies that have created computerized brain improvement games claim to improve IQ and help take even the cognition of non-autistic children "to the next level." However, they have recently come under fire for their claims of improving IQ in all customers. Following customer complaints even the Federal Trade Commission has come down on their claims pretty harshly. Researchers seem to disagree on the efficacy of such programs. But it's easy to see why it may not work very well in the general population. These programs need to be tailored to address specific deficits in individuals like auditory memory, audiovisual sensory integration involving dedicated continuous practice over long periods of time.

Neurofeedback Therapy

Biofeedback therapy is a technique used by therapists to train people to improve their health by controlling certain bodily processes that normally happen involuntarily, such as heart rate, blood pressure, muscle tension, and skin temperature. An individual's response to certain external stimuli is measured with a measuring device and the individual is trained to respond differently in an attempt to improve health. Electrode patches are placed on different parts of the body to measure nerve or muscle response, heart rate, blood pressure or other function. The electrodes are connected to a monitor that displays the measures. With help from a biofeedback therapist, patients are trained to consciously control their responses, thereby helping them practice certain types of responses over others.

Neurofeedback is a type of biofeedback where brain waves are used to produce a measurable signal that is used as feedback to teach self-regulation of brain function. This is useful in autism and ADHD therapy where the subject is relatively verbal and understands the need to work with the equipment and train him or herself to self-regulate brain response. Electrodes are glued on to target areas of the scalp and the other end connected to measuring equipment and a monitor displaying brain activity.

There can be variations in how brain training can be achieved. For example, the subject may be asked to watch a movie or video and based on the brain wave activity the monitor is programmed to dim down or the volume drops in response to types of brain activity that reflect a lack of focus. This becomes a reward system with focus and concentration being rewarded with good picture quality and sound. Alternatively, a game could be played where the subject controls an object on the screen using his brain waves.

It should be pointed out that neurofeedback is not a cure for the underlying condition but an effort to train the brain to overcome its shortcomings. The outcomes depend on the techniques of the therapist, the patient and the equipment used, the ability of the therapist to filter noise from real brainwave activity, etc. While some parents report incremental positive changes for kids on the spectrum, this might typically help higher functioning kids on the spectrum or perhaps typically developing kids with minor shortcomings.

Key Take Away: Neuroplasticity or the ability of the brain to learn new skills remains a very important aspect of treatment for spectrum kids. However, the level of benefit depends on the extent of damage a kid starts with and the expertise of the personnel handling the treatment. The ability of the brain to learn slows down with age and early intervention of expert therapists can make a difference, although outcomes are not guaranteed as learning is only one aspect of the overall brain damage recovery picture.

CHAPTER 18

Biomedically Based Treatments

These are treatments directed toward creating a brain environment conducive to repair and recovery. It could be antiviral medication to reverse vaccine and other viral effects, neurotransmitter-based medication for calming the brain or supplements to help the gut and brain. Based on the severity of brain damage, biomedical interventions are marginally effective but have been far from the cure they are sometimes touted to be. It is easier to cure a diseased organ than to fix an organ that is damaged permanently. Still, armed with knowledge of what really is causing the issue you could sort through the mechanisms of how a certain cure might work and make an informed decision about pursuing it. Most of these treatments I go over in this chapter do not help cure autism altogether, but they help alleviate certain aspects of behavior or help verbalization or help with better coordination or any one of the many brain functions that are impacted by autism. All this is handled by pediatricians specializing in treating Autism, as the mistakes made by the Ob/Gyns become the challenges for the pediatricians to solve.

The DAN Protocol

Dr. Bernard Rimland (1928-2006) was an American psychologist and researcher whose son Mark was diagnosed with autism. He set out to correct a lot of myths surrounding autism in the 1960s and led the movement that dispelled the now preposterous refrigerator mother theory. He wrote a book on Infantile Autism and founded two organizations: the Autism Research Institute (ARI) and what is now the Autism Society of America (ASA). He has had the single biggest influence in autism research, directing research toward both neurological and biomedical interventions.

The DAN protocol was originally a program from the Autism Research Institute. It is based on the belief that autism is a disorder caused by a combination of a lowered immune response, external toxins from vaccines and other sources, and problems caused by certain foods. The Autism Research Institute has discontinued the DAN protocol since 2011 (apparently due to their inability to control individual practitioners and their quality of service).

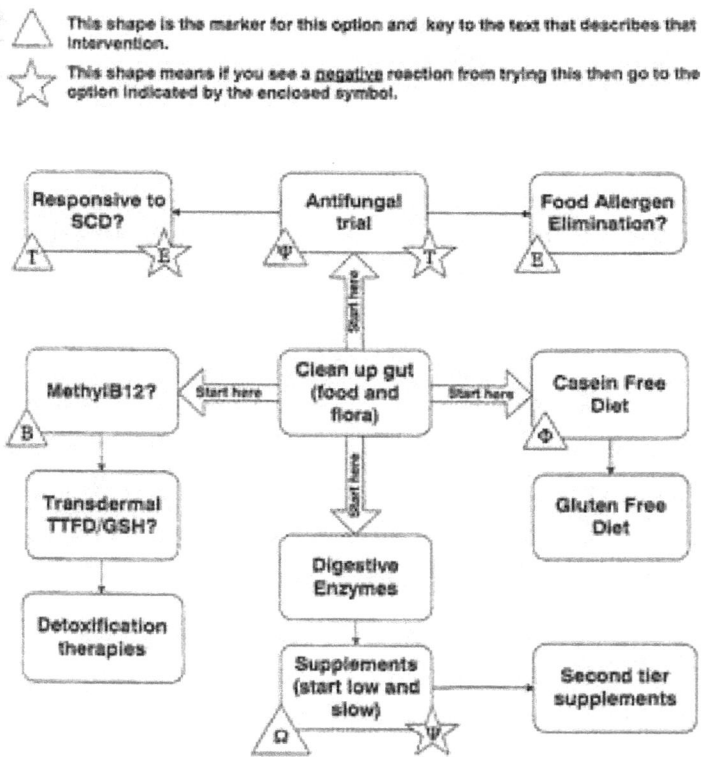

Fig. 18.1: The discontinued DAN protocol.

A summary list of treatments under the DAN protocol include Actos, amino acids, anti-inflammatories for inflammatory bowel disease (Rx), anti-yeast diets, antifungal pharmaceuticals, antiviral medications, chelation, chelation (oral), chelation (rectal suppositories), chelation (transdermal products), colostrum, diet avoiding food allergens, digestive enzymes, essential fatty acids supplementation, Feingold diet, glutathione, gluten and casein free diet, heavy metal detoxification, hyperbaric oxygen therapy (hard chamber), hyperbaric oxygen therapy (soft chamber), intravenous immunoglobulins (IVIG), low dose naltrexone, low oxalate diet, methylcobalamin (B12 injection), nutraceuticals, probiotics, secretin, specific carbohydrate diet, spironolactone, transfer factor, vitamin/mineral supplementation, and vitamin C and/or minerals (IV).

While many of these treatments offered under the DAN program have been incrementally useful in the vast majority of autism impacted kids, none of these seem to help completely recover from the condition in most cases. Some aspects of the DAN approach remain valid, particularly the need to rule out the low hanging fruit like Lyme disease, PANDAS, PANS and food allergies that produce autism symptoms in a small fraction of kids that receive the autism diagnosis. In my experience and the experience of most parents I have talked to, the DAN approach can be summarized as follows.

Effective treatments in the DAN approach include:

▸ Detection and treatment of Lyme, PANDAS, PANS.
▸ Antiviral drugs (acyclovir, valacyclovir)
▸ Gluten free diets
▸ Food allergy identification and avoidance.
▸ Yeast(candida) overgrowth reduction (low sugar diets, antifungal treatment)
▸ Supplement deficiencies in Vitamins, Minerals, Essential fatty acids, Amino acids, Enzymes and co-enzymes.

In summary, treatments of the DAN approach targeting immune and viral effects and gut dysbiosis proved to be their most effective approaches while some of the other treatments like heavy metal detection and chelation (with no obvious exposure), GcMAF, Secretin etc., are often either ineffective or very subjective where clear patterns cannot be established.

With the Autism Research Institute (ARI) taking a reputational beating after the loss of the vaccine omnibus trials and the repeated attacks by medical boards on DAN doctors for trying out experimental and off-label use of drugs in their attempts to treat Autism, the DAN protocol was discontinued in 2011. But this only meant, for autism parents, things were back to square 1, as the regular medical community could not offer anything more than ABA, Occupational and speech therapies. These therapies are only partly effective as kids on the spectrum tend to suffer retrogression of skills with every viral infection, even a common cold sends progress into a tailspin, which means lasting progress is mostly never achieved, without the support of the biomedical interventions.

Medical Academy of Pediatric Special needs – MAPS (medmaps.org)

The discontinuation of the DAN protocol in 2011 left a vacuum in terms of the wholistic approaches to manage autism. There were no alternate protocols, guidelines or evidence-based methods for doctors interested in specializing in autism biomedical treatment options. Some of the doctors practicing DAN previously, put together medmaps.org. The MAPS program was originally developed by Dan Rossignol, M.D., to address the unique issues that play a huge role in the symptoms we describe as autism. Dr Rossignol is himself a parent of 2 sons on the autism spectrum. He describes in one of his papers the shock, surprise and denial he felt when his older son Isaiah was diagnosed with autism in 2002. Later his second son Joshua was also diagnosed. His story, very similar to mine, makes me think the cause of his kids' autism might be similar to mine, one of Pitocin abuse birth injury. I haven't had the chance to meet him personally after I discovered the true cause of my kids' autism after the MRI report in late 2016. Being a parent created program, the MAPS is a reliable biomedical approach that pretty much helps maintain and manage the multi-decade or even lifelong battle for recovery from birth injury. Since its creation in 2012, MAPS has morphed to involve all of integrative pediatrics (including ADHD, other neurodevelopmental delays, asthma, autoimmunity, gut issues, immune dysfunction, and many other chronic pediatric conditions). MAPS has also expanded to address the unique issues faced by these children as they transition into adulthood.

This organization now offers a comprehensive education & fellowship program to medical professionals for the care of children with autism spectrum disorders and

BIOMEDICALLY BASED TREATMENTS

related chronic complex conditions. With an objective very similar to that of the DAN doctors these MAPS doctors continue to provide valuable service to the Autism community, sharing biomedical approaches to treat the gut dysbiosis, gut allergies and associated root causes for autism behaviors and autism related symptoms. The Medmaps organization conducts annual training conferences for practitioners and pretty much continues the work of the prior DAN organization, without getting into the more controversial chelation and some other therapies under DAN that were found ineffective and sometimes harmful. The focus of MAPS treatments is geared towards addressing the supposed mitochondrial dysfunction in autism. Approaches common to most biomedical treatment plans and some other treatments are outlined in the upcoming paragraphs.

Antiviral and Neuro Medications

Viruses known and unknown can wreak havoc in the brain, particularly a damaged one, with a leaky barrier, both by their direct impact and by the impact of immune responses including inflammation. Even viruses that exist in almost 100% of the human population which don't affect individuals with normally functioning brains can introduce detrimental effects in someone with brain damage. As explained in the chapter on vaccines some viruses routinely cross the blood brain barrier and others don't. An illness with viruses that cross the blood brain barrier always causes retrogression of skills in kids with autism. Your doctor might be able to order antibody testing to identify any viral excesses in your child's body. When treated with the appropriate antiviral medication the outcome tends to have an incrementally positive effect in reducing behaviors and helping the development of a child on the autism spectrum.

Neurotransmitter-based drugs that are known to calm down individuals might prove effective in controlling and calming down autistic children with behavioral, anxiety, sleep, OCD and even seizure issues. Working with a trusted MAPS doctor or a neurologist would be the best course of action in this case to narrow down the drug that might help best. Ideally, it is advisable to avoid drugs where possible, but in the worst of cases, where the benefits outweigh the risks, they might be an important ingredient that could be of incremental help in bringing about positive outcomes.

Food Restrictions

When done right food can truly be medicine, and food restrictions help kids on the autism spectrum to the extent that brain healthy foods tend to improve focus and awareness in everybody. The vital role of food in maintaining mental health is finally being recognized by science and has led to the burgeoning new field of nutritional psychiatry.

While not a miracle remedy, in many cases avoidance or inclusion of certain foods can work like medicine and such effects are particularly pronounced in kids on the autism spectrum. These kids have a lot of digestive issues and food allergies, thanks to viruses latent and hiding in their damaged brains and enteric nervous system.

Gluten Free / Casein Free Diets: The most common among these diet restrictions is the gluten free casein free diet (GFCF) diet. Glutamate is a neurotransmitter in the brain that is excitatory. Foods with gluten content are seen to have a significant excitatory effect for many kids on the ASD. Gluten is a protein commonly found in many protein rich foods including meats, dairy, wheat, rye, barley, soy, couscous, semolina and many others. Like all other types of protein, the digestion process breaks down the gluten protein into amino acids in the body. One such amino acid resulting from protein breakdown is called glutamine and glutamine in turn can switch to becoming glutamate in the brain (in what is called the glutamine – glutamate cycle). Excessive glutamate in the brain results in excitatory overload and hyperactive behavior.

Of all gluten containing foods, wheat, soy and dairy products seem to contain the most glutamine content and so it makes sense for ASD kids to avoid them. Unfortunately, in our world of processed foods, gluten proteins are used as the glue that gives the consistency and chewiness to most processed foods, making avoiding gluten a difficult task. But the results of avoiding it can be worth it in many cases, particularly where there is a gluten allergy involved alongside the ASD and hyper-activeness.

Food allergies avoidance: Children on the autism spectrum in many cases are not verbal and so do not complain verbally about any discomfort to parents. Sometimes it might look like they are crying for no reason, but it is likely due to some discomfort that they can't verbalize. It's up to parents to play sleuth to discover what the underlying reasons could be. Hence the IgG, IgE and skin prick allergy testing panels tend to be important tools in the hands of parents trying to get at possible allergies in their kids (particularly all the gut allergies that kids on the spectrum typically suffer from) that might be causing them pain. The IgG is a particularly convenient panel test that has become popular, although it often can come up with some false positives, particularly for foods consumed regularly and frequently. But it also indicates sensitivity to other rarely eaten foods as well which tend to be correct. It gives parents a good starting list of foods to watch out for. Removal of these food allergens can help symptoms up to a certain extent. These are efforts aimed at reversing the harmful effects of processed foods, food allergies and fighting the impacts of residual viruses from the live vaccine doses hiding in the brain and gut neurons of autistic kids.

Low Carb Diets: High amounts of sugar in the diet can be the enemy in hyper-active kids. It can introduce silly behaviors like uncontrolled giggling and stim-ming while worsening restlessness and causing hyperactivity (among other disruptive behaviors). These effects might be due to intestinal dysbiosis of sugars where they end up promoting candidiasis and other undesirable gut biome issues.

High carb diets can generally be more inflammatory than lower carb diets. Such inflammation can in turn be part of the problem causing the adverse effects on kids with ASD. Of the various diets out there for that show promise for vari-ous health conditions, the Keto diet has become popular among autism parents after a recent study[18.2] at the University of Honolulu, Hawaii seems to have found significant improvement in about half of the 15 participants that were on a keto diet after 3 months.

The keto diet involves restricting diet to 70% fats, 25% proteins and 5% carbohydrates. This switches the body to using the ketogenic digestive pathway that is designed to use fats as the main source of fuel for body processes. It is a difficult diet to follow as it involves removal of processed foods altogether.

Simple Carbohydrate Diets: The simple carbohydrate diet is an elimination diet prescribed in the DAN protocol. It works for kids on the autism spectrum and others with very significant gut allergy issues. It proposes limiting diets to simple carbohydrates containing nothing more than a single glucose molecule. Typical complex carbohydrates contain polysaccharides or multiple glucose molecules which are considered harder to digest and absorb for kids with Crohn's disease or irritable bowel syndrome with or without autism symptoms. It is indeed helpful for a certain segment of those impacted with autism symptoms, but it can again be a hard diet to follow particularly in kids.

Stem Cell Treatments

Stem cells are precursors of all living cells in mammals. After the initial embryonic stage where the entire embryo is made of stem cells, these differentiate into other cells creating the entire body composed of hundreds of cell types. However, stem cells continue to exist in various parts of the body throughout life. These cells have the ability to divide symmetrically into 2 stem cells or asymmetrically into one stem cell and another body cell. Thus, they have properties of self-renewal and multipotency.

Use of these cells in treating various diseases has been a subject of controversy particularly around the use of stem cells from human embryos. But not all research involves embryos. It is possible to harvest stem cells from other body parts like the bone marrow and grow them indefinitely in laboratory settings. Stem cell treatments are not an FDA approved option in the US for the treatment of autism, although they seem to have some marginal positive effects in many kids. There are concerns regarding safety, efficacy and standardization that need to be addressed. However, there have been instances where there has been miraculous recovery, where a kid goes from marginally verbal to fully verbal after stem cell treatment. For reasons already explained, the younger the child (particularly children under 6) the better the probability of seeing some positive changes. The useful properties of stem cells in these cases are thought to be their immune modulatory effects rather than the potential to differentiate into neuron cells.

As of early 2020 two types of stem cell therapies are available to patients for autism treatments based on where the stem cells are sourced from. Autologous stem cell treatment is where stem cells are used that are harvested from the bone marrow of the hip bones of the patient. The stem cells are multiplied and re-injected into the patient a few hours later. The challenge with this treatment is the torture you have to put the child through to extract bone marrow and deal with the after effects of rejection of cells by the immune system, which happens most of the time.

Another type of treatment involves use of stem cells sourced from umbilical cord derived stem cells from own preserved cord or donors. These cells are then multiplied in a lab. This only needs a limited amount of donor cells that are then re-used to create more stem cells in the lab and injected into the patient. These cord stem cells are more primitive than stem cells derived from bone marrow. The treatment typically involves four injections of stem cells over a period of four days. While considerably less painful, this process has the same probability of success as the autologous route.

Both these current processes owe their efficacy (if any) to their immune modulation effect, which in turn can result in reduced inflammation in the brain. It might work in cases where constant brain inflammation is the cause of the autism symptoms. But the ability of these stem cells to differentiate into neurons and grow in the brain is very low or unknown and as a result the efficacy remains low. What might really work is if the stem cells can be directed toward becoming neurons for repairing the damaged brain. Such a possibility exists with neural stem cells (NSC). Neural stem cells are specialized stem cells that generate radial glial cells that give rise to the neurons and to the glia of the central nervous system. They are under research for their ability to help recovery from stroke and ischemic damage. While these could most certainly help with autism, they are not commercially available to patients due to challenges with sourcing neuronal stem cells. These are found in localized brain regions called "niches" such as the sub granular zone of the hippocampal dentate gyrus, the subventricular zone of the lateral ventricles, and the external germinal layer of the cerebellum. Extracting and growing these cells in laboratory settings remain a challenge. The efficacy of any such method in treating autism particularly from traumatic injury and ischemic injury needs to be evaluated. But this kind of treatments hold out a lot of hope for kids and adults in the autism spectrum in the years to come.

HBOT – Oxygen Therapy

Fiscus religiosa (commonly called the sacred fig or the Peepal tree) is a large dry season-deciduous or semi-evergreen tree that grows up to 30m tall and is native to the tropical and semi-tropical climates of India and Southeast Asia. In the eastern traditions this tree is considered very sacred. Gautama Buddha, the originator of the Buddhist religion, is said to have attained enlightenment while meditating underneath a Ficus religiosa. The leaves of this tree move continuously even when the air around is still and no perceptible wind is blowing. Walking around this tree in the morning and evening has traditionally been suggested as a remedy for mental retardation. The modern explanation to this is that this tree gives out copious amounts of oxygen which helps the damaged brain heal and work better.

In a medical context, hyperbaric oxygen chambers therefore could serve as a remedy for traumatic brain injury. There are known cases of people with traumatic brain injury doing better with HBOT therapy. However, HBOT therapy has mostly fallen short when it comes to treatment of kids on the autism spectrum. Only very slight improvements (if any) are seen even in kids that are treated on a regular basis. This might be due to the fact that this treatment may only work in cases where there is currently existing, festering brain damage and inflammation from it. Unfortunately, those with damaged but healed and scarred pathways in the brain (like seen in many spectrum children) may see limited to no improvement from this therapy.

Perhaps use of medically induced hypothermia which has proven to be successful in newborns, if successfully adapted to older children and adults, might prove to be more effective. Since both HBOT and Hypothermia are based on oxygenation of the brain they could perhaps be used in conjunction to come up with a treatment protocol that might work better.

Key Take Away: Biomedical interventions can help promote better bodily functions which can help improve brain functioning. The DAN movement and treatment protocol was among the first efforts towards identification of true causative factors of autism. DAN has since given ways to the MAPS program. Elimination of inflammatory processes and promoting of healing mechanisms are the main hallmarks of biomedical interventions and can bring incremental relief to many kids on the spectrum. But these methods do not bring complete recovery from autism symptoms and those with the least impacted brains see the most significant improvements from these treatments.

CHAPTER 19

Potential Future Treatments

Up and Coming Technologies

For parents impacted by autism in their kids, current medical science has no options to treat the condition. The issue is further compounded by the fact that autism researchers have bought into the story of genetic causes of autism. They have been hard at work trying to find genetic causes for the malaise, looking for evidence that doesn't exist, wasting valuable time and resources that could have been deployed to look at brain damage recovery instead. Now that we understand that autism is caused almost entirely by traumatic or hypoxic brain injury, happening mostly during birth, it stands to reason that parents can look towards current research in the field of traumatic brain injury recovery for answers. And looking at the symptoms and directions of research for traumatic brain injury (TBI) provides even more evidence for the fact that autism is caused by traumatic brain injury. The latest research in TBI recovery[19.1] seems to be focused on stem cell treatments and use of hypothermia, while also investigating mitochondrial dysfunction, gut dysbiosis, microglial activation, cerebral microcirculation impairment that seem to follow TBI exactly like it happens in autism. Mitochondrial dysfunction and gut dysbiosis might follow TBI, directly as a result of a compromise in the blood brain barrier by injury even in adults. I have previously mentioned in chapter 14 that mitochondrial dysfunction could be a result of viral latencies when certain viruses get past the blood brain barrier and establish a latency in the neuronal cells of the brain.

Neuron cells in the central nervous system (CNS), typically do not regenerate or regenerate enough once they are damaged. Decades of research into the possibility of regeneration of neurons has turned out to be fruitless this far. Current research into brain damage, particularly Chronic Traumatic Encephalopathy (CTE), Stroke, Multiple Sclerosis, Alzheimer's and Parkinson's, might provide useful information leading to the next breakthrough in autism treatment. Any treatments that can address neuron regeneration, scar tissue removal, reversal of neuronal viral latencies can be of particular help for autism. The open sourcing of gene-editing with CRISPR and the evolution of bio-hacking might even hold out hope to speed up research in this area, not only for genetic diseases causing autism symptoms but also for brain healing from trauma by methods unknown to us at this time. Some of the current research showing promise are discussed below:

Neuron regeneration: Any treatments that have the potential to add additional neuron supply to the brain can be of potential benefit to autism patients. Neuronal stem cells (NSC) is a technology currently under study for brain damage in stroke patients. NSC's are capable of differentiating into neurons, astrocytes, and oligodendrocytes, and adding an additional dose of these cells into the brain might help further natural healing. But immune rejection and long-term functional integration of such cells into the brain continue to be challenges to overcome Such technology might offer help to autism patients in future if successful.

In similar fashion, another possible solution is tissue nano transfection (TNT), where skin cells are teased into growing other cell types capable of repairing damaged organs. TNT involves use of a nanochip to deliver a biologic payload to skin cells in the target area, reprograming these cells to create another targeted type of body cell. This kind of technology is currently successful in lab animals. If successfully applied to the human brain, such a technology would be a boon for numerous kids and adults on the autism spectrum.

In vivo reprogramming: This is an emerging strategy for repairing hard to heal organs like the brain that consists of converting resident tissue-specific cells into the cell types that have been lost due to disease or damage by a process called in vivo lineage reprogramming. Even in areas of damage like in a transected spinal cord, the bridges of healing tissue that develop seem to contain radial glial cells[19,7]. If glial cells in the brain can be repurposed to become neurons, then they could be used to help the CNS heal from damage. A payload of retroviral protein capable of such reprogramming when ingested could accomplish this feat. It has been demonstrated in lab animals, and if successfully reproduced in humans it could hold the promise of a cure for brain damage.

Scar dissolution and removal: In the case of trauma scarring is necessary to quickly isolate dead tissue, re-establish the blood brain barrier and repair broken capillaries. But it is widely believed within the scientific community that the scar tissue formed in response to brain and spinal injury inhibits regrowth of neurons. Some new technologies such as using rapid acoustic pulses to reduce scar volume have been promising. If such types of technology could be used to reduce scarring in the brain and spinal injuries they might help with healing and recovery from injuries of the central nervous system. (Recently there have been some studies that seem to suggest that scarring actually helps regrowth, but it is hard to give them credence knowing that scarring represents both a physical and chemical barrier to regrowth.)

Reversing of Neuronal viral latencies: As mentioned before, viral latency in the body and its physiological effects can be a huge unknown. A latent virus can impact cellular processes. When the latency is inside of neuron cells, the effects can be even more profound due to the possible impacts on complex brain processes. During a latency, the viral genome is maintained as a separate genetic entity (an episome) within the neuronal cell nucleus. It can then re-activate when the conditions are right or create ongoing chronic conditions, which can be the effects of the virus itself or the antibody response. The Herpes Simplex Virus (HSV-1) is one such virus that is believed to establish a neuronal latency. Other viruses capable of infecting neuron cells and establishing a latency include the measles and polio viruses. These viruses take advantage of the differentiated functioning of brain immunity to impair the body's self-healing abilities to recover from trauma. Hence, removal of viral latency in neurons (if possible) represents one of the best ways to help the body heal itself from damage. In fact, of all the research into traumatic brain injury recovery, this viral latency removal might represent the lowest hanging fruit. Not to say it is easy by any means, but with current technologies like CRISPR protein and gene-editing have put this type of treatment in the realm of possibility.

Advances in brain research and treatments for healing injury have been gaining traction in recent times. For autism parents these offer a ray of hope. Given the right directions of research and funding soon there might come a time when brain damage will become treatable and completely reversible.

Cytotron – Quantum Magnetic Resonance Therapy

The Cytotron is a medical device that utilizes Rotational Field Quantum Magnetic Resonance (RFQMR) technology, employing precisely focused radio frequency waves and magnetic fields, and has been explored for various medical conditions, including brain tumors. The Cytotron was created by Dr. Rajah Vijay Kumar, a scientist from Bangalore, India. Kumar began his research into creating the machine as far back as 1987 and produced the first prototype in 1999. It began its commercial utilization in 2006 as a tool for tissue engineering.

The purported mechanism involves altering the transmembrane potential of cells, aiming to trigger apoptosis in cancerous cells or stimulate tissue regeneration in degenerative conditions. RFQMR utilizes non-thermal, non-ionizing radio frequency waves and hence does not have any known adverse side effects. It has received a "Breakthrough Device Designation" from the FDA for certain cancers. In 2012, Cytotron was approved for clinical use in Europe under the CE (Conformité Européenne) Mark. It is mainly used for musculoskeletal disorders and cancer, its use in brain treatment, particularly for tumors, remains investigational. Some clinical studies, including a compassionate study on pediatric brain tumors in Mexico, have been conducted, but the broad efficacy and safety of Cytotron for brain-related conditions are still under evaluation, and it is not yet an approved standard treatment in many parts of the world, including the United States.

The Netflix movie "Lucca's World" recounts the true story of Lucca, a Mexican boy who has cerebral palsy due to a challenging birth, and his family's arduous journey to India for specialized "cytotron therapy" treatment. This film, along with the "cytotron" treatment it features, has garnered significant attention from parents of children with autism. The promise of tissue regeneration using this machine offers hope for those whose children's autism stems from brain damage caused by hypoxic or traumatic birth events. More details are available from shreis.org and gliaihc.com

The Age of AI – Companions for Social Well-Being

In the evolving landscape of assistive technologies, artificial intelligence is poised to offer a profound and transformative form of support for individuals with intellectual disabilities: the AI social companion. Imagine a future where personalized AI bots seamlessly integrate into daily life, acting not as mere tools but as genuine companions, tailored to the unique needs and communication styles of each individual. These digital companions could patiently navigate the nuances of communication, employing simplified language, visual cues, and repetition as needed, fostering understanding and reducing the frustration that can sometimes arise in human interactions. They could become steadfast conversational partners, engaging individuals in discussions about their specific interests, thereby alleviating feelings of loneliness and isolation that can often be a significant challenge.

Furthermore, these AI companions could serve as invaluable tools for social learning and skill development. By simulating various social scenarios in a safe and non-judgmental environment, individuals could practice essential social skills, from basic greetings to more complex interactions, building confidence before venturing into real-world social situations. For those with significant communication barriers, AI could even act as a bridge, interpreting gestures, vocalizations, or AAC device outputs, facilitating smoother communication with caregivers and the wider community.

Beyond social interaction, AI companions hold the potential to significantly enhance emotional well-being. Advanced AI could be trained to recognize and respond to emotional cues, offering empathy, comfort, or suggesting appropriate coping strategies. The consistent presence of a non-judgmental AI could provide a safe space for individuals to express their feelings, potentially leading to improved emotional regulation and reduced anxiety. Moreover, by continuously monitoring communication patterns and emotional indicators, these AI companions could potentially detect early signs of distress, alerting support systems for timely intervention.

The capabilities extend to fostering greater independence and structure in daily life. AI bots could provide personalized reminders for tasks and appointments, offer step-by-step guidance for complex activities, and help manage individualized daily schedules, promoting predictability and autonomy. They could also serve as interactive educational tools, delivering tailored content and reinforcing learned skills at a pace and style that suits the individual's needs.

However, the integration of AI social companions must proceed with careful consideration of ethical implications. Ensuring data privacy, preventing over-reliance, and maintaining the crucial role of human connection are paramount. Accessibility, affordability, and the mitigation of potential biases within AI algorithms are also critical to ensure equitable access and fair outcomes. Recognizing the diverse spectrum of intellectual disabilities and tailoring AI companions to meet individual needs will be an ongoing endeavor.

In conclusion, the future of AI as a social companion for intellectually disabled individuals, presents a remarkable opportunity to enhance their lives in profound ways. By offering personalized interaction, fostering social engagement, supporting emotional well-being, promoting learning, and encouraging independence, these digital companions hold the potential to unlock new avenues for connection, growth, and a significantly improved quality of life, provided that development and implementation are guided by ethical principles and a deep understanding of individual needs.

Key Take Away: The similarity of symptoms between autism and traumatic brain injury in adults further underscores the fact that one major cause of autism is indeed traumatic brain injury. Gut dysbiosis and mitochondrial dysfunction are consequences of damage to the blood brain barrier. Treatments that can reverse these aftereffects might be critical in finding permanent recovery from TBI. Numerous mechanisms capable of regenerating damaged neurons and healing brain damage are currently under investigation. Some of these have shown promise in animal studies, and could become viable options for autism treatment in the future. Drugs currently under research for brain injury recovery, Alzheimer's, Multiple Sclerosis etc., might also hold out hope for kids and adults on the spectrum. The age of AI is expected to usher in an era of AI social companions which could benefit and enable kids and adults on the autism spectrum.

PART V

The Legal Recourse

M alpractice by a medical practitioner is defined as a deviation from the accepted standard of care, particularly if that deviation resulted in injury. Pitocin abuse by prolonged induction of labor beyond labelled contra-indication is a perfect poster child for a birth injury lawsuit. Yet the defeat of autism cases in vaccine court in 2010-11 and the court pointing at genetic causes poured cold water on lawyers' willingness to undertake any 'autism' cases. Lawyers who might be willing to take on birth injury cases balk at the possibility once the word autism comes into the picture. Turning that attitude around is the goal of this final part.

There is unfortunately one other shift that happened in 2018 that sabotages the possibility of legal action by individual parents, thanks to a disruptive move by the ACOG.

CHAPTER 20

The Impact on the Family

Many autism parents have written media articles and some even entire books detailing the challenges parents face and live through as a result of their kids' autism. Some even describe how they have been suicidal at times, even contemplating taking the lives of their kids along with themselves. While such extremes might be construed as weakness and desperation, I can totally understand how those kinds of thoughts might come about. Watching a 10-year-old child scream and throw tantrums, unable to verbalize the reason for their outburst and explain the pain they're going through can bring on those feelings of helplessness and desperation to the extreme. It can easily make someone hate their lives and pity the existence of their suffering child. It's possible to go through suffering and stay strong if you know there's light at the end of the tunnel. Unfortunately, for parents of kids on the autism spectrum (particularly lower functioning kids), there's not been much to hope for in the past, although the emerging technologies of the future described in the previous chapter, do hold out a lot of promise for the future.

Sometimes ignorance is bliss. From the moment we found out what had actually happened to our cute little kids (thanks to the MRI scan of my second son) things have never been the same again. In our case our pain multiplied a few times and was joined by anger when we found out that the condition of our kids was not natural but the result of obstetric malpractice at birth. Previously, my wife and I would jokingly blame each other's cranky moments as the reason why the kids had turned out the way they did. She blamed my lineage and I would tease her about her family history, but neither had any real clue. Life went on, challenging and frustrating, but without the nagging sense of having been wronged for life by the doctor we had counted on so much.

Stalled Development

Initially we weren't surprised when we heard the autism diagnosis, thanks to prior research we had done on our boys' hyperactive behavior but weren't sure of what to expect. We were not expecting this was going to turn our whole lives upside down. But that is exactly what happened, and we were caught totally unprepared. The impacts have been felt not just by us, but by the extended family, relatives and close friends as well.

At first there is the denial of any deep issues with your child. I simply couldn't believe anything would go wrong with our kids. Unfortunately for most parents, this state of denial depending on how long it lasts, results in the loss of valuable time in the life of the damaged child. Like in our case, it takes a while for parents to come around to the realization that something is wrong with their child and they need to act quickly to help their child. For me it has been particularly difficult after I learned about all the disinformation being shared out there on the internet, effectively ensuring other parents stay in the dark about the root causes of their children's misery.

Outwardly, there was truly nothing wrong with our kids when they were infants and toddlers. But we came to realize later the brunt of these impacts are truly all-round and we had to adjust our lives and priorities around the kids. Most of the ill-effects became more and more obvious with time as the kids grew up. Unfortunately, autism is a problem which tends to only get worse with time. As our kids grew up, the divergence between them and the rest of their peers got more and more manifested. Regular pediatricians are not equipped to deal with such cases. They address the problem in the typical symptomatic shotgun approach of modern allopathic medicine, and all they are able to come up with is only speech therapy and Applied Behavior Analysis (ABA). Our experience in this regard has been very typical of most parents out there suffering the consequences of labor induction brain damage.

The brain controls all human behavior and all the complex higher-order functions, including speech, verbal ability, cognitive processing and the complex social interactions that we take for granted as humans. When the brain is damaged, the first impact is to these higher cognitive functions which typically only develop outside the womb as a baby grows up in the first few years of life. The gap in development between undamaged kids and those with brain damage begins to show between the ages 2 and 3. That is when kids start taking off with their verbal ability and social interactions, while kids with damaged brains tend to be in their own world. Progress from that point becomes an uphill battle for the entire family as this gap only gets worse with age if left unattended and hard to fix even with a lot of effort.

After about 6 months old our older boy became a tough baby to carry and hold onto. He was always squirming and wiggling, trying to jump out of my hands with no fear of falling down. Once he started walking, he always ran to get from one place to another, sometimes unable to maneuver around obstacles and bumping into them. I took it to be precocious development and was generally happy he was so fast. However, hidden beneath this veil of apparently extreme motor skills were some really serious deficiencies. My son was always throwing up a lot. He would refuse to stand in place long enough to learn words to talk. He refused to be potty trained, and stayed in diapers until he was about 4.

Our 2nd boy was a little slower and only learned to stand up and walk with support at 11 months old. He didn't become proficient at walking until he was about three years old. Just before age 3 he was beginning to show signs of talking and becoming a typical kid. But his third-year vaccination did him in and he retrogressed into losing the interest and ability to talk.

While both boys did learn to walk and run on their own, there were some serious deficiencies in how our boys progressed. Both lacked the ability to pay attention to my directions. I could never train either of them to stand still long enough or listen long enough to play any games. The lack of response to simple yes/no questions even at age 3 seemed to get in the way of learning anything. They lacked the motor coordination, focus and strength in their hands and fingers to hold onto simple objects like pencils, preventing them from even drawing in a meaningful way. Then there was repetitive behaviors like looking at the wheels of toy cars and spinning them all the time. This became so bad that we had to take away all toy cars.

Most people, even those with high functioning kids on the spectrum, cannot quite understand what life is like on the lower end of the spectrum. An easier way to imagine what it is like, is to think of a teen or adult that behaves like 2- or 3- year-old. The lack of fine motor control at various levels makes even simple functions like blowing the nose, rinsing the mouth or swallowing a tablet quite a challenge. Doctors' visits and injections can be a nightmare, with them twisting, turning, and screaming, making it practically impossible to get a needle in at the right spot even with 2 or 3 attendants holding them down. Having to put them through medication and injections, knowing that their condition was caused by birth malpractice only adds to the trauma of the parents.

The only redeeming factor is they retain their innocence and cuteness for much longer. But for the most part they simply destroy toys or play with them inappropriately, put objects in their mouths, and have no concept of dirty versus clean. There's constant vocal stimming and hand flapping all day. They are unable to follow stories even in the simplest of pre-school cartoons. Essentially, it's the terrible twos with the weight, strength and reach of an older 10 plus year old with no end in sight. A typical special needs parent can expect weekends to be taken up mending and fixing things that have seen the wrath of a low-functioning child.

Kids on the autism spectrum are otherwise regular kids that are lacking certain higher-order functions like speech, memory, etc. That means they come into this world capable of the same feelings and emotions as all others. Unfortunately, their main issue is the ability to express themselves verbally as their brains don't process information at conversational speed. They are full of thoughts, feelings and desires that they would like to express but simply cannot do so with words. With time this inability to express themselves turns into nervousness and social anxiety that is amplified to a much greater degree than would otherwise. The result is they try to shut themselves out from the outside world. Combined with their basic inability to focus on what their eyes see and their ears hear imprisons them in their own mind.

Having difficulty talking is usually due to an inability to pay attention, which in turn to a lack of environmental learning which is critical for any sort of higher-order social development and a key aspect that makes up the complex social interactions of humans. If kids on the spectrum can't copy what the adults or peers do due to their lack of focus, it just means they can't learn anything by themselves or be taught anything very easily. While attention deficiency is rampant even in the regular peer groups of children, such extreme lack of focus is typical in the spectrum. This results in an inability to learn language or express their needs and even share little things like "my tummy doesn't feel well."

The Future of Autistic Kids

Like every other aspect of our lives, even family vacations were impacted and subjected to constraints. The very few vacations we've managed in the past few years we take during odd off-peak times so that we don't run into overcrowded situations in tourist destinations. The sounds and chaos can be overwhelming and our kids don't take well to crowds and don't enjoy all that sensory overload. On one such early November off peak season visit to the theme parks of Orlando, Florida, we came across a large group from a special needs caretaker home sporting 'autism' T-shirts. They had probably picked the same times to visit for the same reasons we picked ours. We saw older otherwise normal looking men in their 40's and 50's and even older having to be helped around the park. They were mostly not talking, just following directions and mostly zoned out, being helped around by caregivers as if they had just turned 3 years old.

Until that moment my wife and I had been living in this bubble that autism kids mostly end up recovering and held on to the hope that our kids would eventually be alright. Every blog and story out there was from parents relating their positive success stories and we never heard of the alternative. Not having had any previous experience with autism in our family circle, we never knew any better. Our boys look normal and we had come to expect they would eventually grow out of their problems. We were suddenly hit with the alternate reality of what would happen if our boys didn't make the recovery we had come to expect.

It's really hard to fathom, but it's true that your birth plays a very crucial role in how your life turns out. The way you came into this world can determine your brain function, which in turn determines a significant amount of how your life turns out. As modern living continues to shift us away from agricultural subsistence-based occupations to more industrial and technological occupations, the reliance on mental faculties for participating in the workforce have become increasingly critical. Brawn-work based occupations are being replaced more and more with brain work. Even schools have over the years shifted focus to improved vocabulary and comprehension as the key ingredients of all their study programs. There tends to be more emphasis on independent study versus the more directed study that has been the norm for many decades.

Unsurprisingly, this puts kids on the autism spectrum at a further disadvantage. With their damaged brains they tend to become adept at doing certain things with narrow areas of focus at best. While such jobs existed in the past, they risk getting left behind more and more as societal expectations change and their condition becomes more and more of a problem. While advances in medical technology might eventually might help these kids, the societal advancements and expectations that accompany such technological changes puts them at an even bigger disadvantage and unable to keep up with the expectations of the world around them.

The future of their children is what worries autism parents the most. What will they do when they get out of school? Will they be able to become self-sufficient? Will they be able to hold on to a job or keep themselves happy, healthy, active and become contributing members of society? Will they be able to have a family of their own? How will they survive in that fast-changing world out there after the parents are gone? Unfortunately, the answers to these questions have not been very promising so far.

While as human beings we are wired to be social beings, we also seem to be wired for ganging up on those of us that fall outside of the norms that we have established for ourselves. The result is these kids can be subjected to a lot of bullying when they don't socialize like others. Worse still, they can have stimming behaviors (giggling, flapping, talking to themselves, etc.) that make them the subject of ridicule and bullying.

Modern society is a social system based on rewarding creativity, logic and social and emotional intelligence. Most successful people succeed because of their intelligence even if a high IQ is not really a pre-requisite to what they do. Higher acumen is amply rewarded in our society, but this is more pronounced in modern times where most opportunities are tuned toward people that excel in a field due to their abilities combined with intellect. This is where kids and adults on the autism spectrum including ADD, ADHD and the like are seemingly doomed for failure. For no fault of theirs, they are destined to not achieve their full potential that could have been had their birth process not damaged their brains.

Lives Changed Forever

For people not used to taking care of a special needs child, it is hard to imagine the mental stress and agony that special needs parents go through. Most people consider autism as something that happens to other people, so they simply don't have a need to understand it. This is perhaps due to the genetic connotation that's commonly associated with a condition like autism. Such an attitude is also what gives rise to the stigma toward autism and other mental health issues in general.

For example, slowly but surely the parents of autistic children (just like their kids) become social outsiders as well. You notice after a while that your friends' kids are not interested in playing with your kids, simply because these kids will not engage in any social play. Soon the parents follow suit and you stop meeting up as much as you used to and your own friends have less and less time for you. Your social circle might shrink down to the closest of friends. And it goes both ways: you don't have time for socializing much either, as social situations are taxing on the kids and you don't want to deal with people who don't understand your kids. Soon the main social group becomes a circle of other special needs parents who are the only other people who can comprehend your situation by virtue of being in a similar situation themselves.

Yet special needs parents are a group that has experienced exceptional trauma and suffers from severe time challenges, which leaves very little time for social meetups. Only the strongest parents manage to persevere, continuing to try to keep the kids engaged. Unfortunately, we live in times where the time you have is money you don't have and vice versa. The autism problem is a double-edged sword in that it takes both time and money to even attempt fixing the problem. In spite of the fighters that we are, most autism parents are too busy fighting for our kid's future that we have not had the time to sit back and think about the root cause of our current situation.

Acceptance of kids with autism is at present hit or miss. In popular culture PBS recently launched a character with autism called Julia that appears on Sesame Street, and the Disney movie 'Finding Dory' was about a fish born with memory disorders. But for every story you hear about families that adopt special needs kids there is a story about hate groups seeking to "cure" the world of autism by killing off children with autism. One popular Google auto complete search term was "people with autism should be killed" and it was only after a protracted fight by impacted parents and good Samaritans of the world that Google finally removed it.

Your kids being called autistic does give you a different perspective in life. All the little trivial things that people complain about all the time, talking about them as these huge challenges in their lives sound trivial, even stupid to you, when autism is on the back of your mind all the time. In our case (as with many other impacted parents) we've leaned into our faith and spirituality. Being believers in the idea of karmic influences in our lives, we console ourselves assuming what happened to our kids was the agenda of the almighty, perhaps part of a grand plan that we have no idea of at the moment. It gives us the strength we need to get through every day of our lives without breaking down. It is very draining to be autism parents and we figured early on that focusing on positives and planning out things a little more conservatively on what we could accomplish with our kids went a long way to reducing frustration and improving our actual accomplishments. We recognized that we need to be around for these kids for longer and letting the stress get to us was not helping our cause.

However, there is a glimmer of hope from the work of some non-profit organizations at the local level who, by blazing new trails in totally unchartered territory of handling grown kids who have turned into adults with autism, have shifted the attention of many others in this direction. More programs like these are needed to help these unlucky victims of the birth process that become collateral damage in the modern society's fight against pandemics using vaccines.

The one thing parents cannot afford to do is to give up on their child, particularly when the whole world around them wants to move on and give up trying to help. For kids on the spectrum, their parents are their only friends, their only true support system in the fast and busy world around them. This is why a coordinated legal response is an absolute necessity, to help secure the future of these kids and to offer some respite to impacted parents.

> **Key Take Away:** The suffering of autism parents knows no parallel as it is a daily fight with no hope for change and no end in sight, particularly on the lower functioning end of the spectrum. Even great motivational quotes from great people like this one from Winston Churchill – "When you are going through hell, keep going" – don't really capture the kind of hell autism parents go through and bring no solace. The only possible redemption is some kind of medical breakthrough to cure brain damage.

CHAPTER 21

The Managed Narrative Online

The Biased and Active Management of the Messaging

E verybody who's followed the news cycles in recent times knows how it's possible to manage the messaging online by hiring public relations or online reputation management firms. In fact, many of these firms have gotten online image management down to a science. For example, the Arab Spring in North Africa and the Middle east in the 2010-2012 timeframe represented a remarkable example of how people were able to organize online on Facebook and Twitter to create mass movements large enough to bring about political changes in entire countries. Some succeeded others failed. Ever wonder why we haven't seen any such movements online on any such scale ever since? The reasons are fairly straightforward, these movements awakened governments and other entities to the scope of such possibilities and they have learned how they can manage the messaging with trolls, bots and cyborgs very effectively such that online opinion cannot be swayed against them very easily.

The messaging of the safety of Pitocin and its role in causing autism, unfortunately, seems to be one of the pioneering cases of such active message management. The first thing that I noticed about online forums, is there seems to be a horde of obviously hired trolls waiting to go ballistic on any parent casting a genuine doubt on the safety of labor induction based on what they are seeing first hand with their kids. There is this diversionary tactic that seems to be a very deliberate (and thus far hugely successful) attempt to confuse the issue with other possible causes, and they all talk about a genetic pre-disposition. Such pre-disposition is a concept unknown to science, but very well known only to these trolls. They blame genetics while vouching for the safety of induction, citing sup-posedly hundreds of cases of successful inductions. Upon closer scrutiny, these trolls are mostly fake profiles manned by total know nothings with no knowledge of autism but trained on a set of standard talking points to blame genetics and environmental factors, which is unfortunately, also the official line. Here I was, looking at these forums, reading these deceptive messages, while sitting with solid evidence of an MRI scan and now clear recollection of the events that lead to my children's condition.

All this makes it clear that there is very active management of the messaging about Pitocin by one or more public relations firms or a legal organization. There are delib-erate efforts to deflect people from finding out the true birth injury causes of autism. They hang around in these forums only to create confusion in the minds of people and they move around between forums and coordinate between them to descend on any thread where there is a voice of reason pointing to the birth injury etiology of autism. Any forum that ranks higher on google is fair game for these trolls. The search engines are being manipulated by some internet reputation management firms such that the pages supporting Pitocin's safety rank higher than any others that raise ques-tions about its safety. Reading through some of these forums I have seen the same opinion echoed by many impacted parents in such forums, who find themselves shouted down by hordes of hired hands.

Search for Pitocin Autism on Google and you will see what I mean. Figure 21.1 is a screenshot of a Google search for the words Pitocin Autism. See what came back in early 2017. Nine out of the top 10 search results vouch for the safety of Pitocin. Trying the same search 3 years later in 2020 brings back a few different results. However, it's the same number of results in support of Pitocin, i.e. 9 out of 10. The same query with the advent of generative AI, in 2025 the answers that come back, are simply non-committal and ask you to discuss with your care provider. This way the AI bots go for the diplomatic answer. But you mostly know what care providers would say. They will pretty much vouch for the safety of labor induction given the official line of the ACOG and their new fall guys the SMFM. And if they say otherwise, they put themselves at risk of losing their license to practice and their reputation.

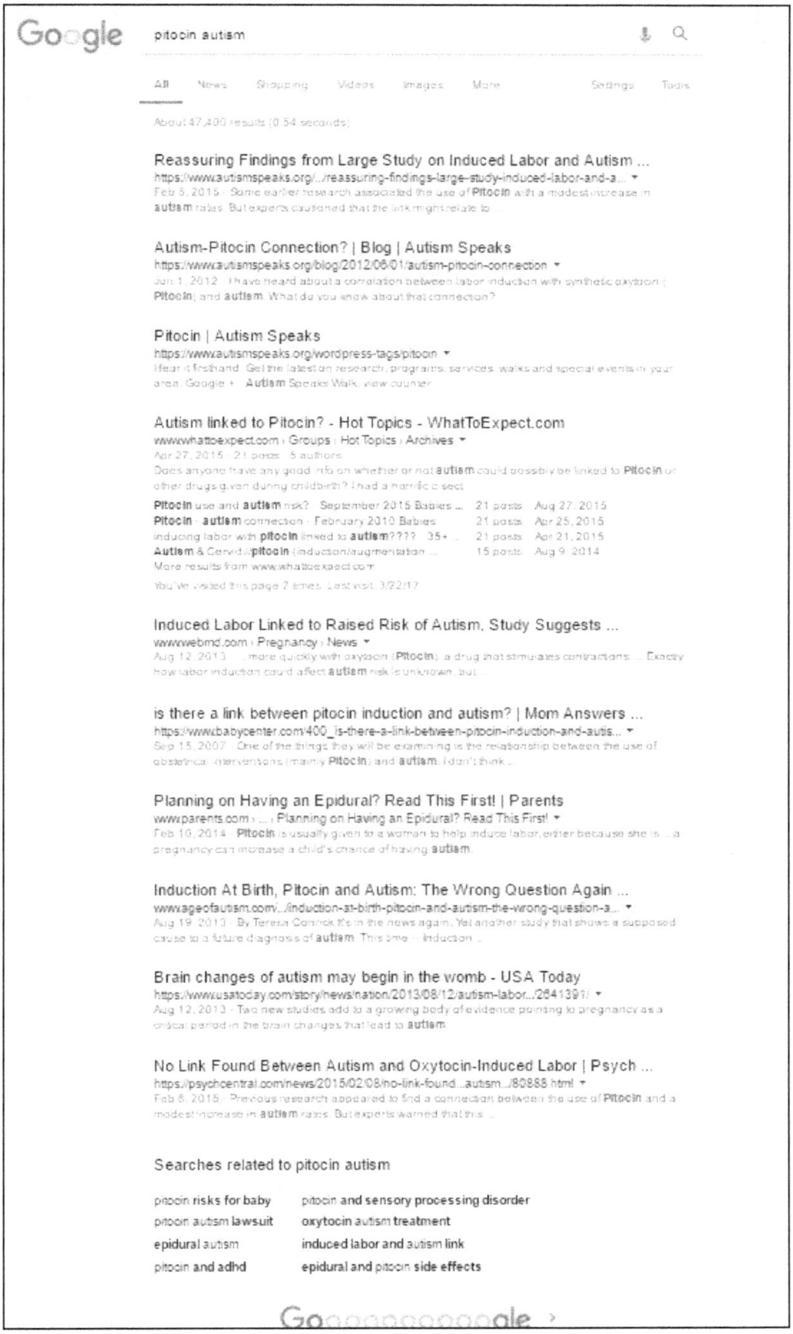

Fig. 21.1: Google search result for 'Pitocin autism' in 2017

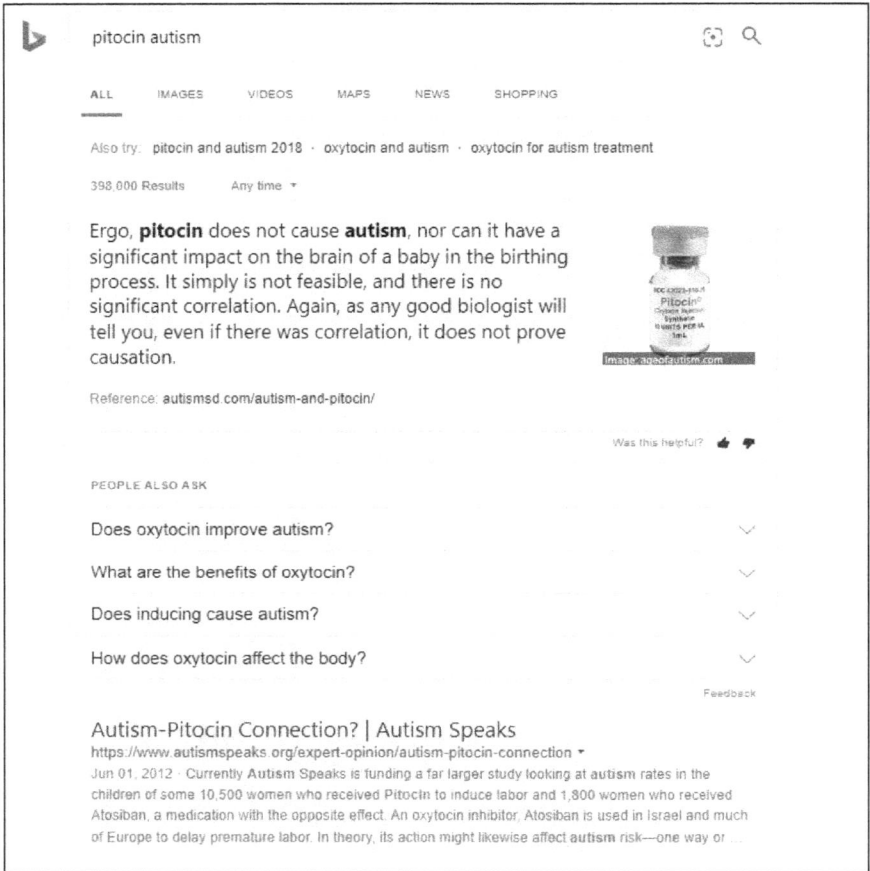

Fig. 21.2: Pitocin Autism search results on Bing in 2020.

The Bing search engine from Microsoft brings back as its top result in early 2020 a blog by name autismsd.com from an anonymous author with the picture of a vial of Pitocin for added effect, forcefully vouching for its safety by someone claiming to be a biologist (Figure 21.2). If you have read through the previous chapters, you know that the safety of Pitocin is not a question a biologist could answer, but one for a biomechanics expert to speak to. Only the latter can speak to the kind of contraction forces crushing a baby's brain and the placenta in the absence of the protection of amniotic fluid causing traumatic/hypoxic damage on a baby's brain. This is one of thousands of examples of how an innocent blog from a well-meaning blogger is being manipulated by special interests. The dates on some of these posts also provides a clue as to when this active messaging started. They all seem to have started around the year 2018. Fast forward to 2025, the Autismsd site seems defunct, and other sites seem to have taken their place. Parent discussions have now moved, consolidating from individual sites to Facebook groups, Reddit groups and the like. This has obviously made the lives of trolls a lot easier.

I haven't been able to find a single blog or forum out there where a parents' genuine comment casting doubts on Pitocin's role in autism is not being diverted or outright discredited with a fake fact from an egregiously fake account. This historical example in Fig 21.3 provides a classic explanation of how it all unfolds. One parent complains about Pitocin causing her child's autism and another comes by 2 years later to claim genetic predisposition to autism when no such thing has ever existed or been proven. The second account obviously throwing out some rubbish was clearly done after this blog started ranking higher in the searches and was probably flagged by a bot that one of the hired social media companies might be using. This is just one example; this is the case universally on the internet. It is hard to find any high-ranking blog where legitimate Pitocin concerns are not being misled or drowned out in a flurry of lies. The large topic-based Facebook groups on autism have been overrun by trolls who have taken over even as admins helping manage these groups. Try telling them autism is the result of birth injury and they will boot you out. Even those groups run by popular autism organizations have been unfortunately overrun by these hired trolls. To this day I see parents' posts questioning the causes of autism, questioning the safety of labor induction all getting deleted from these forums the moment they start gaining attention.

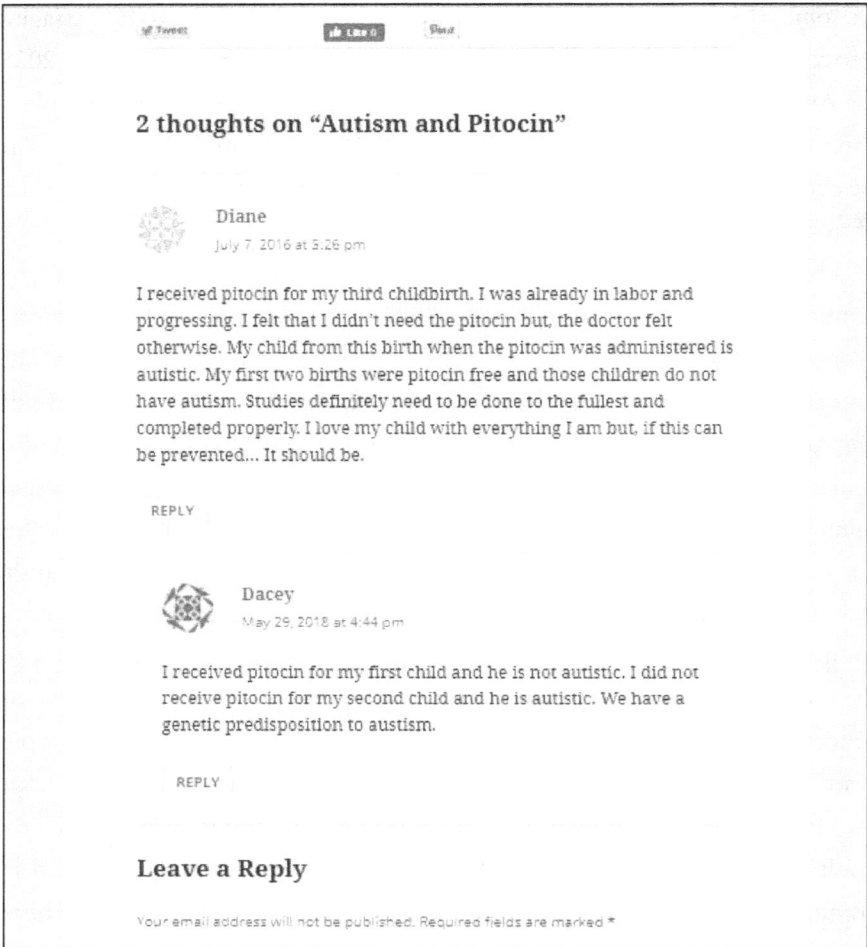

> **2 thoughts on "Autism and Pitocin"**
>
> **Diane**
> July 7, 2016 at 5:26 pm
>
> I received pitocin for my third childbirth. I was already in labor and progressing. I felt that I didn't need the pitocin but, the doctor felt otherwise. My child from this birth when the pitocin was administered is autistic. My first two births were pitocin free and those children do not have autism. Studies definitely need to be done to the fullest and completed properly. I love my child with everything I am but, if this can be prevented... It should be.
>
> REPLY
>
> **Dacey**
> May 29, 2018 at 4:44 pm
>
> I received pitocin for my first child and he is not autistic. I did not receive pitocin for my second child and he is autistic. We have a genetic predisposition to austism.
>
> REPLY
>
> **Leave a Reply**
>
> Your email address will not be published. Required fields are marked *

Fig 21.3 One example of legitimate Pitocin concerns being shot down with rubbish in online blogs.

Thankfully beginning in late 2020 a paper titled "Increased Risk of Autism Development in Children Whose Mothers Experienced Birth Complications or Received Labor and Delivery Drugs" by Smallwood et. al[8.11] from the Neuroscience Program, Trinity University, San Antonio, TX, USA, have started ranking higher on Google searches, a good 4 years after publication in 2016. Their data is from parent surveys and another dataset from the Southwest Autism Research and Resource Center (SAARC - autismcenter.org San Antonio

TX / Phoenix AZ). Their study is hard to refute, considering that it is based on numbers and numbers don't lie. But the facts are that autism is a consequence of Pitocin-abuse not Pitocin-use and chances are there will soon be a counter study from someone claiming safe Pitocin numbers. Unfortunately, that is the state of studies these days and short of concerted action from impacted parents, even such evidence often falls by the wayside when faced with the true complexity of the facts involved in Pitocin abuse. It is the length of time of induction after amniotic rupture that truly counts, and the correlation is clear in the cases of the healthiest mothers and the contra-indication is defined in the Pitocin label, but it is hard for scientific studies to collect that kind of data, without creating a whole movement around it, like some of us parents are trying to do with the AutismPI.org retrospective research data collection initiative.

The Entities Behind the Online Message Management

Synthetic oxytocin is now a generic drug that is manufactured around the world by many big and small pharmaceutical companies in the US and in other countries. Some of the bigger names include Pfizer and Novartis. Cheaper generic pricing has meant most manufacturers have razor-thin margins and make little or no money on it. Some have decided to stop manufacturing it, resulting in shortages for what is a widely used drug all over the world for its post-partum use in stopping blood loss after delivery. Manufacturing has also moved to cheaper destinations outside the US. The manufacturer's liability for the product is limited to their accountability to physicians and warning them of the side effects. The other applications of the drug outside of induction, including abortions and stopping post-partum bleeding, ensure a very steady demand for Pitocin. It's hard to imagine manufacturers or even large suppliers being involved in any internet messaging scam to promote its use in induction, although they are the ones with the kinds of budget to do it. While their hand cannot be totally ruled out their chances of involvement remains low as their exposure in this case remains low.

The other major party that might stand to benefit from not revealing obstetric malpractice is the malpractice insurance companies that insure OB/GYNs. They are probably aware that it could be a challenge to their survival if they are hit with large numbers of malpractice suits against OB/GYNs they insure. Compensation in these types of cases could run into multiple millions per case as it comes down to what is fair compensation for ruining someone's entire life starting at birth and the damage caused to their entire family. Malpractice insurers are also the people that will be aware of birth injury lawsuits from Pitocin abuse in extreme cases, where the birth injury was caught immediately after birth and ended up paying out compensation. When they settle out of court, they tend to make parents sign nondisclosure clauses, shutting them up from disclosing the possible pathway to autism.

The involvement of OB/GYN organizations namely the ACOG and more recently the SMFM who have made totally flawed recommendations about the primary suspects. They might themselves be guilty of birth malpractice, by way of abusing Pitocin and could be very much aware of the damage they have caused. It is in the interest of these medical practitioners to not get sued for their past mistakes. It's also in the manufacturers /marketer's interest to hide the unsafe side effects of the drug, particularly when the cause can be easily hidden. Pitocin itself is not a major moneymaker for big pharma and most manufacturers are out of the business, but sometimes it's amazing how much influence even small players can have on the messaging when it comes to the internet. The malpractice insurers have everything to gain from keeping the causes of autism from Pitocin abuse under wraps. Such attempts at suppression of the truth on the internet could be the result of collusion by some or all of these actors. Whatever it is, it seems to be a devious conspiracy that has potentially kept the truth hidden from the public for decades.

The outcome is one where those involved in the deception are riding a tiger, afraid to let go for fear of retribution, while the crime continues to be committed by some OB/GYNs who in their zeal to avoid the 'intrusive' C-section continue to promote a drug to patients as 'safe and natural' when in fact it is causing irreparable damage to millions of babies over the years in the US and around the world. Unfortunately, this 'modern' method of child delivery is spreading rapidly in other parts of the world causing autism there as well.

While Pitocin can be a useful tool in the hands of an expert OB/GYN, there are many others in whose hands it has manifested as this dangerous weapon causing irreversible brain damage, which when not caught immediately is later labeled autism. Most experts would accept these dangers of Pitocin in private, and express their concerns from time to time, but their voices are muted in the face of this massive messaging to the contrary about 'autism'.

Following the Money

Most obstetricians I have come across are mostly decent folks who believe they're doing a good job at obstetrics. They might even be willing to own up to their mistakes if they are made to realize the true extent of the damage they have caused. But when it comes to a wide-ranging practice where most of them have caused brain damage at some point in their careers, it is often out of an individual obstetrician's hands. While it might make sense to hold the ACOG responsible for mismanagement of the messaging around Pitocin brain damage and autism causation, it is almost guaranteed that they are doing it under pressure from hospital systems and insurance conglomerates to keep it under wraps. In this case as in every good investigation of wrong doing, it's important to follow the money. When obstetricians commit mistakes and get sued for it, the party that pays the compensation and legal bills is the malpractice insurance company. Hospitals typically carry their own liability insurance. Thus, the parties really interested in suppressing the truth about autism could be the powerful insurance conglomerates who might have billions, even trillions in exposure if the truth about autism causation comes out. These are obviously the folks that have been managing the narrative on autism online constantly diverting the topic to genetics, while the true cause remains hidden in plain sight.

Social Media and the Autism Over Diagnosis Problem

Autism by definition is a disorder which is a collection of a vast array of possible symptoms resulting in it being called a spectrum. Due to this symptomatic definition, which has gotten expanded over the years, it has degenerated into disarray causing the trivialization of symptoms over time. The neurodiversity nonsense that has gotten associated with the condition has further diminished the public perception of the suffering, and it is instead being celebrated as a gift. Inability to put your thoughts into words, inability to pay attention for longer than a few seconds due to a restless mind, inability to process spoken words and inability to maintain a conversation with others due to slow processing is not a gift, but a curse. The distortion of autism on social media has given rise to the autism is cute crowd. While it is true that impacted individuals remain at a cute childlike level of maturity in many cases in spite of having physically grown up, it is probably not a desirable trait to not have age-appropriate level of maturity. They can easily get taken advantage of, in most cases they are unable to advocate for themselves. One of the other main traits of autism that gets forgotten by the social media crowd is the sensory overload factor that is most common with autism. It is associated with brain damage and inability to process information being received by the senses, most noticeable with auditory and visual senses. Auditory overload results in inability to cope with noisy environments, inability to process the words they hear fast enough to keep up a conversation. Slow visual processing is the reason they gravitate towards noticing stationary inanimate objects better than people, people's faces or other moving and animate objects.

The neurodiversity insanity is also responsible for this strange phenomenon of self-diagnosed autistics on social media. This is almost like the third-year syndrome formally called the "Medical Student Syndrome", a widely recognized phenomenon where medical students, while learning about various diseases and their symptoms, begin to perceive themselves as experiencing those very symptoms. This is mostly the case with these self-diagnosed autistics, who pick on some of the autism behaviors they misunderstand as trivial and notice such habits in themselves ending up claiming they are autistic. For example, obsessive compulsive disorder (OCD), to me means my 2nd boy, at 16 years old will throw a tantrum, hit himself in the head and cry for a full 2 hours or more because he didn't find mom at home upon returning from school. His expectation is for everybody to be home when he gets back home from the bus, if one of us is missing (and he makes it a point to go looking around the house), he will throw a tantrum which simply continues uncontrolled until that order he expects is restored and whoever was missing returns home. Contrast that with the meaning associated with OCD by the folks who have never experienced autism and this level of OCD. They simply assume habits they create for themselves as OCD, vs the reality of it is complete loss of functioning, when a certain self-imposed order is lost.

But these self-diagnosed autistics hit up social media, claiming they are autistic and that they are fully functional having overcome their issues and even start questioning why it is not possible to live a normal life with autism. This behavior is also common to trolls and even regular folks on social media who haven't truly been impacted by autism. People try to laugh it away as a not so debilitating problem. That unfortunately is the curse of social media, where anybody can blurt out any opinion on anything and trolls rule the roost, overwhelming commonsense and logic. People forget that most real autistics are not on social media because they are simply can't, because they're intellectually disabled or simply not social, or because they lack the skills to keep or follow conversations anywhere, even on social media. The consequences of this trivialization and over-diagnosis are significant, particularly for those on the lowest end of the autism spectrum who require substantial or very substantial support (DSM-5 Level 2 and Level 3). When autism is casually adopted as an identity marker for minor social differences, it simply diminishes the profound daily struggles faced by individuals with high support needs. Of course, I do not want to take away from the few cases of misdiagnosis, particularly in girls and young women who may have been misdiagnosed with other conditions like anxiety, depression, ADHD, or even personality disorders instead of autism, or those that developed ways of masking their disabilities at the expense of great personal distress. But such girls are not the ones out there on social media trivializing their struggles.

Key Take Away: Online forums that impacted parents turn to for help have been overrun by trolls and people working on behalf of vested interests trying to hide the birth injury causes of autism. The neurodiversity fad and self-diagnosis phenomenon have only served to sow further confusion in the autism scene. The most active participants on online autism group forums are people who have no personal impact from the true autism epidemic, who are trying to trivialize the suffering of the impacted individuals.

CHAPTER 22

Practical Difficulties with the Legal Case

W hen I first discovered what had caused my children's development issues, I was naive enough to think that I would seek justice in courts for the egregious malpractice that had happened, which had pretty much ruined the rest of their lives. I was angry, overcome with grief that it had all happened right under my watch. I had let these children down, allowed a clueless obstetrician to harm them, right as they were coming into this world. My experience with the nurses and pediatrician Dr Joe made me think this is not a widespread occurrence. I knew the truth in the conclusions I had arrived at based on my experience with not one, but two kids brain damaged exactly the same way by the same obstetrician. Afterall, it is backed up by the FDA sanctioned label on the Pitocin drug which clearly states it is capable of causing traumatic brain injury, as a by-product of the uterine movements it brings about. I had even discovered details of the protocol ACOG recommends and is used in hospitals to avoid this kind of damage. However, I had little clue I would be stirring the pot on a sinister cover up. I was under the impression, that once I threw the cause out on a Face-book group or somewhere online, the idea would catch on like wildfire. Instead, what I saw was an army of trolls descending on me, telling me why I didn't know what I was talking about. I noticed that I wasn't the only one, they were doing the same to every parent out there, questioning the safety of labor induction. That's how I figured these must be hired hands working for a social media public relations outlet of some kind that must be hired by folks wanting to keep their nasty secret hidden from public view. They obviously don't want anybody to even get the idea of suing their obstetrician for labor drug abuse. Unfortunately for parents like me, their line "autism is genetic" is the official line taken by the unwarranted comments out of the judgements from the vaccine omnibus trials and the position being held by the CDC. So, these scumbag trolls are technically toeing the official line. And worse still, I have watched these trolls use their active engagement on some of these groups to get elevated as admins in most of these groups. Even the groups owned by popular autism non-profits like Autism speaks and TACA haven't been spared.

The real impact of all this is that it discourages lawyers and expert medical witnesses from coming forward to support birth injury cases once the word "autism" enters the picture. A legal case against a medical practitioner is typically an uphill battle, but it is made particularly difficult when the consequence of a doctor's indiscriminate use of a drug is brain damage which can come about in multiple ways. Pitocin abuse can cause hypoxic injury, traumatic injury or both and because similar damage can be caused by some natural causes like nuchal cords and numerous other birth complications the cause-effect connection for autism has remained obscured for years. Only the most egregious medical blunders ever see the light of day in court, and it is even rarer for victims to emerge victorious in a court of law. Years of Tort reform and aggressive efforts to curtail frivolous litigation have also meant it is much more difficult for legitimate but complex cases like birth malpractice leading to autism to even make it to court, no matter the merits. In fact, it's much easier to sue for injury in an auto accident or an injury at a business/place of work than to sue for obstetric malpractice.

The Complexity of Obstetric Malpractice Lawsuits

Obstetric malpractice lawsuits are some of the most complex and most expensive lawsuits to undertake. For parents it often follows a period of immense personal hardship, grief, and a growing sense that an obstetrician's negligence or lack of knowledge has caused significant harm to their child, harm that lasts a lifetime. But the steps involved in a lawsuit can be daunting, but knowledge is power and looking into the details of the process might help overcome initial hesitation. The first step is to find an attorney that takes the case. Birth injury attorneys take up cases on a contingency basis. They invest money upfront into cases that they think they can win or perhaps settle for a good payout so they can make a profit on their upfront investment. The risk is all on them.

For most attorneys it only makes business sense to take up cases with situations that have a precedence of winning. Most states within the last decade have instituted rules that require that a medical doctor in the same field as the MD being sued, provide a certificate of merit confirming that the defendant did not follow the standard of care in the case. Many states, thanks to their recent tort reforms don't allow filing of a case without this certificate of merit. Hence, any malpractice attorney even before they take up a case, they try to find an MD that can provide this certificate. Then a complaint is drafted and filed in court. The defendants are then served by certified letters notifying them of the lawsuit. A discovery phase then begins where demands are made for records and information is exchanged between the 2 parties to the suit. Then there are depositions under oath between the parties which includes doctors that might serve as expert witnesses on the case. There is then attempts to find an out of court negotiated settlement. If that fails then the case proceeds to a jury trial, with jury selection, arguments and a jury verdict on the case.

When an attorney takes up a birth injury case, they hope they can settle for a good sum as injury compensation as it involves permanently altered lives. The best shot at doing it is if they take up cases where there is a precedent of winning. It is a business decision to maximize returns given the high upfront investment from the attorney's side in these contingency fee cases. I have heard it takes anywhere between $100k - $300k from various firms to even file a birth injury case properly. Unfortunately, in cases of prolonged labor induction without fetal distress, most of the precedent set, has been that of losses in court, not because the plaintiffs were wrong but because they did not have the right arguments. However, given the backdrop of losses, in multiple such cases, attorneys have become very hesitant to take up cases like this. Another issue is that courts only listen to doctors serving as expert witnesses that can vouch that the defendant obstetrician did not follow the standard of care. After tort reforms, doctors from other fields such as pediatrics cannot testify against an obstetrician, attorneys need obstetric witnesses to come forward and testify to prove causation. After the ACOG's acceptance of the dog and pony show of the ARRIVE trial, even the standard of care has shifted to ignore the previous "Failure to progress diagnosis point". All this part of the sinister plan to get out from underneath this big skeleton in the obstetric cupboard of abusive labor induction causing hidden traumatic brain damage leading to Autism, ADD, and ADHD in the US and around the world since 1980. After this change in official stance, it has become even more difficult for obstetric witnesses to quote deviation in standard of care in these cases. Obviously, they are doing all this in the hope that impacted parents and attorneys are not going to be able to pull them to court given the protections afforded by the tort reforms. But they are forgetting that the Pitocin label still carries multiple warnings, all of which talk about brain damage outcomes and its not going to be possible to hide it for too long. But in the immediate term, it has made lawsuits even more difficult for parents impacted by this malpractice.

The only cases with wins in the context of Pitocin abuse, involve cases where there was fetal distress that was ignored. These are cases where Pitocin abuse caused hypoxic distress from tachysystole or placental abruption or extreme brain trauma resulting in observable fetal distress. For this reason, lawyers only want to deal with cases where there was a NICU stay, so they know there was some kind of hypoxia involved. Most such cases do win jury awards, upwards of 10 million dollars for the lifetime of suffering inflicted on the victims. A lot of times, the awards are paid by the malpractice insurance of the provider, and sometimes the hospital depending on the finding of fault in the case. When we take on a malpractice suit, we're really taking up a case against the malpractice insurance companies, that mostly have deep pockets to pay for legal representation which again makes fighting a case so much harder and more expensive.

Medical Malpractice Insurance

Claims of malpractice against a doctor are mostly settled by malpractice insurance companies as per the limits of liability set by the policy carried by the insured doctor or their practice group. Usually, it is not possible to sue the hospital itself unless the doctor was an employee of the hospital. In most cases OB/GYNs are independent contractors with their own practice that use the hospital facilities for birth services. Depending on how much they were insured for, compensation payable by these companies might be limited and not commensurate with the damage done in case of autism. Going after the personal wealth of the Doctors may or may not be fruitful as well.

The hospital may be liable for doctors using their facilities, following their policies and for informing the patients of the risks, but that again might be more complex to prove negligence with many OB/GYNs involved and could be a secondary approach once the offending OB/GYNs are singled out. However, when cases are settled by insurance companies out of court, they often do it without admission of guilt and nondisclosure conditions, which make it possible for the perpetrators to continue their practice with no consequence for their actions.

Medical malpractice insurance is the primary mechanism for resolving financial claims against healthcare providers. Doctors and medical practices pay premiums to these insurance companies in exchange for coverage against potential lawsuits. The insurance policy has a "limit of liability," which is the maximum amount the insurance company will pay out for a single claim or over a policy period. This limit can vary significantly depending on the doctor's specialty, location, and the level of coverage they choose (or are required by their practice or hospital to carry).

Insurance companies are incentivized to settle claims within the policy limits to avoid the risk of a larger judgment at trial, which could potentially exceed those limits and expose the doctor's personal assets. It's important to note that the policy limits may or may not include the costs of defending the lawsuit (attorney fees, expert witness fees, etc.). Some policies have limits that cover both damages and defense costs, which can further limit the amount available for settlement.

Hospitals may or may not be directly liable. If the OB/GYN is a direct employee of the hospital (receives a salary, benefits, and is subject to the hospital's direct control over their practice), the hospital can often be held vicariously liable for the doctor's negligence under the legal doctrine of "respondeat superior" ("let the master answer"). In most cases, OB/GYNs are independent contractors with their own practices who have "privileges" to use the hospital's facilities for delivering babies. In this scenario, it's generally more difficult to directly sue the hospital for the doctor's malpractice. However, there are exceptions where a hospital can be held liable even for the actions of independent contractors: If the hospital holds out the independent contractor as its agent or employee, the hospital can be held liable. This often depends on factors like signage, admitting paperwork, and the patient's understanding of the relationship. Direct negligence of the hospital, negligent credentialing, negligent provision of facilities or staff, failure to adequately warn of risks associated with independent contractors using their facilities and most importantly, not properly implementing or enforcing its own safety protocols and policies that could have prevented the harm. Hospitals often have significantly more substantial insurance coverage than individual practitioners, and for lawsuits involving catastrophic injuries like brain damage it's important for plaintiffs to sue the hospital for not enforcing the Pitocin protocols that all of them had in place between the mid 90's to 2018.

The policy limits of the OB/GYN's insurance may be insufficient to fully compensate for the significant and lifelong damages associated with a child born with autism due to medical negligence (e.g., ongoing care, therapy, lost earning potential, emotional distress). Families can find themselves in a situation where the insurance payout is far less than the actual cost of care and lost quality of life. Pursuing the personal wealth of the doctor is a possibility, but OB/GYNs, like other professionals, often have legal strategies in place to protect their personal assets from lawsuits. And it's usually not considered the most ethical strategy.

Insurance companies often prefer to settle cases out of court for various reasons including cost control by avoiding expensive trials, risk management by limiting the potential for a larger jury verdict and negative publicity and increased efficiency by resolving claims more quickly. A standard clause in many settlement agreements is that the defendant (doctor or hospital) does not admit any fault or negligence. This protects their professional reputation and can have implications for future legal actions. Settlements frequently include NDAs that prevent the plaintiff and their attorneys from publicly discussing the details of the settlement, including the amount and the specific findings of negligence. The combination of no admission of guilt and NDAs can create a situation where healthcare providers who have committed malpractice can continue practicing without any public record or professional repercussions. This can be deeply frustrating for patients and advocates seeking accountability and systemic change. It can also hinder the ability of other patients to make informed decisions about their healthcare providers. NDAs can also make it more difficult for future plaintiffs to discover patterns of negligence by the same provider or institution, as past settlements are often kept confidential.

The role of malpractice insurance is central to how these cases are handled. While it provides a mechanism for compensating injured patients, the limitations of policies, the complexities of hospital liability for independent contractors, and the common use of no-admission-of-guilt and nondisclosure clauses in settlements can create significant challenges for plaintiffs seeking full accountability and just compensation, especially in cases involving severe and lifelong conditions like autism. Understanding these dynamics is crucial for families navigating the difficult terrain of a medical malpractice lawsuit.

In conclusion, the case of autism from traumatic brain damage by Pitocin abuse, the stakes are too high for malpractice insurance companies. Its an existential threat for them if all parents become aware of the true cause of their child's autism and start suing their obstetricians for it. The damages could be in the trillions, much larger than these companies themselves. Hence these companies have a vested interest in keeping this hidden from parents and in my opinion some of them that are hospital plus insurance conglomerates might be involved in the social media suppression and misinformation, potentially with the covert endorsement of every player in the industry.

The Role of State Medical Boards in the US

State medical boards are government agencies empowered to investigate complaints about doctors and when warranted take action against them. The state medical board is tasked by the state legislature with granting licenses, administration of exams and oversight of medical practice in general within that state. Physicians are licensed to practice in a state by that state's medical licensing board. The federation of state medical boards is an organization that helps the 70 different medical boards (including the 14 osteopathic medical boards) in the US by providing guidelines, standards and best practices for the boards themselves.

Malpractice judgments against a physician in court may or may not have an impact with a state medical board depending on which state the ruling is in. Interestingly, even in the same state, in spite of the fact that courts on many occasions take the advice of the boards, the board may not agree with the court's decision. While the court can order malpractice compensation, it's the boards that regulate whether the practitioner continues his practice. Thus, even OB/GYNs with proven malpractice cases with the court system can continue to practice in many jurisdictions unless such judgments reach abnormally high proportions. Disciplinary action against a physician by a state medical board can be very much consequential since boards have the power to revoke their license to practice, impose fines not covered by malpractice insurance, etc. It is also easier to lodge a complaint against a physician with a state medical board, but harder to prove malpractice as the boards are not typically swayed by just a single report of negligence as such.

The boards are typically comprised of distinguished physicians appointed by state governors and confirmed by state legislature. Being physicians themselves, it's understandable that they tend to be more understanding of other physicians and tend to come down harshly only on the most egregious of malpractice. Since Pitocin usage has been so common in maternity wards in the US for decades, it's even possible some boards have OB/GYNs who have abused Pitocin in the past, who might be sympathetic to peers, or want to protect themselves from past malpractice for their own abuse of the drug. It's not easy to predict the kind of support Pitocin abuse cases might get from state medical boards if they are called on for help. Even though the labelling on Pitocin is clear, even other 'experts' in the field that a court might call upon could be compromised.

A lot of tort reform was justified by their proponents based on the assumption that complaints to the medical boards would be cheaper and more effective in enhancing patient trust and safety. Unfortunately, this has turned out to be an empty promise. Medical boards do absolutely nothing, when they get a patient complaint about a provider. Case in point, I had complained to the State medical board of the state where my children were born, about our obstetrician A.S. I had attached my second sons MRI scan report as evidence. The website promised they would look into the matter and even reach out if they had additional questions. Nothing like that happened. They just closed the complaint exactly a month later saying they need medical or legal evidence against the practitioner, that they broke state law, to take action. Now how is that any different from the requirements of a lawsuit? How does that reduce the burden of proof on patients more than a lawsuit would. Their boiler plate answer even went on to say that sometimes a single reported case may not warrant action. However, this same state medical board was quick to jump on a medical doctor accused of being anti-vax. This physician's only fault was she had refused to toe the official line on covid and some other vaccinations. This MD's license was revoked indefinitely without even a case or a hearing. In short, medical boards have pretty much become instruments of power to stifle patient rights and protect establishment medical doctors and bringing down an iron fist on voices of dissent. Unfortunately, institutions like these have also become part of the reason why the cause of the autism epidemic has remained hidden for 45 years from 1980 as of the time of this writing.

Hurdles to Autism Research – Deficient Data & Sham Research

We live in the age of information, where data has come to be the foundation of all logical reasoning. It could easily turn into the golden age of healthcare if data pertaining to millions of individuals can be mined to find the cause and effect of numerous conditions, their treatments and effectiveness of medications and results. Tech companies with the best of intentions have tried making an impact in healthcare, but to no avail. While hospitals are big businesses, they are mostly not billion-dollar corporations capable of putting in a lot of money toward their IT infrastructure. Hospitals with their smaller and tight budgets are torn between maintaining their IT systems and paying for doctors and medical equipment and still turn a profit. Hospital IT systems continue to be locked-in by a select group of vendors with their proprietary systems that restrict the adoption of next generation IT systems. Strict privacy requirements have also meant there has never been any incentive for data sharing for any purpose whatsoever. Billing systems are truly the only IT systems with any decent data in hospitals. They may have disease codes and treatments, but deriving meaningful history of patients from invoices is next to impossible. There is no single consistent personal health record that even doctors can access. Add to this the fact that people change care providers or consult multiple providers and specialists.

The result is it is impossible to decipher meaningful information about individual disease histories and treatments and arrive at correlations that might be beneficial to all, in a case like this. Government initiatives in the US like HITECH, EHR mandate, etc. are steps in the right direction, but they have only scratched the surface when it comes to creating systems capable of sharing data in any meaningful way.

On the flip side, insurance companies have been trying to get their hands on consolidated patient history information for ages, but for their totally devious purposes of jacking up rates or denying coverage at the slightest hint of disease. This has disincentivized individuals from sharing their information, and as a result stifling any possibility of making data available for research. While individual patients can request their records from various places and put a case together, it is not possible to seek out impacted cases from hospital records from any other angle. This makes discovery in any legal case so much harder as it is almost impossible to gather data to prove a pattern of malpractice by a given doctor.

Autism research has instead depended exclusively on observational studies. These are not clinical trials of drugs, but passive observations collected over time from various sources. Running medical studies involves a lot of time and resources. They are mostly done by academic researchers and funded by industry with specific goals in mind. With autism, the problem itself is not clearly defined. With the possible vaccine connotation, it's the last thing anybody in the field wants to touch, simply because nobody wants to dive into a field so controversial, where coming up with any conclusions only puts you at odds with the vast majority of other researchers. Unfortunately, this has been the reason it has taken this long to pinpoint the causes of autism.

Proving medical malpractice and getting into legal complications is something any academic or scientific research program would want to avoid at all costs. Hence even if they touch on the topic, their results always come up as inconclusive and end up pointing to the need for further research. As a result, autism studies have been focused on what could be the most non-controversial cause, which is finding genetic roots for autism. When a deficit in the body is not traceable to viral or bacterial disease, looking for genetic reasons seems to be the default fallback for contemporary science and unfortunately, autism has fallen into that same rut. When a study like the Duke Autism study sponsored by the department of environmental sciences points at use of Pitocin, there is immediately sham research emerging from the premier institutions in the US like Harvard and even funded by the NIH that are put up to debunk the findings using false assumptions (discussed in Chapter 8 – Almost Outed - section of this book). Disgracefully, in numerous health fields plagued by economic and commercial pressures, researchers are reduced to mere puppets, handed predetermined outcomes and tasked with fabricating evidence to support them. The same is true of autism research, where fabricated research is used to hide the truth whenever a research team like the Duke researchers come up with a finding that is right on the mark. The current state autism research is so skewed toward finding genetic reasons that even researchers seeing white matter integrity issues in MRI scans of people with autism wonder what the genetics behind it is, rather than identify it for the traumatic brain damage it actually represents! On the other hand, it would have been fairly straightforward to debunk Dr Rutters genetic basis theory exactly like I have in chapter 9. And if I can do it, it shouldn't take researchers any amount of time at all. But the genetic theory is being kept alive by news headlines from sham research looking for genetic roots to autism that doesn't exist.

The Perpetrators

Meaning well does not equate to doing good. Unfortunately, in the case of Pitocin abuse and brain damage, numerous OB/GYNs – in their zeal to avoid the 'dreaded C-section' – have ended up causing autism. Their incompetence and lack of understanding of the dangers of Pitocin induction and inability to direct the treatment as per the labeling on the drug being administered has caused an epidemic. They tend to believe that Pitocin being a naturally occurring hormone is 'safe and the most natural way' to deliver a baby. Their ill-conceived notion that neuroplasticity would help babies recover from any brain damage has resulted in thousands of victims. By their negligence and beliefs contrary to the drug labeling, each of these autism perpetrators has made suffering the only way of life for hundreds of families they have victimized. They tend to be serial Pitocin abusers impacting multiple families the same way, while their malpractice has remained hidden for years, with some of them even rising in power and stature to become part of the powerful medical board committees that wield ultimate power in their fields.

Medical insurance companies that try to push doctors to do fewer C-sections are part of the problem too. Their primary motive is the cost factor that comes with C-sections compared to regular vaginal deliveries. The cost of a typical hospital delivery in the US is almost impossible to guess, with estimates for 2019 ranging from $15,000 to $32,000 for normal deliveries and $30,000 to $52,000 for C-sections (these numbers are the amount hospitals charge insurance companies and most people with insurance end up paying much less). Being one of the most common procedures done in hospitals it's a pity the price would be so high in the first place, but suffice to say C-sections cost approximately 50% more than a normal delivery due to anesthesia, surgery and additional care expenses involved. I see stories on the internet where insurance companies have resorted to shaming obstetricians for doing more C-sections in an effort to curb costs while claiming better outcomes for mothers. Unfortunately for parents of babies impacted by Pitocin abuse, the price of trying to fix the mistake of not doing a C-section runs into millions over the lifetime of the child while the affliction still cannot be fixed. A kid on one-on-one ABA therapy costs approximately $120,000 per year, and that's not counting the pain, suffering and other incidentals that parents and the child have to go through. The long-term costs of supporting a kid with autism far exceeds anything insurance companies might have paid for a few additional C-sections.

But the primary culprits in this story are the people who have engaged in manipulation to hide the risks from the messaging. Take for example what happened in 2013 when a large widely reported study from the Duke Center for Autism by Dr Simon Gregory and his colleagues[8,9] for the first time established a correlation between induced labor and an autism diagnosis by analyzing North Carolina birth records with educational records. Their conclusion of the association between augmented labor and autism is perfectly on the money. But a lack of data regarding induction indications and methods effectively stopped them from being able to establish a causal relationship. They did not have duration of induction in their data, which would have been the best pointer to causation. They also got misled by research out there during that time describing Oxytocin's role as a neurotransmitter on the inside of the blood brain barrier (BBB) vs its hormonal role in causing contractions of the uterus. It is important to note that oxytocin does not cross the BBB and so has this dual role as a neurotransmitter inside the BBB and hormone on the outside as mentioned previously in chapter 5. Unfortunately, the Gregory team in their attempt to explain their findings ascribed plausible cause to a totally flawed hypothesis in the autism research world that oxytocin exposure of the fetal brain could somehow be responsible for autism. Sadly, this nonsensical hypothesis seems to have hijacked conventional scientific belief, despite the fact that oxytocin doesn't last in the maternal blood stream for any significant time (that's the reason you have to use it as a continuous drip to induce contractions). Anything that reaches the fetal brain is potentially 1000's of times diluted, and whatever does find its way there is blocked by the baby's fully functional blood brain barrier.

It was obviously not possible for the Gregory study to look at the malpractice involved due to lack of actual hospital treatment records in their data set. Nevertheless, there's been an almost immediate torrent of misdirected rebuttals of these results from other studies, who themselves erroneously stick to the oxytocin chemical effects thesis and fault the Gregory study for not looking at the possible use of other concoctions of drugs used in labor induction by then, particularly the off-label use of prostaglandins. Somehow it doesn't occur to these experts that this could be traumatic brain injury by the force of contractions and abuse by the use of excessive contractions, which the fetal monitors – designed to pick up hypoxia – do not detect.

What is alarming is the volume of immediate counter studies and rebuttals which seem to have been established solely for the purpose of discrediting the original Duke study. And they all used flawed methods to achieve their objective, like the Sara Oberg et al paper looking at the Swedish data that added a genetic twist to forcibly break the correlation between autism and labor induction in their data. OB/GYN organizations like the ACOG (www.acog.org) seem to be all too eager to embrace these counter arguments that go egregiously overboard defending labor induction.

The case against Pitocin and other labor drug abuse is complex simply because of the numerous other factors that can impact the brain. While fingers have been pointed at induced labor multiple times in the past, nothing has come out of it. However, the time for redemption has arrived. Increasing numbers of parents are now able to trace their kid's brain issues to their birth. My expectation is that this book will cement their knowledge and take away the diversion of vaccines and environmental factors since they are truly a secondary add-on effect arising out of their interaction with a damaged brain with a compromised blood brain barrier.

It is time for impacted parents to lose their dependence on 'studies' and 'experts' and trust what they see with their own eyes and experience. What is needed is a movement by impacted parents to clear the smokescreen once and for all and stop the genetic nonsense being parlayed about autism for years. Outsiders that are not impacted by autism cannot understand it, the way the parents of impacted individuals do. Only impacted parents can bring out the truth that most autism is caused by birth trauma sometimes naturally and at other times by the labor induction drugs, which are living up to the Pitocin warning label, causing traumatic brain injury at the hands of OB/GYNs lacking the expertise to handle them.

Key Take Away: Labor drug abuse should be easy to establish, but it is a difficult undertaking nevertheless, due to the complex nature of the cases and the backlash to past successes in courts. Heavy-handed tort reform as response to past attempts has resulted in a loss of moral courage to take on these cases among the legal community. The unwillingness of the scientific community to delve into issues of malpractice and their eagerness to embrace genetic reasons to autism that do not exist, has not been very helpful.

CHAPTER 23

Establishing Serial Pitocin Abuse

G iven the uphill task of proving individual malpractice cases in court, further complicated by a legal 'catch-22' when it comes to finding expert witnesses (as I will explain in the next chapter), a faster and more efficient approach would be to demonstrate multiple instances of Pitocin abuse by a single practitioner. At our new non-profit, AutismPI.org (more details in upcoming pages), our strategy is to establish class-action lawsuits against individual OB/GYN practitioners exhibiting patterns of abuse. Our fundamental premise is that these Pitocin abusers are serial perpetrators, having caused numerous cases of autism by inducing excessive contractions and disregarding the drug's contraindication limits. Our retrospective data collection initiative aims to establish this relationship, thereby providing much-needed proof of serial Pitocin abuse. Before delving into that, let's examine some key factors in legal history that have led us to this point.

The Court Cases and Precedents

For special needs families already battling chronic shortages of time and money, the prospect of litigation can feel overwhelming. Some find solace in faith, while others are simply exhausted by their circumstances, lacking the emotional forti-tude to pursue legal action alone. Conversely, a segment of parents is eagerly awaiting the results this data collection will provide and are poised to initiate lawsuits. Understanding the outcomes of past autism litigation is crucial to ex-plaining the strategic rationale behind pursuing a class action, and why it might achieve success where individual efforts have faltered.

Vaccine-Autism Omnibus hearings: Beginning with British gastroenterologist Dr. Andrew Wakefield's 1998 publication of case studies implicating the MMR vaccine with the rise of developmental disorders including autism and inflammatory bowel disease in children, the notion that vaccines were the cause of the astronomical rise of autism since the 1980s started gaining traction. However, several subsequent epidemiological studies ostensibly debunked his theory, and Dr. Wakefield was dealt with firmly by the British medical establishment, and his publisher (the respected Lancet journal) was forced to retract his statements in 2004. Due to his unflinching advocacy of his findings, after years of deliberation Dr. Wakefield was ultimately stripped of his medical license in 2010. But the popularity of the theory among the general population only increased due to it being corroborated by actual parental observations.

The "Defeat Autism Now" (DAN) movement of Dr. Rimland had accepted the notion that vaccines were the cause of autism, particularly the mercury in the thimerosal adjuvant used as both a preservative and enhancer to improve the effectiveness of vaccines. Mercury poisoning can lead to brain damage and cause symptoms similar to autism and the correlation sounded plausible. This resulted in over 5600 claims being filed against the National Vaccine Injury Compensation Program (NVICP). The vaccine court selected 6 test cases to represent the different circumstances of usage, including vaccines containing thimerosal, MMR and combinations of the two. These consolidated cases constituted the Omnibus Autism Proceedings (OAP) that began in 2007. The court found no evidence of any causative relationship to autism in any of the cases and consequently no compensation was paid in any of the 5600 cases when they were adjudicated in 2009–10, and the future of making a vaccine autism relationship in vaccine court looks bleak.

To make matters worse, the experts called on by the court and the special masters at the Omnibus proceedings argued future research needed to focus on genetics and that research into environmental causes should only be considered as part of gene–environmental interactions. This ended up badly damaging the credibility of anti-vaxxers and their medical community sympathizers and it enabled the government, the medical boards and their media supporters to promote a heavy-handed approach to quell the genuine concerns of parents regarding vaccines. This judgement also resulted in the government redirecting valuable research dollars into looking for genetic causes that don't exist. As a result, the underlying cause of most autism – birth injury – remains hidden to this day because it is not even remotely related to genes or the chemicals in the environment.

John Edwards and Electronic Fetal Monitoring: The advent of electronic fetal monitoring in the 1960s opened up the possibility of detecting hypoxia happening during birth. Electronic fetal monitors are the reason induction of labor is even possible. As part of managed labor in a hospital, fetal monitoring has since become standard practice in the US and most other nations. The cardiotocograph uses a monitor placed on the mother's abdominal wall to monitor contractions and fetal heart rate. The fetal heart rate typically drops with every contraction and quickly recovers in the interval between contractions. Fetal distress can be detected when the heart rate doesn't recover quickly enough or stays low for a longer time interval. Yet as straightforward as it sounds, there are complexities that need considered, including a moving baby, change in monitor position, the complexity of signals getting through the abdominal and uterine wall, and so on. A second more reliable but more invasive monitor is the fetal scalp electrode (FSE) which can be used after at least 3cm dilation of the cervix is achieved. The scalp electrode is placed under the fetal skin in the head and among other risks carries the possibility of causing an infection but is credited to be more reliable. But even this apparently is not considered a very reliable predictor of fetal hypoxia.

John Edwards, former US Senator and one-time presidential and vice-presidential candidate, was a birth injury lawyer who excelled in winning obstetric malpractice claims for his victim clients. His cases were mostly about kids that ended up with cerebral palsy from hypoxic injury. John Edwards is said to have successfully argued his cases based on the electronic fetal monitor readings. Furthermore, he went one step further and not only sued the doctors, whose malpractice insurance settled the claims, but also the hospitals for letting this happen in their facilities, holding them liable for millions in additional compensation. Wikipedia estimates John Edwards won about 208 million in compensation for his various clients in the 1980's.

However, these suits by John Edwards and other astute birth injury lawyers of that era in the 1980's ended up being instrumental in unleashing a backlash of heavy-handed tort reform in most states by way of limiting jury awards and putting time limits of less than 18 years and many such actions to severely curtail birth injury lawsuits. These ill-advised tort reforms have further complicated the possibility of winning malpractice suits for birth injury. People have been accused of pointing to a squiggly in electronic fetal monitor graph as cause for brain damage in their baby and claiming compensation. Numerous subsequent cases against prolonged induced labor have since been lost in courts. Unfortunately, this has emboldened a new generation of OB/GYNs who in their excessive zeal to please insurance companies by avoiding C-sections have brought on Pitocin abuse, raising autism levels to unprecedented highs.

The Autism Parents Initiative: Autismpi.org

The Autism Parents Initiative or AutismPI (pronounced autism π – autismpi.org) is an organization founded by a group of autism-impacted parents, including myself. Our core mission is to help track down all causes of brain damage and autism. In cases involving Labor induction abuse, our specific aim is to assist with the formation of class-action lawsuits against individual OB/GYNs responsible for such misconduct. Our website serves as an online Pitocin abuse injury registry, allowing parents to securely register their children's case details. This retrospective data collection and information dissemination effort is crucial for supporting successful legal initiatives against Pitocin-related injuries.

Pitocin Abuse and Other Autism Data Collection

by Autism Parents Initiative - AutismPI.org

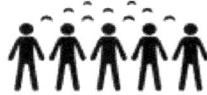

Parents suspecting Pitocin abuse or any other causes of autism defined here register at autismpi.org website

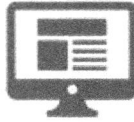

Web registry clusters the cases around specific OB/GYN's for Pitocin abuse and specific causes in other non-Pitocin cases.

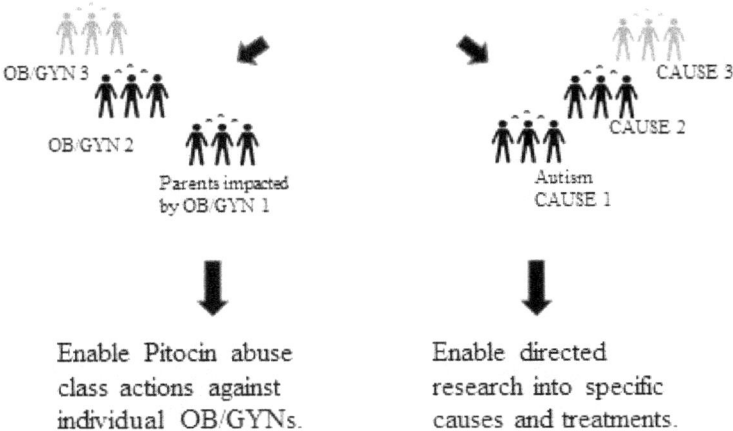

OB/GYN 3

CAUSE 3

OB/GYN 2

CAUSE 2

Parents impacted by OB/GYN 1

Autism CAUSE 1

Enable Pitocin abuse class actions against individual OB/GYNs.

Enable directed research into specific causes and treatments.

We intend to collect this information and report back to parents when we identify clusters of autism linked to labor induction abuse by specific OB/GYNs. This will provide impacted parents with the grounds for a successful class-action lawsuit. Our goal is to help every autism parent similarly affected by Pitocin abuse during induced labor to demand and receive compensation for the injustice inflicted upon them and their children. Given the history of attempting to prove autism causation in court, a legal case against a medical practitioner for Pitocin abuse is only feasible when multiple instances of abuse per OB/GYN are identified. The prospects of direct lawsuits have been seriously diminished by tort reforms and the legal "catch-22" I describe in the next chapter (unless there's some form of government intervention).

As the first step of our strategy, we seek to identify serial Pitocin-abusing obstetricians who have profoundly impacted our lives and those of our children. This is an open website where anyone can register with just an email. We hope to run this data collection campaign for two years or more across the U.S. The site is designed to eliminate the last barrier between parents and the elusive proof required to win a case in a court of law. AutismPI.org is a quest to prove autism caused by labor contraction abuse through the numbers, backing up the conclusions reached in this book with clear, logical arguments. I know for a fact that every impacted parent reading this book who has gone through the induced labor process has a story similar to mine, as this has been corroborated by many. Our stories are real, but in the face of schemes designed to thwart us from finding the truth, we'll need to band together to bring that truth to light.

It is no longer necessary for autism parents to accept autism as a fact of life that happened to them. With this book, I have provided the real reasons for this scourge. Labor drug abuse by using excessive contractions to hammer a baby headfirst against a mother's cervix has been the major causation factor in autism and the solution can't be any clearer. Severely restricting the practice of using induced labor after amnion rupture can have a significant impact on autism occurrence. If waiting and traditional remedies (enemas, sexual stimulation) don't produce the desired results, then making the C-section as the main and only alternative will go a long way in eliminating the incidence of autism. Such changes can only happen if parents rally around and identify the obstetricians responsible for serial Pitocin abuse malpractice. Clustering autism data by OB/GYN and hospital can allow us to isolate specific OB/GYN's that are routine Pitocin abusers and the hospitals allowing them to continue unchecked. These folks are responsible for large numbers of autism cases. The data collection effort by AutismPI.org (pronounced autism pie/π) is designed to bring out the evidence of malpractice against individual practitioners and their hospitals.

There are bound to be people trying to put down our voices and discredit our analysis, perhaps some with great credentials. They do it for the news headline value in discrediting challenges to their authority. But this is a topic where researchers have been thwarted by a sinister scheme and diverted into looking in the wrong places, at the wrong types of data and coming up empty-handed for ages and the people trying to put us down are people with malevolent vested interests. We have irrefutable evidence hidden in plain sight right in the Pitocin label that is being deliberately overlooked for decades. Parents being the closest observers of their kids are the best judges of their individual situations. As you may have realized, this book is not just about the ideas that have been put forward. There is going to be action to back it up. To help eradicate the scourge of autism and to seek compensation for impacted parents' woes and it is important for impacted parents to band together and pursue legal recourse using all remaining avenues in spite of multiple doors being closed on us.

A Retrospective Research Data Collection Effort.

At autismpi.org we believe proof of birth injury as the true cause of autism needs to be based on solid foundations and irrefutable evidence. Given the enormous diversity of conditions and mechanisms that can cause brain damage at birth, extensive data collection is crucial to cover these varied circumstances. I invite all impacted autism parents in the U.S. to join the Autism Parents Initiative today. Our retrospective research at AutismPI.org is a no-obligation data collection effort aimed at cataloging the various birth causes of autism as observed by parents. For cases involving Pitocin abuse, a separate registry is intended to provide proof of obstetric malpractice at birth. Register your child's autism-causing birth conditions at our parent-founded organization at **https://autismpi.org** and participate in bringing forth overwhelming evidence to prove the diverse birth injuries causing the autism epidemic. This evidence could also make a difference in potential legal action if we can assemble a class-action lawsuit against your individual obstetrician.

I recognize that most autism parents would rather see their children "fixed" than seek monetary compensation. Unfortunately, the court system can only offer financial compensation. There are no guaranteed "fixes" on the horizon, and even if a treatment eventually emerges, there's no reclaiming the years lost in this struggle. Focusing on this legal initiative is vital to securing the financial future of these children and addressing the problems caused by this tragedy. It's essential to bring these cases to court to deter future Pitocin abuse and reduce autism's occurrence.

Beyond legal avenues, this new retrospective data collection could offer other significant benefits. Insights obtained from parent-side surveys can lead to more focused research and the development of better treatments for brain damage at birth resulting from hypoxia, ischemia, and other natural causes. We can even assess other impacts of induced labor. For example, do induced mothers face a higher risk of uterine cancer? Without a centralized effort to track this data, there's no way to find out. A lack of data is precisely why this birth injury has remained hidden, but together, we can dismantle this final barrier to ending autism in this world.

Our appeal to all impacted parents: please participate in this autism parents birth data collection effort at autismpi.org today so that together, we can bring this malady of autism to an end and seek compensation for the birth injury that has been hiding in plain sight for more than four decades. Now that we understand the benefits of the retrospective research at AutismPI.org, let us delve into the factors that have been instrumental in keeping the causes of the autism epidemic hidden.

Reasons why Autism's Cause has Remained Hidden

Just as autism causation is considered multifactorial, so too are the reasons its origin has remained a mystery. While a sinister cover-up by those with knowledge is the primary driver, various other factors that have facilitated this hush-up.

1. There are multiple ways the fetal/infant brain can be damaged during the perinatal period, in-utero, during birth and immediately after birth. Hypoxic brain damage can happen in all these 3 listed stages while traumatic damage from labor induction happens during birth. Having such multifactorial causes has contributed to confusion.

2. The collusion by the obstetric organizations, hospitals and malpractice insurers deceiving the public by diverting to the chemical neurotransmitter effects of Pitocin (supposed downregulation of oxytocin receptors in the brain) rather than acknowledging the risk of traumatic brain damage from its known physical effect of uterine stimulation and use of excessive contractions beyond known limits.

3. The failure of the ACOG to come out openly about their protocol to address contraindication #5 and the brain damage warning on the Pitocin labelling upon prolonged labor induction. Their protocol of 72 contractions limit has been kept a closely guarded secret resulting in it being kept secret even from practicing obstetricians.

4. The Arrive trials by rookie members of the Society for Maternal fetal medicine focused on short term neonatal outcomes like still birth and neonatal death within 7 days to arrive at faulty conclusions without taking into account the previously discovered brain damage consequences, the fools exposure paradox that followed, was actually gamed by the obstetric establishment and hospitals to their advantage, to get out from under the liability for prior mistakes committed.

5. The extreme suppression of the parental voices of reason on popular online social media platforms, potentially by hospital and insurance

conglomerates using hired social media management agencies, have successfully diverted popular opinion away from birth injury causes of autism onto more easily blamed, but non-existent genetic causes.

6. The switch to using unapproved prostaglandins for inducing live births in most hospitals has meant there are no warning labels against hidden traumatic brain injury that practitioners get to see, unlike the Pitocin label. This is an illegal practice that has become so commonplace, that nobody even understands that these abortion drugs are being abused for live births off-label.

7. The fact that the brain doesn't feel pain upon injury to itself and there is no other visible indication of trauma during birth. Plus, the fact that if pushing is involved any scarring sustained during the cervical dilation stage gets erased during the deformation of the head in the pushing stage causes this injury to go invisible in ordinary MRI scans and unnoticed by neurologists.

8. Radiologists do not directly consult with patients, but radiology remains crucial for assessing brain damage. However, the lack of direct interaction with parents and limited access to comprehensive patient history leads neuro radiologists to attribute findings like scarring, gliosis, and other artifacts to 'non-specific' causes instead of correlating these to birth situations and injuries as the causative factor.

9. Years of heavy handed and unjust tort reform in almost all states in the US have made it difficult for parents and lawyers to obtain any significant compensation, even in cases where malpractice completely ruined the entire lives of patients. There is limited avenue for legal challenges in other parts of the world with their universal health care systems.

10. Years of failed lawsuits that didn't correctly strike at the root of the problem have made lawyers wary of taking up anything not involving NICU stays. Thus, the legal feedback which has invariably become the necessary driver for effecting changes in medical practices has been missing.

11. The judgement from the vaccine omnibus trials in 2009 pointed to genetics instead of saying it was known to be from birth injury, which was

the known truth at the time of these trials or they should have just stated they did not understand or know what caused autism.

12. The presence of universal health care systems in other high-income countries of Europe and elsewhere in the world has meant avenues for legal recourse in these countries is very limited if not nonexistent. The small minority of cases where the issue with prolonged induction happens often goes unnoticed.

13. The cause and effect in these cases are separated by at least 2 years or more, by which time the birth circumstances are mostly forgotten. Other factors like the complexities of childhood development, viral infections, vaccines, gut dysbiosis etc., tend to obscure the picture from the traumatic brain injury cause of autism.

14. The larger-than-life influence of some researchers like Dr Michael Rutter continuing to back the genetic origin theory of autism using research that was obviously flawed due to only taking into account zygosity and not the more important shared placenta (chorionicity) and the folly of projecting high risk twin pregnancy results to a situation involving low risk pregnancies targeted for labor induction simply hijacked the conversation from the true cause.

15. The sponsorship and use of phony research by the conspiracy apparatus involved in hiding the truth from the public including the ability to use the credibility of top-notch schools and secure NIH funding on a whim have allowed them to hide behind such flawed research.

While this list is still not exhaustive, the most consequential of it all with implications for the current and future concealment of autism causation is the legal catch-22 situation created by the about-face by the ACOG on their labor induction protocols. In 2018, the ACOG dropped their contraction limits from their labor induction protocols, thus getting out from under their liability for past mistakes while abandoning the babies of the future to a matter of chance as to whether they run into labor drug abuse during birth or not. The legal tangle this creates for the victims is discussed in the next chapter.

Key Take Away: Pitocin contra-indication and doctors exceeding labelled limits ought to be a straightforward and clear-cut legal case. Yet, years of tort reform, have made things a lot more complicated. Establishing a pattern of abuse against individual obstetricians makes these cases a lot easier. AutismPI.org is a parents' organization dedicated to collecting data on autism causes and of all pathways with strong advocacy for brain damage and regeneration research. AutismPI.org is also running a data collection initiative to catalog causes of autism. This retrospective data collection is also aimed at clustering malpractice data on obstetricians and hospitals, thus making the cases a lot easier to pursue as class actions against individual practitioners and hospitals. If you are a parent of a child with autism, it is very important to register your data with AutismPI.org.

The Legal Catch-22 & the Path to End the Epidemic

Autism has been a problem that has confounded the scientific community for over a century. In the 1880's and 1890's initial clinical descriptions linked difficult births and signs of "asphyxia" (lack of breathing) with subsequent neurological issues years before the term autism was coined in 1908. In the mid 1900's with the development of tools to assess fetal and newborn status (like Apgar scores, introduced in 1952), the correlation between low oxygen levels at birth and neurological outcomes became more quantifiable. Research began to explore the specific ways oxygen deprivation impacted the developing brain. The late 20th century brought significant advancements in understanding the pathophysiology of hypoxic-ischemic encephalopathy (HIE). Studies using animal models and clinical observations in newborns detailed the cascade of cellular events leading to brain injury following oxygen deprivation. The importance of the duration and severity of hypoxia in determining the extent of brain damage became clearer. The modern era research focuses on early identification, prevention, and therapeutic interventions (like hypothermia therapy) to mitigate the effects of hypoxic brain injury in newborns. Advanced neuroimaging techniques have further refined our understanding of the specific brain regions affected by hypoxia at birth.

The advent of modern birth interventions and the abuse of these interventions have introduced a new component of traumatic brain injury into the mix. The use of forceps beginning in the 1900's up to the 1970's introduced the possibility of traumatic brain injury at birth when they were used ineptly. Use of forceps has since declined in favor of vacuum extraction which comes with its own risks. With the approval of Pitocin for elective labor induction in 1980 obstetricians gained unprecedented control of the uterus and another avenue for possible traumatic brain injury opened up. This one has been a lot more consequential due to the injury being literally covered up by the birth process itself, with damage caused at the cervical dilation stage being covered up by the pushing stage, causing it to stay hidden. There is no indication of damage as the brain doesn't signal pain upon damage to itself. For parents the labor induction process itself is made to be painless and the entire traumatic birth of the baby is seemingly uneventful for the mothers that undergo this intervention.

During this time the field of psychiatry was also evolving alongside and started to deal with adults with neurological conditions. These folks who might have otherwise survived unnoticed in a rural society, found themselves out of place in a society where logic and higher learning began to be rewarded more. Dealing with adults and older children with neurological conditions, birth trauma as the cause was lost on these psychiatrists and researchers. This was also a time when the field of genetics started evolving and psychiatrist Dr Michael Rutter came up with a novel idea of looking at twins who share genes and had a higher incidence of autism. While in his papers he does acknowledge perinatal brain injury related to what he called biological hazards including kernicterus, perinatal apnea of more than 6 minutes, neonatal convulsions and takes out that data, he also removed twins with congenital abnormalities (i.e. actual genetic diseases) from consideration and still claimed a genetic influence on autism. While it brought a new sense of compassion towards individuals suffering from autism, it hijacked attention from the true hypoxic birth injury cause of autism at that time. As I have pointed out, Dr Rutters research did not take into consideration the effect of a shared placenta in certain types of twins. Autism incidence in twins is fully explained by chorionicity and placental insufficiency in cases of shared placenta causing autism in both twins rather than genes.

I have shared our story of how a clueless OB/GYN turned a perfectly healthy 'low risk' pregnancy into a case of Autism not once but twice in our life. I have shared the MRI evidence of damage and the clear evidence of malpractice where the OB/GYN went against established norms at the hospital causing MRI visible brain damage. I have met numerous other parents with similar stories – in fact it's a story that is repeated all too often in maternity wards. It's a story only impacted parents would know from start to finish, from birth to the autism diagnosis. The best judges of this situation are the impacted parents, but many of them in their desperation to help their children have become overly dependent on the scientific community to give them the answers. They are forgetting that as the people spending the most time with these kids, they have front row seats to years of observation that science is not privy to. The scientific community has been caught in the crossfire between true research consistently turning up birth injury as the cause of autism and the forces trying to cover it up, who seem to be capable of getting NIH funding on a whim and come up with phony "research" of their own to contradict everything that true research turns up. Genuine researchers are torn between conflicting professional and economic interests and the results have been confusing signals, and a deliberate lack of clarity in conclusions of studies for fear of repercussions to any statements they make on this emotionally charged topic. Privacy laws have worked out in favor of some special interests to further stifle the truth for years.

I have shown how traumatic brain damage has remained hidden in most cases due to damage at the first cervical dilation stage of labor being literally 'erased' by the pushing stage of labor as seen in the MRI evidence of my own boys. We have seen how the damaged blood brain barrier from birth TBI leads to gut dysbiosis and mitochondrial dysfunction in many cases of autism and how the same symptoms are shared even by adult victims of TBI. I have shown how certain categories of viruses are known to cross the blood brain barrier (BBB) while others do not. The worst diseases are caused by the viruses that cross the BBB and children with prior TBI at birth show serious retrogression of skills when they fall sick with these viruses. Such regression is also noticed when live virus vaccine variants of these viruses are administered to children with prior TBI causing most parents to point to vaccines as the cause of their children's autism. These viruses are also known to establish neuronal viral latencies interfering with neuron growth factor production, eliminating the ability of the brain to heal itself from the damage thereby making it permanent. Thus, use of vaccines in previously brain damaged individuals has been a contributing factor aggravating the autism epidemic. We have discussed the brain immune deviation called the ACAID phenomenon which can make neuronal viral latencies and gut dysbiosis more permanent by allowing certain viruses to operate freely in the body unimpeded by the immune system.

We have also looked at the contra-indications for Pitocin in its labeling and I have shared my story of exactly how it gets to be abused. I have explained how the abuse of misoprostol for induction in live births effectively hides the brain damage dangers of labor induction drugs from new inexperienced obstetricians who take the routine use of these drugs as a testament to their safety. This alongside the secrecy surrounding the ACOG protocols have created an environment where obstetricians operate in a bubble of unawareness. All this culminated in the flawed "Arrive" trials which pretty much regularized abusive labor induction by not taking into account the not so obvious long term brain damage consequences of its actions.

I have shown how the ACOG's acceptance of the "Arrive" trial completely contrary to their own protocols is potentially a ploy to get out from under years of legal liability for the brain damage they caused over the years. Their move to drop the failure to progress diagnosis point in labor induction and abdicate their leadership in labor induction to the SMFM creates a legal entanglement with no possible solution. By shifting the standard of care, they complete alleviate the possibility of "expert witnesses" supporting a court case against traumatic birth injury by excessive contractions. That combined with the suffocating tort reforms in most states effectively buries the truth from emerging at any point in time, now or in the future.

All this solid evidence is known to many people but has probably not been said the way I have. Sometimes it takes someone to say things the way they are, before change can happen. For the sake of brevity, I have captured the true etiology of the Autism Epidemic mainly occurring because of Pitocin abuse in Fig 24.1.

Etiology of the Autism Epidemic

1980 - Pitocin was approved with a label that limited its use to a certain number of contractions - beyond which its starts causing fetal brain damage.

MID 1990's – Time by which ACOG realized they were causing Traumatic Brain Injury leading to autism in cases requiring excessive contractions for cervical dilation and came up with a directive to establish protocols in hospitals to limit contractions to 72 for labor induction.

MID 1990's to 2018 – While labor induction protocols were in place in hospitals, the ACOG were very secretive about it, as they were already sitting on a large liability situation, in the initial decade plus of abuse of the drug. However, newbie and ignorant obstetricians continued the abuse, unchecked during this time.

2018 – ACOG.org capitalized on the opportunity offered by the flawed ARRIVE trials to get out from under the legal liabilities for the historical birth injuries that had been caused by their flock over the years, by abandoning their contraction limits and abdicating their leadership in labor induction to the SMFM.org. This has paved the way for the autism epidemic to continue unchecked thanks to the legal tangle it creates.

Fig 24.1 – Timeline showing the etiology of the Autism Epidemic.

Pitocin abuse as the true cause of the autism epidemic, while being the truth, will be a tough truth to face and people not impacted by it could have a hard time understanding how something like this could ever happen. It will probably need validation by a decisive victory in a court of law. The challenge lies not in demonstrating the scientific veracity of this argument but in the monumental hurdle of confronting deeply entrenched societal beliefs and vested interests.

The public trust in the medical system, medical boards, other governing bodies and self-governing institutions all take a beating, in the light of what has really happened with autism in the last four plus decades. This truth is a truly bitter pill for the public to swallow, as it shatters a fundamental sense of security and implies a systemic betrayal of trust. Medical professionals and institutions involved will potentially refuse to acknowledge their involvement and culpability for past mistakes. Chances are the bigger institutions will throw everything at their disposal to defend themselves and try to escape blame for this malaise.

Unfortunately, the very mechanism for achieving this societal acceptance – the legal system – has historically proven to be a double-edged sword. The previous legal undertaking, specifically the vaccine omnibus trials, tragically ended in a judgment that not only failed to acknowledge the observation of thousands of parents or establish the link I have cited between vaccines and autism but, based on the defendants' arguments, issued unwarranted statements pointing to genetics as the primary cause. This court-sanctioned redirection was catastrophic. It inadvertently legitimized an alternative, unproven etiology, thereby diverting substantial research funding, public attention, and scientific inquiry away from the genuine birth injury causes of autism. This legal precedent solidified a false narrative, making it exponentially harder now to shift public perception and bring the focus back to the true underlying factors. The public is often swayed by authoritative pronouncements, and a legal ruling, even if based on incomplete or manipulated information, can solidify a 'truth' in the public consciousness, making subsequent challenges incredibly difficult.

To make matters worse, medical protocols have been abusively redesigned to defend professionals from lawsuits rather than safeguard patients from injury. This perilous shift has caused this legal catch 22 situation described in Fig 24.2.

The Legal Catch 22

Medical tort reforms implemented by almost all US states in the 90's, 2000's and 2010's severely restricted patient protections and ability to sue for legitimate injury. Malpractice lawsuits are a crucial feedback loop highlighting fringe scenarios, systemic failures and dangerous flaws in the system. Heavy handed tort reform has left the very protocols of care unchecked and, in some instances, totally flawed.

In the adjudication of medical malpractice claims, courts rely on other practitioners serving as "expert witnesses" to explain the instances where the defendant failed to adhere to the standard of care, to bring clarity to protocols and medical jargon.

In the case of traumatic brain injury from excessive contractions, pretty much the entire obstetric community is compromised with everybody having abused Pitocin at some point in their career, most of them before they understood its effects and some to this day because they don't know better.

Emboldened by the lack of legal consequences for their labor drug abuse in the past, thanks to tort reforms, the ACOG completed a legal master stroke in 2018 after the flawed ARRIVE trials. They abandoned their failure to progress diagnosis point in labor induction protocols, abdicating leadership in labor induction, to their new found fall guys William. A. Grobman and the SMFM.org.

With the protocol intended to safeguard against traumatic brain damage abandoned, the standard of care has shifted, effectively shielding obstetricians from legal challenges for not stopping inductions at the 72-contraction limit. No obstetric expert can now come forward as "expert witness" to support a lawsuit against excessive contractions causing traumatic brain injury – a true Catch-22 that is perpetuating the autism epidemic.

Fig 24.2 – Proving Autism Causation – The Legal Catch 22.

The Turning Point in 2024 -2025

As you can see, one way to overcome the legal "catch-22" is by creating class actions against individual practitioners, as discussed in the prior chapter. I first suggested this approach in my previous book, *Autism Answers and Action – by Dinesh Danny*, in April 2021. While that has been a difficult undertaking and remains a work in progress, lady luck may have smiled upon us, the parents impacted by autism, in late 2024 or early 2025. With the re-election of President Trump and his alliance with Robert F. Kennedy Jr., we finally have an administration that is genuinely serious about ending the autism epidemic. Those behind the apparatus attempting to hide the true cause of autism could not have imagined in their wildest dreams the possibility that an administration would attach so much importance to finding its true cause. This is precisely what inspired me to rewrite my previous book, incorporating new, clearer details that debunk the genetic origin theory, clarify contraction limits, analyze the ARRIVE trial, and provide other crucial insights not featured in my earlier work.

Considering how the new administration might help solve the autism causation question, two possible avenues come to mind:

1. Launch an inquiry into ACOG's labor induction history: This would involve scrutinizing their committee opinion on labor induction and autism, along with their diversionary tactics that point to the chemical neurotransmitter effects of Pitocin rather than its primary uterine motility effect.

2. Investigate the research fraud committed in the name of the ARRIVE trial: This trial failed to consider the contraction count limits necessitated by the labeling of Pitocin, the only drug approved by the FDA for live birth labor induction.

I believe this could be part of a congressional or HHS investigation. Some questions ACOG would have to answer are listed in Fig 24.3, which would make their intentions and mistakes very clear to the public.

Questions for the ACOG to Answer in Public

Which year was the brain damage effect of excessive induced contractions first identified by the ACOG?

When was the failure to progress diagnosis contraction limit established as hospital labor induction protocols.

Why did the ACOG drop the failure to progress protocol, fully aware that the brain damage is a function of the contraction count no matter what the drug.

Knowing the rising autism rates and the ARRIVE trial's disregard for contraction limits, why did ACOG cede leadership in labor induction to the SMFM?

Fig 24.3 – Questions to prove ACOG guilt in autism causation.

A quick and easy way to re-confirm autism causation with excessive contractions would be to examine the Arrive trial participants who underwent long hours of labor induction, particularly those who were subjected to prolonged induction (excessive contractions) after the loss of amniotic fluid. A cross reference to school records of these individuals could be a quick way to establish causation by the specific obstetricians involved in the Arrive trial.

Another possibility is to check the birth circumstances of participants in CDC's SEED trials (Study to Explore Early Development) to identify the birth trauma involved in each case and how much of it was caused by induced labor. Some other objectives of such investigations would be:

- ▶ Investigating and bringing the perpetrators to justice.
- ▶ Breaking the legal catch 22
- ▶ Institute care improvements to end the Autism epidemic.

Investigating and Bringing the Perpetrators to Justice

It is essential to investigate and publicly identify malpractice insurance companies, hospitals, their social media management clients, who may have been involved in organizing and funding disinformation campaigns aimed at suppressing parental concerns about a potential labor induction-autism link on social media. This investigation should scrutinize the funding of research designed to counter claims against Pitocin and evaluate potential phony research into genetic causes, assessing whether the primary motivation was to manipulate media narratives. Any companies and institutions found to have deliberately suppressed truthful information on social media must be held accountable for their actions, and individuals who orchestrated these campaigns should face appropriate legal repercussions. Transparency and accountability are crucial to addressing these potential attempts to conceal information and the resulting harm.

The ARRIVE trial was a profound deception, and it is alarming that such a large-scale trial, involving multiple obstetricians and hospitals, was even permitted to proceed when these "researchers" were actively disregarding prevailing labor induction safety protocols that had its roots in the labeling of the drug. This trial yielded no actionable outcome, yet it was used to dismantle established safety protocols by employing a methodology that did not even consider long-term brain damage outcomes – the very reason those protocols were originally established. The protocol mandated a contraction count limit that was intended to remain constant, regardless of the drug used to induce contractions. That said, the off-label use of misoprostol for live labor induction in hospitals warrants immediate regulatory attention. This practice should either be discontinued, or if the drug's purported superiority is substantiated, the FDA should approve it for this indication with comprehensive labeling that includes a definitive contraction count for the "failure to progress" diagnosis with emphasis on cervix preparation before induction. My second son, who is more severely impacted and whose MRI scan shows visible brain damage, was induced for 18 hours with both misoprostol and Pitocin. Hence, I believe any claim of misoprostol superiority is false propaganda. It is inconsistent that autism care providers like the DAN doctors were penalized for off-label and "experimental" treatments, yet the off-label hospital administration of misoprostol in live births appears exempt from similar enforcement.

Someone like Dr. Andrew Wakefield was effectively annihilated by the health authorities (in the U.K.) for merely explaining a correlation he saw between live vaccines and their impact on brain development and gut dysbiosis—and he was, in part, correct. This is a common observation among most autism parents, who notice that their children suffer a regression of skills not just after vaccines but also after viral illnesses involving viruses capable of crossing the blood-brain barrier. As I have explained previously, live vaccines remain a secondary cause of autism as they make pre-existing brain damage more permanent by inhibiting recovery, thanks to neuronal viral latencies, the brain immune deviation called the ACAID phenomenon, and the gut dysbiosis that follows any traumatic brain damage. But Dr. Wakefield did not cause autism in anybody, contrary to what the ARRIVE trial proponents have probably done. They have likely been directly responsible for the causation of autism in hundreds of cases and indirectly responsible for countless more. What consequences do they deserve?

Breaking the Legal Catch 22

To navigate the current legal deadlock, two key approaches could be considered. First, it would be beneficial for hospitals to reinstate and rigorously enforce the ACOG labor induction protocols that were in effect prior to 2018. Furthermore, it might prove crucial for these protocols to be widely disseminated throughout the obstetric and medical communities, ensuring they become common knowledge rather than remaining obscure. Reinstating these guidelines could provide a clear standard of care against which to assess cases of Pitocin misuse, thereby allowing related lawsuits to proceed. Any other standard of care changes implemented as a result of the flawed ARRIVE trial may also need to be reversed, particularly the interventionist induction at 39 weeks recommendation. The period of harm between 2018 and the present would then require a separate, but equally determined, legal strategy.

Second, the establishment of a distinct legal framework, perhaps a specialized court or arbitration process, could be considered to address claims for compensation resulting from traumatic brain damage due to obstetric malpractice that has devastatingly impacted individuals with autism. These cases, particularly those arising from induced labor, might warrant a dedicated approach, drawing parallels with the Omnibus Autism Proceedings. It is crucial to recognize that many of these mothers experienced healthy pregnancies and would likely have delivered healthy infants naturally, were it not for the unnecessary and potentially abusive intervention of labor induction, often targeting "low-risk nulliparous" women. The resulting brain damage has profoundly affected these children's lives and inflicted immense emotional distress on their families. Malpractice insurance companies should be compelled to provide fair compensation that transcends their current inadequate limits for the extensive suffering endured by these patients due to the actions of their insured obstetricians.

States might need to be encouraged to dismantle their restrictive tort reforms, at least in critical areas where the effects of malpractice lead to lifelong devastation, such as in obstetrics. They could be made to understand that significant improvements in medical standards of care often necessitate legal action to drive meaningful change and compel the medical community to learn from its mistakes. State-level tort reforms essentially suffocate that avenue. For example, surgeons only truly understood that operating on patients with high blood sugar levels caused death after lawsuits, following the deaths of a few individuals, made headlines. There are many such examples in vascular and neurosurgery where surgeries failed and young, healthy patients died, but it was the subsequent lawsuits and headlines that brought lasting change in medical practices in these areas. Tort reforms that impose unnecessarily low caps on compensation for malpractice that irrevocably changes someone's life are, in my view, outright evil, a human rights violation, and have no place in modern society.

Care Improvements Necessary to End the Autism Epidemic.

Addressing the autism epidemic will likely require a paradigm shift in the standard of perinatal obstetric care. Elective induction of labor, as an intervention, might benefit from severe restrictions. Cervical dilation strategies might need to be prioritized over labor induction in healthy pregnancies. Both excessive and hypertonic contractions resulting from labor-inducing drugs should ideally be openly recognized for the significant brain damage threat they pose. This risk exists with full induction as well as augmentation when labor stalls. It could be considered that when labor gets stuck, it is sometimes because the mother's body instinctively senses a potential for brain damage to the baby if further contractions are initiated. At such junctures, in the absence of other immediate risks, the mandate could shift towards watchful waiting rather than promptly administering labor drugs. If other risks are present, a C-section might often be the safer option.

The notion that post-term pregnancy is inherently a complication deserves re-evaluation. In our current era of prenatal vitamins and excellent pregnancy care, healthy mothers can often safely continue pregnancies well beyond 42 weeks, even extending to 46 or 47 weeks or more, culminating in natural deliveries of healthy babies. The historical case of Beulah Hunter in Los Angeles, CA, whose pregnancy lasted over 53 weeks in 1945, serves as a powerful reminder of this physiological reality. The obstetric community might consider recognizing that healthy women with high bone density are often naturally post-term and capable of carrying their pregnancies for much longer than 42 weeks, while still delivering healthy babies vaginally. In these cases of postdating, obstetricians could be encouraged to recommend natural home remedies like enemas and sexual stimulation of the mother as alternatives to hospital labor induction. Tragically, these supposedly "low-risk nulliparous women" are frequently targeted for labor induction before 42 weeks. Their calcium-sensitive bodies often do not respond effectively to Pitocin or prostaglandins, leading to prolonged and traumatic labors that result in brain damage in otherwise healthy infants—a direct consequence of unnecessary birth interventions. The perceived risk of stillbirth in these carefully monitored, post-term healthy pregnancies appears demonstrably exaggerated. Furthermore, it could be beneficial to mandate that every pregnant couple create and discuss a birth plan emphasizing minimal interventions, with any intervention undertaken only in the presence of genuine complications.

Consider establishing a standard score for birth trauma and possible brain damage during birth. Rather than relying solely on the Apgar score, which measures a baby's health as perceived by a care provider, this new measure could estimate an actual birth trauma score, considering maternal complications, prematurity, breech birth, nuchal cords, fetal distress, planned C-section, and other relevant factors. Newborns with higher trauma scores might benefit from being maintained in incubators on higher oxygen for a week or more than current norms.

It might be prudent to delay vaccines for children known to have had a traumatic birth based on the new trauma score, or who have experienced life-threatening hospitalizations within the first six months of birth. This could include children delivered by C-section due to fetal distress, and those who experience significant viral illnesses in the first six months of birth involving substantial brain-damaging fevers, respiratory distress, and similar conditions.

A mandate for a post-natal MRI scan could be considered when certain criteria are met, such as when the duration of active labor has exceeded eight hours, birth interventions have been involved, or the trauma score is high for any other reason. The MARBLE (Magnetic Resonance Biomarkers in Neonatal Encephalopathy) study by Imperial College London and the NIH concluded that magnetic resonance spectroscopy of the thalamus region, measuring N-acetylaspartate levels, can reliably predict neonatal brain damage. This could be a valuable addition to every hospital birth where feasible, particularly in cases of hypoxic injury.

Mandating the use of cooling therapies to induce medical hypothermia might significantly help the brain heal faster in neonates where neurological damage is suspected. This could potentially alleviate the risk of long-term neurological disorders. Cooling blankets and therapies, unfortunately, are not yet widely used in the U.S., but they have been proven helpful in hospitals that utilize them, and they should ideally become part of the standard of care.

A Final Word

If you have read this far, you likely now understand why the primary cause of autism has remained hidden since 1980. Birth injury compensation claims and settlements are among the most expensive in the realm of malpractice suits, precisely because they devastate the the rest of the lives of newborns. All children injured by hypoxia or contraction trauma at birth often end up on the autism spectrum, whether their birth injury is acknowledged or not. Autism doesn't merely impact the individual; entire families, extended families, and society at large suffer the consequences. Hence, the substantial claims are, in fact, justified.

However, it is beyond comprehension to consider that money and fear of reputational damage have driven something as inhumane as the autism epidemic to be inflicted upon patients by the leadership within the obstetric community and the broader medical system across multiple countries. Tort reforms have been instrumental in suppressing patient rights and concealing this truth from the public. Equally incredible is the enormous apparatus behind this suppression. I never imagined such a truth could be hidden in the dark shadows of obstetric malpractice, in the free world, for a full 45 years. I've been working since about 2018 to uncover this reality, peeling back the layers of deception one at a time, and I'm still unsure if I've revealed its full extent.

Now that I have exposed the truth about the autism epidemic, it is imperative for impacted parents to come forward, join the fight for justice, and give voice to our children who cannot stand up for themselves. Change must come from the highest levels of government to truly end this epidemic. While lawsuits and compensation could help alleviate some of the suffering our families endure, parental involvement is also vital to propel further research into brain damage recovery. Several promising developments are on the horizon, but they require support to be accelerated. With your help, the days of complete brain damage recovery are not far.

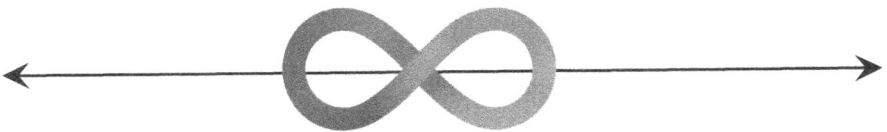

REMEMBER

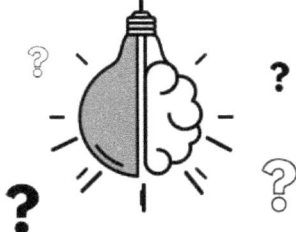

Autism is mostly the result of hypoxic or traumatic birth injury historically.

If it wasn't a known trauma or condition like, premature birth, tight nuchal cord, breech birth, known congenital birth defects, maternal infection in pregnancy, planned or emergency C-section and the mother was induced, then traumatic brain injury from abusive labor induction was the cause of Autism in your child, particularly severe non-verbal childhood autism.

IRREFUTABLE FACTS

This book is based on the following undeniable facts.

1. The Pitocin drug carries a traumatic brain damage warning on its FDA required label/package insert.

2. Contraindication #5 on the Pitocin label relates to excessive contractions causing brain damage.

3. ACOG instituted labor induction protocols to address contraindication #5 by restricting induction to 72 contractions, sometime in the mid 90's and these were in place were in place until 2018 although some OB/Gyns never followed it.

4. The brain does not signal any pain upon damage to itself.

5. Traumatic brain injury is almost always followed by gut dysbiosis months later.

6. Synthetic oxytocin by names Pitocin/Syntocinon is the only FDA approved drug for labor induction in live births.

7. Most hospitals have transitioned from Pitocin to the off-label use of misoprostol, a prostaglandin originally approved only for abortions, to induce labor in live births.

8. ACOG denies autism labor induction link by pointing to the chemical effect that downregulation of oxytocin receptors in the fetal brain from oxytocin exposure during induction is not proven.

9. The contraindication #5 on the Pitocin label remains unaddressed by the current standard of care after 2018.

10. The updated standard of care since 2018 precludes the possibility of lawsuits for brain damage caused by excessive contractions.

WWW.AUTISMPI.ORG

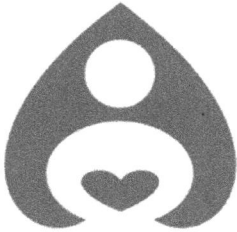

Autism Parents Initiative

The retrospective data collection effort at autismpi.org is like the SEED effort by the CDC, but for birth circumstances of impacted children.

Register your autism birth data there now to enable research and legal discovery.

APPENDIX - PITOCIN LABEL

Pitocin®
(Oxytocin Injection, USP) Synthetic

DESCRIPTION

Pitocin (oxytocin injection, USP) is a sterile, clear, colorless aqueous solution of synthetic oxytocin, for intravenous infusion or intramuscular injection. Pitocin is a nonapeptide found in pituitary extracts from mammals. It is standardized to contain 10 units of oxytocic hormone/mL and contains 0.5% Chlorobutanol, a chloroform derivative as a preservative, 1.65 mg acetic acid and 0.16 mg ammonium acetate as buffers, and with the pH adjusted with acetic acid to achieve a targeted pH of 3.5. Pitocin may contain up to 16% of total impurities. The hormone is prepared synthetically to avoid possible contamination with vasopressin (ADH) and other small polypeptides with biologic activity. Pitocin has the empirical formula $C_{43}H_{66}N_{12}O_{12}S_2$ (molecular weight 1007.19). The structural formula is as follows:

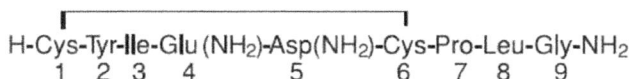

$$\text{H-Cys-Tyr-Ile-Glu(NH}_2\text{)-Asp(NH}_2\text{)-Cys-Pro-Leu-Gly-NH}_2$$
$$\quad\;1\quad\;2\quad\;3\quad\;4\qquad\quad\;5\qquad\;\;6\quad\;7\quad\;8\quad\;9$$

CLINICAL PHARMACOLOGY

Uterine motility depends on the formation of the contractile protein actomyosin under the influence of the Ca^{2+}-dependent phosphorylating enzyme myosin light-chain kinase. Oxytocin promotes contractions by increasing the intracellular Ca^{2+}. Oxytocin has specific receptors in the myometrium and the receptor concentration increases greatly during pregnancy, reaching a maximum in early labor at term. The response to a given dose of oxytocin is very individualized and depends on the sensitivity of the uterus, which is determined by the oxytocin receptor concentration. However, the physician should be aware of the fact that oxytocin even in its pure form has inherent pressor and antidiuretic properties which may become manifest when large doses are administered. These properties are thought to be due to the fact that oxytocin and vasopressin differ in regard to only two of the eight amino acids (see PRECAUTIONS section).

Oxytocin is distributed throughout the extracellular fluid. Small amounts of the drug probably reach the fetal circulation. Oxytocin has a plasma half-life of about 1 to 6 minutes which is decreased in late pregnancy and during lactation. Following intravenous administration of oxytocin, uterine response occurs almost immediately and subsides within 1 hour. Following intramuscular injection of the drug, uterine response occurs within 3 to 5 minutes and persists for 2 to 3 hours. Its rapid removal from plasma is accomplished largely by the kidney and the liver. Only small amounts are excreted in urine unchanged.

INDICATIONS AND USAGE

IMPORTANT NOTICE

Elective induction of labor is defined as the initiation of labor in a pregnant individual who has no medical indications for induction. Since the available data are inadequate to evaluate the benefits-to-risks considerations, Pitocin is not indicated for elective induction of labor.

Antepartum

Pitocin is indicated for the initiation or improvement of uterine contractions, where this is desirable and considered suitable for reasons of fetal or maternal concern, in order to achieve vaginal delivery. It is indicated for (1) induction of labor in patients with a medical indication for the initiation of labor, such as Rh problems, maternal diabetes, preeclampsia at or near term, when delivery is in the best interests of mother and fetus or when membranes are prematurely ruptured and delivery is indicated; (2) stimulation or reinforcement of labor, as in selected cases of uterine inertia; (3) as adjunctive therapy in the management of incomplete or inevitable abortion. In the first trimester, curettage is generally considered primary therapy. In second trimester abortion, oxytocin infusion will often be successful in emptying the uterus. Other means of therapy, however, may be required in such cases.

Postpartum

Pitocin is indicated to produce uterine contractions during the third stage of labor and to control postpartum bleeding or hemorrhage.

CONTRAINDICATIONS

Antepartum use of Pitocin is contraindicated in any of the following circumstances:

1. Where there is significant cephalopelvic disproportion;

2. In unfavorable fetal positions or presentations, such as transverse lies, which are undeliverable without conversion prior to delivery;

3. In obstetrical emergencies where the benefit-to-risk ratio for either the fetus or the mother favors surgical intervention;

4. In fetal distress where delivery is not imminent;

5. Where adequate uterine activity fails to achieve satisfactory progress;

6. Where the uterus is already hyperactive or hypertonic;

7. In cases where vaginal delivery is contraindicated, such as invasive cervical carcinoma, active herpes genitalis, total placenta previa, vasa previa, and cord presentation or prolapse of the cord;

8. In patients with hypersensitivity to the drug.

WARNINGS

Pitocin, when given for induction of labor or augmentation of uterine activity, should be administered only by the intravenous route and with adequate medical supervision in a hospital.

PRECAUTIONS

General

1. All patients receiving intravenous oxytocin must be under continuous observation by trained personnel who have a thorough knowledge of the drug and are qualified to identify complications. A physician qualified to manage any complications should be immediately available. Electronic fetal monitoring provides the best means for early detection of overdosage (see OVERDOSAGE section). However, it must be borne in mind that only intrauterine pressure recording can accurately measure the intrauterine pressure during contractions. A fetal scalp electrode provides a more dependable recording of the fetal heart rate than any external monitoring system.

2. When properly administered, oxytocin should stimulate uterine contractions comparable to those seen in normal labor. Overstimulation of the uterus by improper administration can be hazardous to both mother and fetus. Even with proper administration and adequate supervision, hypertonic contractions can occur in patients whose uteri are hypersensitive to oxytocin. This fact must be considered by the physician in exercising his judgment regarding patient selection.

3. Except in unusual circumstances, oxytocin should not be administered in the following conditions: fetal

distress, hydramnios, partial placenta previa, prematurity, borderline cephalopelvic disproportion, and any condition in which there is a predisposition for uterine rupture, such as previous major surgery on the cervix or uterus including cesarean section, overdistention of the uterus, grand multiparity, or past history of uterine sepsis or of traumatic delivery. Because of the variability of the combinations of factors which may be present in the conditions listed above, the definition of "unusual circumstances" must be left to the judgment of the physician. The decision can be made only by carefully weighing the potential benefits which oxytocin can provide in a given case against rare but definite potential for the drug to produce hypertonicity or tetanic spasm.

4. Maternal deaths due to hypertensive episodes, subarachnoid hemorrhage, rupture of the uterus, and fetal deaths due to various causes have been reported associated with the use of parenteral oxytocic drugs for induction of labor or for augmentation in the first and second stages of labor.

5. Oxytocin has been shown to have an intrinsic antidiuretic effect, acting to increase water reabsorption from the glomerular filtrate. Consideration should, therefore, be given to the possibility of water intoxication, particularly when oxytocin is administered continuously by infusion and the patient is receiving fluids by mouth.

6. When oxytocin is used for induction or reinforcement of already existent labor, patients should be carefully selected. Pelvic adequacy must be considered and maternal and fetal conditions evaluated before use of the drug.

Drug Interactions

Severe hypertension has been reported when oxytocin was given three to four hours following prophylactic administration of a vasoconstrictor in conjunction with caudal block anesthesia. Cyclopropane anesthesia may modify oxytocin's cardiovascular effects, so as to produce unexpected results such as hypotension. Maternal sinus bradycardia with abnormal atrioventricular rhythms has also been noted when oxytocin was used concomitantly with cyclopropane anesthesia.

Carcinogenesis, Mutagenesis, Impairment of Fertility

There are no animal or human studies on the carcinogenicity and mutagenicity of this drug, nor is there any information on its effect on fertility.

Pregnancy

Teratogenic Effects

Animal reproduction studies have not been conducted with oxytocin. There are no known indications for use in the first trimester of pregnancy other than in relation to spontaneous or induced abortion. Based on the wide experience with this drug and its chemical structure and pharmacological properties, it would not be expected to present a risk of fetal abnormalities when used as indicated.

Nonteratogenic Effects

See ADVERSE REACTIONS in the fetus or neonate.

Labor and Delivery

See INDICATIONS AND USAGE section.

ADVERSE REACTIONS

The following adverse reactions have been reported in the mother:

Anaphylactic reaction	Premature ventricular contractions
Postpartum hemorrhage	Pelvic hematoma
Cardia arrhythmia	Subarachnoid hemorrhage
Fatal afibrinogenemia	Hypertensive episodes
Nausea	Rupture of the uterus
Vomiting	

Excessive dosage or hypersensitivity to the drug may result in uterine hypertonicity, spasm, tetanic contraction, or rupture of the uterus.

The possibility of increased blood loss and afibrinogenemia should be kept in mind when administering the drug.

Severe water intoxication with convulsions and coma has occurred, associated with a slow oxytocin infusion over a 24-hour period. Maternal death due to oxytocin-induced water intoxication has been reported.

The following adverse reactions have been reported in the fetus or neonate:

Due to induced uterine motility:	Due to use of oxytocin in the mother:
Bradycardia	Low Apgar scores at five minutes
Premature ventricular contractions and other arrhythmias	Neonatal jaundice
Permanent CNS or brain damage	Neonatal retinal hemorrhage
Fetal death	

Neonatal seizures have been reported with the use of Pitocin.

For medical advice about adverse reactions contact your medical professional. To report SUSPECTED ADVERSE REACTIONS, contact Par Pharmaceutical at 1-800-828-9393 or FDA at 1-800-FDA-1088 (1-800-332-1088) or www.fda.gov/medwatch.

OVERDOSAGE

Overdosage with oxytocin depends essentially on uterine hyperactivity whether or not due to hypersensitivity to this agent. Hyperstimulation with strong (hypertonic) or prolonged (tetanic) contractions, or a resting tone of 15 to 20 mmHg or more between contractions can lead to tumultuous labor, uterine rupture, cervical and vaginal lacerations, postpartum hemorrhage, uteroplacental hypoperfusion, and variable deceleration of fetal heart, fetal hypoxia, hypercapnia, perinatal hepatic necrosis or death. Water intoxication with convulsions, which is caused by the inherent antidiuretic effect of oxytocin, is a serious complication that may occur if large doses (40 to 50 milliunits/minute) are infused for long periods. Management consists of immediate discontinuation of oxytocin and symptomatic and supportive therapy.

DOSAGE AND ADMINISTRATION

Parenteral drug products should be inspected visually for particulate matter and discoloration prior to administration whenever solution and container permit.

The dosage of oxytocin is determined by the uterine response and must therefore be individualized and initiated at a very low level. The following dosage information is based upon various regimens and indications in general use.

A. Induction or Stimulation of Labor

Intravenous infusion (drip method) is the only acceptable method of parenteral administration of Pitocin for the induction or stimulation of labor. Accurate control of the rate of infusion is essential and is best accomplished by an infusion pump. It is convenient to piggyback the Pitocin infusion on a physiologic electrolyte solution, permitting the Pitocin infusion to be stopped abruptly without interrupting the electrolyte infusion. This is done in the following way.

1. **Preparation**

    a. The standard solution for infusion of Pitocin is prepared by adding the contents of one 1-mL vial containing 10 units of oxytocin to 1000 mL of 0.9% aqueous sodium chloride or Ringer's lactate. The combined solution containing 10 milliunits (mU) of oxytocin/mL is rotated in the infusion bottle for thorough mixing.

    b. Establish the infusion with a separate bottle of physiologic electrolyte solution not containing Pitocin.

    c. Attach (piggyback) the Pitocin-containing bottle with the infusion pump to the infusion line as close to the infusion site as possible.

2. **Administration**
    The initial dose should be 0.5–1 mU/min (equal to 3–6 mL of the dilute oxytocin solution per hour). At 30–60 minute intervals the dose should be gradually increased in increments of 1–2 mU/min until the desired contraction pattern has been established. Once the desired frequency of contractions has been reached and labor has progressed to 5–6 cm dilation, the dose may be reduced by similar increments.

    Studies of the concentrations of oxytocin in the maternal plasma during Pitocin infusion have shown that infusion rates up to 6 mU/min give the same oxytocin levels that are found in spontaneous labor. At term, higher infusion rates should be given with great care, and rates exceeding 9–10 mU/min are rarely required. Before term, when the sensitivity of the uterus is lower because of a lower concentration of oxytocin receptors, a higher infusion rate may be required.

3. **Monitoring**

    a. Electronically monitor the uterine activity and the fetal heart rate throughout the infusion of Pitocin. Attention should be given to tonus, amplitude and frequency of contractions, and to the fetal heart rate in relation to uterine contractions. If uterine contractions become too powerful, the infusion can be abruptly stopped, and oxytocic stimulation of the uterine musculature will soon wane (see **PRECAUTIONS** section).

    b. Discontinue the infusion of Pitocin immediately in the event of uterine hyperactivity and/or fetal distress. Administer oxygen to the mother, who preferably should be put in a lateral position. The condition of mother and fetus should immediately be evaluated by the responsible physician and appropriate steps taken.

B. Control of Postpartum Uterine Bleeding

1. Intravenous infusion (drip method). If the patient has an intravenous infusion running, 10 to 40 units of oxytocin may be added to the bottle, depending on the amount of electrolyte or dextrose solution remaining (maximum 40 units to 1000 mL). Adjust the infusion rate to sustain uterine contraction and control uterine atony.

2. Intramuscular administration. (One mL) Ten (10) units of Pitocin can be given after the delivery of the placenta.

C. Treatment of Incomplete, Inevitable, or Elective Abortion

Intravenous infusion of 10 units of Pitocin added to 500 mL of a physiologic saline solution or 5% dextrose-in-water solution may help the uterus contract after a suction or sharp curettage for an incomplete, inevitable, or elective abortion.

Subsequent to intra-amniotic injection of hypertonic saline, prostaglandins, urea, etc., for midtrimester elective abortion, the injection-to-abortion time may be shortened by infusion of Pitocin at the rate of 10 to 20 milliunits (20 to 40 drops) per minute. The total dose should not exceed 30 units in a 12-hour period due to the risk of water intoxication.

HOW SUPPLIED

Pitocin (Oxytocin Injection, USP) Synthetic is available as follows:

NDC 42023-116-25 Packages of twenty-five oversized 1-mL vials, each containing 10 units of oxytocin.

NDC 42023-116-02 Packages of twenty-five 10 mL multiple-dose vial, each containing 10 units of oxytocin per mL (total = 100 units of oxytocin per vial).

STORAGE

Store between 20° to 25°C (68° to 77°F). (See USP Controlled Room Temperature.)

REFERENCES

1. Seitchik J, Castillo M: Oxytocin augmentation of dysfunctional labor. I. Clinical data. Am J Obstet Gynecol 1982; 144:899–905.

2. Seitchik J, Castillo M: Oxytocin augmentation of dysfunctional labor. II. Multiparous patients. Am J Obstet Gynecol 1983; 145:777–780.

3. Fuchs A, Goeschen K, Husslein P, et al: Oxytocin and the initiation of human parturition. III. Plasma concentrations of oxytocin and 13, 14-dihydro-15-keto-prostaglandin F2a in spontaneous and oxytocin-induced labor at term. Am J Obstet Gynecol 1983; 145:497–502.

4. Seitchik J, Amico J, et al: Oxytocin augmentation of dysfunctional labor. IV. Oxytocin pharmacokinetics. Am J Obstet Gynecol 1984; 150:225–228.

5. American College of Obstetricians and Gynecologists: ACOG Technical Bulletin Number 110—November 1987: Induction and augmentation of labor.

Rx only.

Distributed by:

Par Pharmaceutical

Chestnut Ridge, NY 10977

REFERENCES

Too many research papers out there seem to start with the faulty premise that all autism is genetic. Such sweeping generalization makes many of these 'autism' papers irrelevant. But good quality research is invaluable and I am grateful for some very good information and images made available by many educational institutions, nonprofits and some select papers available from the National Institute of Health website. Some of these references used in individual chapters are listed below.

1.1)   Benvenuto A, Manzi B, Alessandrelli R, Galasso C, Curatolo P. Recent advances in the pathogenesis of syndromic autisms. Int J Pediatr. 2009;2009:198736. doi:10.1155/2009/198736

1.2)   Konkel L. The brain before birth: using fMRI to explore the secrets of fetal neurodevelopment. Environ Health Perspect. 2018;126:112001. https://ehp.niehs.nih.gov/doi/10.1289/EHP2268

1.3)   Stiles J, Jernigan TL. The basics of brain development. Neuropsychol Rev. 2010;20(4):327-348. Doi:10.1007/s11065-010-9148-4

1.4)   Paus T, Zijdenbos A, Worsley K, et al. Structural maturation of neural pathways in children and adolescents: in vivo study. Science. 1999;283(5409):1908-1911. Doi:10.1126/science.283.5409.1908

3.1)   Saunders NR, Liddelow SA, Dziegielewska KM. Barrier mechanisms in the developing brain. Front Pharmacol. 2012;3:46. Published 2012 Mar 29. doi:10.3389/fphar.2012.00046.

3.2)   Sudo N, Chida Y, Aiba Y, et al. Postnatal microbial colonization programs the hypothalamic-pituitary-adrenal system for stress response in mice. J Physiol. 2004;558(Pt 1):263-275. doi:10.1113/jphysiol.2004.063388

4.1) Changes in Practice among Physicians with Malpractice Claims, Publication: The New England Journal of Medicine, Publisher: Massachusetts Medical Society, Date: Mar 28, 2019

6.1) Wolf JH. Risk and Reputation: Obstetricians, Cesareans, and Consent. J Hist Med Allied Sci. 2018 Jan 1;73(1):7-28. doi: 10.1093/jhmas/jrx053. PMID: 29240893; PMCID: PMC5892390. https://www.ncbi.nlm.nih.gov/pmc/articles/PMC5892390/

7.1) Macones GA, Hankins GD, Spong CY, Hauth J, Moore T. The 2008 National Institute of Child Health and Human Development workshop report on electronic fetal monitoring: update on definitions, interpretation, and research guidelines. Obstet Gynecol. 2008 Sep;112(3):661-6. doi: 10.1097/AOG.0b013e3181841395. PMID: 18757666. https://pubmed.ncbi.nlm.nih.gov/18757666/

7.2) Lothian, Judith A.. "Saying "No" to Induction." The Journal of Perinatal Education vol. 15,2 (2006): 43–45. doi:10.1624/105812406X107816 https://www.ncbi.nlm.nih.gov/pmc/articles/PMC1595289/

7.3) Budden A, Chen LJ, Henry A. High-dose versus low-dose oxytocin infusion regimens for induction of labour at term. Cochrane Database Syst Rev. 2014 Oct 9;(10):CD009701. doi: 10.1002/14651858.CD009701.pub2. PMID: 25300173. https://pubmed.ncbi.nlm.nih.gov/25300173/

7.4) Bishop, Edward H. (August 1964). "Pelvic Scoring for Elective Induction". Obstetrics & Gynecology. 24 (2): 266–268. PMID 14199536.

7.5) Tenore J (2003). "Methods for cervical ripening and induction of labor". Am Fam Physician. 67 (10): 2123–8. PMID 12776961.

8.1)   Bin Wang et al. Effects of Prenatal Hypoxia on Nervous System
        Development and Related Diseases.
        https://www.frontiersin.org/journals/neuroscience/articles/10.3389/f
        nins.2021.755554/full

8.2)   Barnabei VM, Rasmusson RL, Bett GC. Autism and induced labor: is
        calcium a potential mechanistic link? Am J Obstet Gynecol. 2014
        May;210(5):494-5. doi: 10.1016/j.ajog.2014.01.020. Epub 2014 Jan
        16. PMID: 24440564.

8.3)   Nocon JJ, Coolman DA. Perinatal malpractice. Risks and prevention.
        J Reprod Med. 1987;32(2):83-90.

8.4)   Karl SJ Oláh FRCOG FRCS MRCP(I),a,* Philip J Steer BSc MD
        FRCOGb The use and abuse of oxytocin. -
        https://obgyn.onlinelibrary.wiley.com/doi/10.1111/tog.12222.

8.5)   Young RC, Barendse P. Linking myometrial physiology to intrauterine
        pressure; how tissue-level contractions create uterine contractions of
        labor. PloS Comput Biol. 2014;10(10):e1003850. Published 2014 Oct
        16. Doi:10.1371/journal.pcbi.1003850

8.6)   Sanchez-Ramos, L, Kaunitz, A, Glob. Libr. Women's med., (ISSN:
        1756-2228) 2009; DOI 10.3843/GLOWM.10130 (The global library
        of women's medicine)

8.7)   Cummins G, Kremer J, Bernassau A, et al. Sensors for Fetal Hypoxia
        and Metabolic Acidosis: A Review. Sensors (Basel). 2018;18(8):2648.
        Published 2018 Aug 13. Doi:10.3390/s18082648

8.8)   https://www.acog.org/clinical/clinical-guidance/committee-
        opinion/articles/2014/05/labor-induction-or-augmentation-and-
        autism

8.9)   Gregory SG, Anthopolos R, Osgood CE, Grotegut CA, Miranda ML.
        Association of autism with induced or augmented childbirth in North

Carolina Birth Record (1990-1998) and Education Research (1997-2007) databases. JAMA Pediatr. 2013;167(10):959-966. doi:10.1001/jamapediatrics.2013.2904

8.10)   Kurth L, Haussmann R. Perinatal Pitocin as an Early ADHD Biomarker: Neurodevelopmental Risk? Journal of Attention Disorders. 2011;15(5):423-431. doi:10.1177/1087054710397800

8.11)   Smallwood M, Sareen A, Baker E, Hannusch R, Kwessi E, Williams T. Increased Risk of Autism Development in Children Whose Mothers Experienced Birth Complications or Received Labor and Delivery Drugs. ASN Neuro. 2016;8(4):1759091416659742. Published 2016 Aug 9. Doi:10.1177/1759091416659742

9.1)   Greenberg DA, Hodge SE, Sowinski J, Nicoll D. Excess of twins among affected sibling pairs with autism: implications for the etiology of autism. Am J Hum Genet. 2001 Nov;69(5):1062-7. doi: 10.1086/324191. Epub 2001 Oct 2. PMID: 11590546; PMCID: PMC1274353.

9.2)   Betancur C, Leboyer M, Gillberg C. Increased rate of twins among affected sibling pairs with autism. Am J Hum Genet. 2002 May;70(5):1381-3. doi: 10.1086/340364. PMID: 11951183; PMCID: PMC447617.

9.3)   Folstein SE, Rosen-Sheidley B. Genetics of autism: complex aetiology for a heterogeneous disorder. Nat Rev Genet. 2001 Dec;2(12):943-55. doi: 10.1038/35103559. PMID: 11733747.

10.1)   Simpson, Kathleen Rice PhD, RNC, CNS-BC, FAAN. Trends in Labor Induction in the United States, 1989 to 2020. MCN, The American Journal of Maternal/Child Nursing 47(4):p 235, July/August 2022. | DOI: 10.1097/NMC.0000000000000824

14.1)   Wilcox CL, Johnson EM. Characterization of nerve growth factor-dependent herpes simplex virus latency in neurons in vitro. J Virol. 1988;62:393–399.

14.2)   Siddiqui MF, Elwell C, Johnson MH. Mitochondrial Dysfunction in Autism Spectrum Disorders. Autism Open Access. 2016;6(5):1000190. Doi:10.4172/2165-7890.1000190

14.3)   Emad M. et al. (2017). The soft mechanical signature of glial scars in the central nervous system. Nature Communications.

14.4)   Angoa-Pérez, M., Zagorac, B., Anneken, J.H. et al. Repetitive, mild traumatic brain injury results in a progressive white matter pathology, cognitive deterioration, and a transient gut microbiota dysbiosis. Sci Rep 10, 8949 (2020). https://doi.org/10.1038/s41598-020-65972-4

14.5)   Zhu CS, Grandhi R, Patterson TT, Nicholson SE. A Review of Traumatic Brain Injury and the Gut Microbiome: Insights into Novel Mechanisms of Secondary Brain Injury and Promising Targets for Neuroprotection. Brain Sci. 2018;8(6):113. Published 2018 Jun 19. doi:10.3390/brainsci8060113

15.1)   Peesay M. Nuchal cord and its implications. Matern Health Neonatol Perinatol. 2017;3:28. Published 2017 Dec 6. Doi:10.1186/s40748-017-0068-7

16.1)   Cornette L. Therapeutic hypothermia in neonatal asphyxia. Facts Views Vis Obgyn. 2012;4(2):133-139.

18.1)   Jolles S, Sewell WA, Misbah SA. Clinical uses of intravenous immunoglobulin. Clin Exp Immunol. 2005;142(1):1-11. doi:10.1111/j.1365-2249.2005.02834.x

18.2)   Lee RWY, Corley MJ, Pang A, Arakaki G, Abbott L, Nishimoto M, Miyamoto R, Lee E, Yamamoto S, Maunakea AK, Lum-Jones A, Wong M. A modified ketogenic gluten-free diet with MCT improves behavior in children with autism spectrum disorder. Physiol Behav. 2018 May 1;188:205-211. doi: 10.1016/j.physbeh.2018.02.006. Epub 2018 Feb 5. PMID: 29421589; PMCID: PMC5863039.

18.3) Sequeira S, Ahmed M. Meditation as a potential therapy for autism: a review. Autism Res Treat. 2012;2012:835847. Doi:10.1155/2012/835847

18.4) Siniscalco D, Kannan S, Semprún-Hernández N, Eshraghi AA, Brigida AL, Antonucci N. Stem cell therapy in autism: recent insights. Stem Cells Cloning. 2018;11:55-67. Published 2018 Oct 23. Doi:10.2147/SCCAA.S155410

19.1) Boese, A.C., Le, Q.E., Pham, D. et al. Neural stem cell therapy for subacute and chronic ischemic stroke. Stem Cell Res Ther 9, 154 (2018). https://doi.org/10.1186/s13287-018-0913-2

19.2) Shoichet MS, Tate CC, Baumann MD, et al. Strategies for Regeneration and Repair in the Injured Central Nervous System. In: Reichert WM, editor. Indwelling Neural Implants: Strategies for Contending with the In Vivo Environment. Boca Raton (FL): CRC Press/Taylor & Francis; 2008. Chapter 8. Available from: https://www.ncbi.nlm.nih.gov/books/NBK3941/

19.3) Li H, Chen G. In Vivo Reprogramming for CNS Repair: Regenerating Neurons from Endogenous Glial Cells. Neuron. 2016;91(4):728-738. Doi:10.1016/j.neuron.2016.08.004

19.4) Gao, X., Wang, X., Xiong, W. et al. In vivo reprogramming reactive glia into iPSCs to produce new neurons in the cortex following traumatic brain injury. Sci Rep 6, 22490 (2016). https://doi.org/10.1038/srep22490

19.5) Sun YJ, Zhang ZY, Fan B, Li GY. Neuroprotection by Therapeutic Hypothermia. Front Neurosci. 2019;13:586. Published 2019 Jun 11. 9.

19.6)   Hasan A, Deeb G, Rahal R, Atwi K, Mondello S, Marei HE, et al. Mesenchymal stem cells in the treatment of traumatic brain injury. Front Neurol. (2017) 8:28. doi: 10.3389/fneur.2017.00028

19.7)   Zibara K, Ballout N, Mondello S, Karnib N, Ramadan N, Omais S, et al. Combination of drug and stem cells neurotherapy: potential interventions in neurotrauma and traumatic brain injury. Neuropharmacology. (2019) 145:177–98. doi: 10.1016/j.neuropharm.2018.09.032doi:10.3389/fnins.2019.00586

19.8)   Maas AIR, Menon DK, Adelson PD, Andelic N, Bell MJ, Belli A, et al. Traumatic brain injury: integrated approaches to improve prevention, clinical care, and research. Lancet Neurol. (2017) 16:987–1048. doi: 10.1016/S1474-4422(17)30371-X

23.1)   Decoteau CL, Underman K. Adjudicating non-knowledge in the Omnibus Autism Proceedings. Soc Stud Sci. 2015;45(4):471-500. Doi:10.1177/0306312715600278

23.2)   Decoteau, C. L., & Daniel, M. (2020). Scientific Hegemony and the Field of Autism. American Sociological Review, 85(3), 451-476. doi:10.1177/0003122420922531

MORE REFERENCES

Image Sources and Credits.

Images have been predominantly sourced from Wikimedia, Government and Educational websites and public domain. Some images are created by the author

1.1:   Brain development with age - Smithsonian Dept of Human Origin, by Karen Carr Studios.

1.2:   Brain functional development - https://developingchild.harvard.edu/resources/inbrief-science-of-ecd

1.3:   Structural parts of the brain - Image modified by author from purchased material.

1.4:   Cerebral functional areas - Image created by author.

2.1:   Neuron cell - Wikipedia, "Anatomy and Physiology" by the US National Cancer Institute's Surveillance, Epidemiology and End Results (SEER)

2.2:   Neuron 3D - Wikimedia Commons: public domain image Ladyofhats

2.3:   Neuroglial Cells - Wikimedia Commons: Artwork by Holly Fischer labelled by author.

2.4:   Grey matter -Wikimedia Commons – from public domain.

2.5:   Brain cross section – from public domain - re-labelled by author.

3.1:   Blood Brain Barrier – By Author

3.2:   Immune system – By Author

4.1:   Barriers to birth – By author

4.2:   Labor feedback loop - (Image source: OpenStax https://cnx.org/-contents/FPtK1zmh@8.25:fEI3C8Ot@10/Preface, CC BY 4.0, https://commons.wikimedia.org/w/index.php?curid=30131134)

4.3:   Three stages of labor - http://mstcparamedic.pbworks.com/w/page/21902870/Stages of Labor

5.1:   Uterus - https://upload.wikimedia.org/wikipedia/commons-/9/96/Blausen_ 0399_FemaleReproSystem_01.png (author labelled)

5.2:   Uterus - public domain image

5.3:   Placenta – public domain image with minor modifications by author

5.4:   Cardiotocograph – By Martin Hawlish -German Wikimedia Commons

5.5:   Amniotic fluid and Induction. - Image by author.

7.1:   Adaptive Immunity - Image by author

7.3:   Cervix Stretch and Tear – by author (also 7.2, 7.4, 7.5)

9.2:   Twin Pregnancy - adapted from https://icombo.org/chorionicity

11.1a: Brain sectional planes - Blausen.com staff (2014). "Medical gallery of Blausen Medical 2014". *WikiJournal of Medicine* 1 (2): 10. doi:10.15347/wjm/2014.010. ISSN 2002-4436;

11.1b: Brain sectional planes - case.edu/med/neurology/NR/MRI Basics.htm

11.2:   DAI - Matt Skalski – Radiopedia.org

14.1:   From actual MMR label from internet sources.

14.2:   Autism from TBI compounded by viral interaction - by author.

15.1:   Autism Causes in a Nutshell - by author

15.2:   Sourced from CDC website at https://www.cdc.gov/ncbddd/birthdefects/microcephaly.html

15.3:   Cord complications - Image by author

15.4:   Placenta abruption - Image by author.

15.5:   Pitocin abuse cycle – Figure by author.

16.1a: Brain Gyrification 1 – Cowan WM. The development of the brain. Sci Am. 1979 Sep;241(3):113-33. PMID: 493917.

16.1b: Brain Gyrification 2 – Image by author.

16.2:   Brain ability to learn - Center on the Developing child. Harvard University. Data source Levitt (2009).

18.1:   Dan protocol – Internet sources, from page 67 of the book *"Autism: Effective Biomedical Treatments"*

21.1:   Google search result for 'pitocin autism' in 2017

21.2:   Pitocin Autism search results on Bing in 2020

Useful Web Links

w1.1	American Pregnancy Association	https://americanpregnancy.org/labor-and-birth/
w1.2	Labor – John Hopkins Medicine	https://developingchild.harvard.edu/resources/inbrief-science-of-ecd
w2.1	Brain Architecture	https://developingchild.harvard.edu/science/key-concepts/brain-architecture/
w2.2	Early Childhood Development	https://developingchild.harvard.edu/resources/inbrief-science-of-ecd
w2.3	Queensland Brain Institute	https://qbi.uq.edu.au/brain/brain-anatomy
w2.4	Transmitting fibers in the brain	https://aiimpacts.org/transmitting-fibers-in-the-brain-total-length-and-distribution-of-lengths/
w3.1	State of World Mothers report	https://www.savethechildren.org/content/dam/usa/reports/advocacy/sowm/sowm-2015.pdf
w5.1	Disease Eradication	https://www.historyofvaccines.org/content/articles/disease-eradication
w5.2	ProCon.org History of vaccines	https://vaccines.procon.org/history-of-vaccines/
w5.3	History of Anti-vaccination Movements	https://www.historyofvaccines.org/content/articles/history-anti-vaccination-movements
w5.4	Timeline-History of Vaccines	https://www.historyofvaccines.org/timeline/all
w5.5	Nerve Growth Factor	https://en.wikipedia.org/wiki/Nerve_growth_factor
w6.1	Infectious Disease in Pregnancy	https://www.merckmanuals.com/professional/gynecology-and-obstetrics/pregnancy-complicated-by-disease/infectious-disease-in-pregnancy

w6.2	The Truth About CPD	https://www.bellybelly.com.au/birth/small-pelvis-big-baby-cpd/
w6.3	Diabetes During Pregnancy	https://www.stanfordchildrens.org/en/topic/default?id=diabetes-and-pregnancy-90-P02444
w6.4	Nuchal Cord:	https://www.thebump.com/a/nuchal-cord
w6.5	Cerebral Palsy	https://www.cerebralpalsy.org/about-cerebral-palsy/cause
w6.6	Hypoxic-Ischemic Encephalopathy	https://www.cerebralpalsy.org/about-cerebral-palsy/cause/hypoxic-ischemic-encephalopathy
w6.7	Dyslexia – Symptoms and causes	https://www.mayoclinic.org/diseases-conditions/dyslexia/symptoms-causes/syc-20353552
w6.8	Birth Defects	https://www.cdc.gov/ncbddd/birthdefects
w7.1	About Oxytocin	https://psychcentral.com/lib/about-oxytocin/
w7.2	What is Pitocin?	https://www.bundoo.com/articles/what-is-pitocin/
w7.3	The Truth About PITOCIN	https://pathwaystofamilywellness.org/Pregnancy-Birth/the-truth-about-pitocin.html
w7.4	5 Things Oxytocin does that Pitocin doesn't	https://www.bellybelly.com.au/birth/5-things-oxytocin-does-that-pitocin-doesnt/
w7.5	Induced Labor Malpractice -	https://www.kennerlyloutey.com/birth-injuries/induced-labor-pitocin/

INDEX

WWW.AUTISMPI.ORG

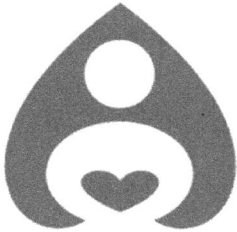

Autism Parents Initiative

Take the first step: Register your autism birth data at www.autismpi.org today. Your contribution will directly power the research and legal discovery needed to make a difference.